The Interdisciplinary Council on Developmental and Learning Disorders

Diagnostic Manual for Infancy and Early Childhood

Mental Health, Developmental, Regulatory-Sensory Processing, Language and Learning Disorders

ICDL-DMIC

Acknowledgements

Most importantly, we'd like to acknowledge that the members of all the Work Groups who contributed to this effort and who are its heart and soul. Their amazing talent and clinical acuity was only matched by their enormous energy and commitment to helping this project reach fruition.

We would like to give special thanks to Jan Tunney whose heroic efforts in helping keep this project organized and going has made this volume possible. We would also like express our appreciation to other individuals who have contributed to the finalizing of this effort. Thanks to Jo Raphael, Jane LaRoque, and Sue Morrisson for their editing expertise; to Jill Sobieski and Gretchen Gerber for their essential support; and to Sharon Markus for all her help.

Interdisciplinary Council on Developmental and Learning Disorders

Diagnostic Manual for Infancy and Early Childhood
Mental Health, Developmental, Regulatory-Sensory Processing, Language and Learning Disorders (ICDL-DMIC)

ICDL-DMIC Work Groups

Stanley I. Greenspan, M.D., Chair
Clinical Professor of Psychiatry, Behavioral Sciences and Pediatrics
George Washington University Medical School
Washington, DC

Serena Wieder, Ph.D., Co-Chair
Associate Chair, ICDL
Director, DIR® Institute
Clinical Psychologist
Silver Spring, Maryland

Neurodevelopmental Disorders of Relating and Communicating and Interactive Disorders Work Group

Serena Wieder, Ph.D.

Stanley I. Greenspan, M.D.

Lois M. Black, Ph.D.
Associate Scientist, Center for Spoken Language Understanding, OGI School of Science & Engineering, Oregon Health & Science University
Beaverton, Oregon

Griffin Doyle, Ph.D.
Clinical Psychologist
Co-Chair, Infant Mental Health Program, Washington School of Psychiatry
Bethesda, Maryland

Barbara Dunbar, Ph.D.
Clinical Psychologist
Atlanta, Georgia

Barbara Kalmanson, Ph.D.
Clinical Psychologist and Special Educator
Clinical Director, Oak Hill School
San Francisco, California

Lori Jeanne Peloquin, Ph.D.
Clinical Senior Instructor in Pediatrics and Psychiatry
University of Rochester School of Medicine and Dentistry
Rochester, New York

Ricki Robinson, M.D., M.P.H.
Clinical Professor of Pediatrics
Keck School of Medicine of the University of Southern California
Co-director, Descanso Medical Center for Development and Learning
La Canada, California

Ruby Moyé Salazar, LCSW, BCD
Director and Senior Clinician
Salazar Associates
Clarks Summit, Pennsylvania

Rick Solomon, M.D.
The Ann Arbor Center for Developmental and Behavioral Pediatrics
Ann Arbor, Michigan

Rosemary White, OTR
Seattle, Washington

Molly Romer Witten, Ph.D.
Licensed Clinical Psychologist
Co-editor, ICDL Best Practices Newsletter
Chicago, Illinois

Stanley I. Greenspan, M.D.

Regulatory-Sensory Processing Disorders Work Group

Lucy Jane Miller, Ph.D., OTR, FAOTA
Executive Director,
KID Foundation, Littleton, Colorado
Associate Professor, Rehabilitation Medicine and Pediatrics
University of Colorado Health Sciences Center,
Denver, Colorado

Marie Anzalone, Sc.D., OTR
Assistant Professor of Clinical Occupational Therapy
Columbia University, New York

Sharon A. Cermak, Ed.D., OTR/L, FAOTA
Professor of Occupational Therapy
Department of Rehabilitation Sciences
Boston University, Sargent College of Rehabilitation Sciences
Boston, Massachusetts

Interdisciplinary Council on Developmental and Learning Disorders

Diagnostic Manual for Infancy and Early Childhood

Mental Health, Developmental, Regulatory-Sensory Processing, Language and Learning Disorders (ICDL-DMIC)

ICDL-DMIC Work Groups *(continued)*

Shelly J. Lane, Ph.D., OTR, FAOTA
Professor and Chairman
Department of Occupational Therapy
Virginia Commonwealth University
Richmond, Virginia

Beth Osten, M.S., OTR/L
Director
Beth Osten and Associates
Pediatric Therapy Services
Skokie, Illinois

Serena Wieder, Ph.D.

Stanley I. Greenspan, M.D.

Language Disorders Work Group

Sherri Cawn, M.A., CCC-SLP
Northbrook, Illinois

Sima Gerber, Ph.D., CCC
Associate Professor, Department of Linguistics and Communication Disorders,
Queens College, City University of New York
New York, New York

Cindy Harrison, M.Sc., SLP, Reg. CASLPO
Ottawa, Ontario
Canada

Diane Lewis, M.A., CCC-SLP
Director, Communication Enrichment Services
Bethesda, Maryland

Jane R. Madell, Ph.D., CCC A/SLP, Cert AVT
Director, Hearing and Learning Center and
Co-Director, Cochlear Implant Center, Beth Israel
New York Eye and Ear Medical Center
Professor, Clinical Otolaryngology
Albert Einstein College of Medicine
New York, New York

Stuart G. Shanker, D.Phil.
Distinguished Research Professor
of Philosophy and Psychology
Director, The Milton and Ethel Harris Research Institute
York University
Toronto, Ontario, Canada

Amy M. Wetherby, Ph.D., CCC-SLP
Laurel Schendel Professor
Department of Communication Disorders
Florida State University
Tallahassee, Florida

Stanley I. Greenspan, M.D.

Learning Challenges Work Group

Pat Lindamood, M.S., CCC-SLP
Director & Co-Founder
Lindamood Bell Learning Processes
San Luis Obispo, California

Robert L. Hendren, D.O.
Professor of Psychiatry
Exec. Director, M.I.N.D. Institute
Chief, Child and Adolescent Psychiatry
University of California
Davis, California

Joan Mele-McCarthy, D.A.
Special Assistant to the Assistant Secretary
Office of Special Education and Rehabilitative Services
Washington, DC

Kytja Voeller, M.D., Ph.D.
Western Institute for Neurodevelopmental Studies & Interventions
Boulder, Colorado

Harry Wachs, O.D.
Director
Vision and Conceptual Development Center
Washington, DC

Paul Worthington, B.A., B.S.
Executive Director of Research & Development
Lindamood-Bell Learning Processes
San Luis Obispo, California

Stanley I. Greenspan, M.D.

Interdisciplinary Council on Developmental and Learning Disorders

4938 Hampden Lane, Suite 800 Bethesda, MD 20814
301-656-2667 www.icdl.com

Advisory Board

Interdisciplinary Council on Developmental and Learning Disorders

4938 Hampden Lane, Suite 800 Bethesda, MD 20814
301-656-2667 www.icdl.com

Advisory Board *(continued)*

Table of Contents

Introduction

Introduction to the DMIC 3

An Interdisciplinary Approach to Classification 4
The Need for a Developmentally Based Diagnostic System 5
The Problem with Symptom-Based Approaches 5
Multidimensional Classification Based on the DIR Model 7
A Clinically Meaningful Approach 7
Unique Features of the ICDL-DMIC 8
Overview of the ICDL-DMIC System 9

A Multi-Axial Approach 11

Selecting a Primary Diagnosis 13
Clinical Thresholds for Diagnosis 14

Making a Diagnosis: Case Illustration 17

Section I - Primary Diagnosis – Axis I

100. Interactive Disorders 31

101. Anxiety Disorder 33
102. Developmental Anxiety Disorder 35
103. Disorder of Emotional Range and Stability 39
104. Disruptive Behavior and Oppositional Disorder 41
105. Depression 45
106. Mood Dysregulation-Bipolar Patterns 48
107. Attentional Disorder 50
108. Prolonged Grief Reaction 58
109. Reactive Attachment Disorder 59
110. Traumatic Stress Disorder 62
111. Adjustment Disorder 64
112. Gender Identity Disorder 65
113. Elective Mutism 66
114. Sleep Disorder 67, 68
115. Eating Disorder 67, 69
116. Elimination Disorder 67, 70

200. Regulatory-Sensory Processing Disorders 73

Sensory Modulation Challenges (Type I) 81
201. Over-Responsive, Fearful, Anxious Pattern 81
202. Over-Responsive, Negative, and Stubborn Pattern 83
203. Under-Responsive, Self-Absorbed Pattern 84
203.1 Self-Absorbed and Difficult to Engage Type
203.2 Self-Absorbed and Creative Type

204. Active, Sensory Seeking Pattern 86
Sensory Discrimination Challenges (Type II) and
Sensory-Based Motor Challenges (Type III) 88
205. Inattentive, Disorganized Pattern 88
205.1 With Sensory Discrimination Challenges
205.2 With Postural Control Challenges
205.3 With Dyspraxia
205.4 With Combinations of 205.1-205.3
206. Compromised School and/or Academic Performance Pattern 89
206.1 With Sensory Discrimination Challenges
206.2 With Postural Control Challenges
206.3 With Dyspraxia
206.4 With Combinations of 206.1-206.3
Contributing Sensory Discrimination and
Sensory-Based Motor Challenges 90
207. Mixed Regulatory-Sensory Processing Patterns 95
207.1 Attentional Problems
207.2 Disruptive Behavioral Problems
207.3 Sleep Problems
207.4 Eating Problems
207.5 Elimination Problems
207.6 Elective Mutism
207.7 Mood Dysregulation, including Bipolar Patterns
207.8 Other Emotional and Behavioral Problems Related to Mixed Regulatory-Sensory Processing Difficulties
207.9 Mixed Regulatory-Sensory Processing Difficulties where Behavioral or Emotional Problems Are Not Yet in Evidence
Case Illustrations 100

300. Neurodevelopmental Disorders of Relating and Communicating 113

301. Type I: Early Symbolic, with Constrictions 118
302. Type II: Purposeful Problem Solving, with Constrictions 120
303. Type III: Intermittently Engaged and Purposeful 122
304. Type IV: Aimless and Unpurposeful 123
Other Neurodevelopmental Disorders (Including Genetic and
Metabolic Syndromes) 125
Children Who Are Difficult to Classify 126

400. Language Disorders 129

401. Self-Regulation and Interest in the World
401.1 In Comprehension
401.2 In Production
401.3 In Both Comprehension and Production
402. Forming Relationships: Affective Vocal Synchrony
402.1 In Comprehension
402.2 In Production
402.3 In Both Comprehension and Production

403. Intentional Two-Way Communication
    403.1 In Comprehension
    403.2 In Production
    403.3 In Both Comprehension and Production
404. First Words: Sharing Meanings in Gestures and Words
    404.1 In Comprehension
    404.2 In Production
    404.3 In Both Comprehension and Production
405. Word Combinations: Sharing Experiences Symbolically
    405.1 In Comprehension
    405.2 In Production
    405.3 In Both Comprehension and Production
406. Early Discourse: Reciprocal Symbolic Interactions with Others
    406.1 In Comprehension
    406.2 In Production
    406.3 In Both Comprehension and Production
Case Illustrations 152

500. Learning Challenges..167

Emerging Learning Challenges with compromises in
    501. Functional Emotional Developmental Capacities
    502. Auditory Processing and Language
    503. Visuospatial Capacities
    504. Regulatory-Sensory Processing Patterns
    505. A Combination of the Above Areas
Early Challenges in Reading and Language Arts with compromises in
    506. Functional Emotional Developmental Capacities
    507. Auditory Processing and Language
    508. Visuospatial Capacities
    509. Regulatory-Sensory Processing Patterns
    510. A Combination of the Above Areas
Early Challenges in Math with compromises in
    511. Functional Emotional Developmental Capacities
    512. Auditory Processing and Language
    513. Visuospatial Capacities
    514. Regulatory-Sensory Processing Patterns
    515. A Combination of the Above Areas
Early Challenges in Reading Comprehension with compromises in
    516. Functional Emotional Developmental Capacities
    517. Auditory Processing and Language
    518. Visuospatial Capacities
    519. Regulatory-Sensory Processing Patterns
    520. A Combination of the Above Areas
Early Challenges in Written Communication with compromises in
    521. Functional Emotional Developmental Capacities
    522. Auditory Processing and Language

523. Visuospatial Capacities
524. Regulatory-Sensory Processing Patterns
525. A Combination of the Above Areas
Early Challenges in Organizing Capacities (Executive Functioning) with compromises in
526 Functional Emotional Developmental Capacities
527. Auditory Processing and Language
528. Visuospatial Capacities
529. Regulatory-Sensory Processing Patterns
530. A Combination of the Above Areas
Case Illustrations 180

Section II - Axes II - VIII

Introduction 193
Axis II - Functional Emotional Developmental Capacities 195
Axis III - Regulatory-Sensory Processing Capacities 207
Axis IV - Language Capacities 209
Axis V - Visuospatial Capacities 211
Axis VI - Child-Caregiver and Family Patterns 225
Axis VII - Stress 229
Axis VIII - Other Medical and Neurological Diagnoses 231

References 235

Appendix I

A Comprehensive Approach to Clinical Evaluation 249

Appendix II

Implications of the ICDL Classification System for a Comprehensive, Developmentally-Based Approach to Intervention 269

Appendix III

Guide for Observations during Clinical Evaluation of Regulatory-Sensory Processing Disorders 289
Record Forms for Regulatory-Sensory Processing Disorders 303-310
Additional Materials and Activities Useful in Assessing Regulatory-Sensory Processing Disorders. 311
Additional Reading Suggestions for Regulatory-Sensory Processing Disorders 315

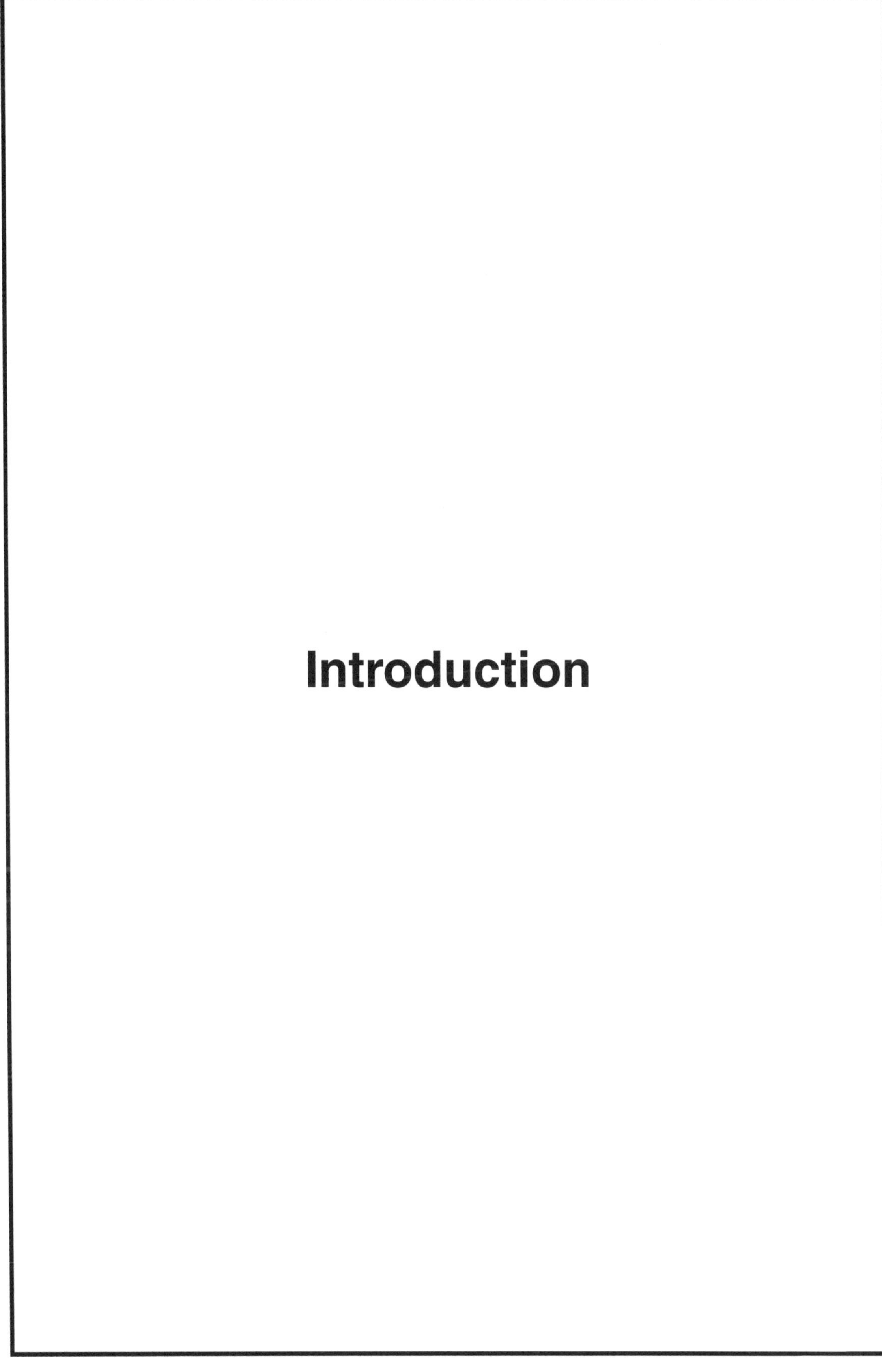

Introduction

Introduction to the ICDL-DMIC

Infancy and early childhood are characterized by dynamic relationships between the different dimensions of human development, including emotional, social, language, cognitive, regulatory-sensory processing, and motor capacities. A comprehensive classification of infant and early childhood disorders must, therefore, describe challenges in each of these areas of functioning and the relationships between them.

A comprehensive classification system is especially important in infancy and early childhood because children with a problem in one area are likely to have problems in other areas. For example, children with severe emotional and social difficulties often have language and/or regulatory-sensory processing difficulties and vice versa.

Yet, such a much-needed comprehensive classification system had not been constructed. Therefore, the Interdisciplinary Council on Developmental and Learning Disorders (ICDL), which represents leaders from all the disciplines that work with infants and young children, created a number of work groups to formulate a developmentally-based classification system for each of these areas of functioning. The goal of this effort was to create a framework to facilitate a more complete clinical description of infant and early childhood functioning. ICDL is now pleased to present this system.

The *ICDL Diagnostic Manual for Infancy and Early Childhood* (ICDL-DMIC) builds on preliminary work dating back to the early 1980s when the co-chairs of this effort (Stanley Greenspan and Serena Wieder) were conducting the Clinical Infant Development Program at the National Institute of Mental Health (NIMH) and brought in a number of leading clinicians to brainstorm on clinical diagnostic and intervention approaches for infants, young children, and their families. The initial working group included Reginald Lourie, Selma Fraiberg, T. Berry Brazelton, Julius Richmond, Ed Ziegler, Katherine Barnard, and many others. This group later expanded and led to the initiation of two organizations–Zero To Three: National Center for Infants, Toddlers, and Families and ICDL.

From the clinical observations, research, and discussions of the original advisory group and the NIMH Clinical Infant Development Programs' longitudinal intervention study of infants and young children and their families, we formulated initial classifications of healthy and disordered functioning and models of intervention. For example, we formulated the concept of "regulatory disorders" involving differences in sensory processing, which were contributing to behavioral and emotional difficulties. We also began to look at the developmental pathways leading to autism spectrum patterns and developed profiles that characterize the child's functional emotional developmental level and sensory processing profile, which led initially to different subtypes of multisystem developmental disorders and, more recently, to a developmentally-based classification of neurodevelopmental disorders of relating and communicating–a new way of sub-typing autism spectrum and related disorders (Greenspan, 1979; 1981; 1992; Greenspan, Wieder et al. 1987; Greenspan & Lourie, 1981).

The framework we constructed was a developmental, biopsychosocial model that provided a system for classifying and treating different groups of infant and early childhood mental health, developmental, and learning disorders. While each child must be understood in terms of his unique developmental profile, we believed it was often helpful to group patterns into broad categories to facilitate research, administrative record keeping, and the overall organization of clinical services. Such grouping also facilitates discussions that can improve the specificity of comprehensive treatment programs.

The two organizations that were an outgrowth of the NIMH program and the initial brainstorming group of pioneers in infant and early childhood mental health are now working to improve the classification of infant and early childhood mental health disorders. These efforts began a number of years ago when we (Greenspan and Wieder) had the honor of chairing the Diagnostic Classification Task Force for Zero To Three: National Center for Infants, Toddlers, and Families. At present, there is an ongoing effort to revise the original classification framework.

In addition, we initiated the Diagnostic Classification Task Force of the Interdisciplinary Council on Developmental and Learning Disorders (ICDL) to expand and further refine the diagnostic system for infancy and early childhood. The ICDL Task Force has expanded the classification system to include language and learning disorders, and a new developmentally-based framework for regulatory-sensory processing disorders and neurodevelopmental disorders of relating and communicating (autism spectrum disorders, multisystem developmental disorders, etc.). Furthermore, the ICDL-DMIC presents a new multi-axial approach, where each primary disorder is additionally profiled in terms of the contributions from functional emotional developmental levels, regulatory-sensory processing differences, language capacities, visuospatial abilities, as well as interactive and family patterns, stressors, and other medical disorders. The ICDL diagnostic classification effort builds on the ICDL *Clinical Practice Guidelines* (Interdisciplinary Council on Developmental and Learning Disorders Clinical Practice Guidelines Workgroup, 2000).

AN INTERDISCIPLINARY APPROACH TO CLASSIFICATION

This classification system integrates all components of development and functioning which traditionally have been addressed by different disciplines. It is intended for professionals of all disciplines working with infants and children and, additionally, can be used as a roadmap to understanding the interactions between the different components of the child's development, family, and environment, as well as to guide assessments and interventions.

The system is designed for professionals credentialed to do diagnoses. It is also intended to provide a systematic approach to describe each child's unique pattern of functioning. This approach can be helpful for all individuals who work with infants and young children. When appropriate, it can augment other existing diagnostic systems such as ICD-10, DSM IV-R, and DC: 0-3. Because the DMIC is an interdisciplinary tool that supports the integration of knowledge from different disciplines, it will, for example, guide the mental health professional to integrate what has been learned about development, regulatory-sensory processing, language, visuospatial, and learning capacities into their mental health expertise. Similarly, pediatricians, occupational, physical, and speech and language therapists, educators, and professionals from other disciplines will integrate understanding of emotional development, interactive disorders, and family and environmental factors on adequate, constricted or disordered functioning.

THE NEED FOR A DEVELOPMENTALLY-BASED DIAGNOSTIC SYSTEM

The need for a developmentally-based classification system in infant and early childhood mental health that includes neurodevelopmental, regulatory-sensory processing, language, and learning disorders is based on a number of challenges that now face clinicians and researchers working with infants, young children, and their families.

As indicated, no system currently exists that includes the most common emotional, social, cognitive, motor, sensory, language, and learning disorders in the first five years of life. The ICDL-DMIC profiles each disorder from multiple perspectives, including emotional, sensory processing, and language dimensions. Also, new understanding of developmental pathways for both healthy and disordered development now makes it possible to formulate a truly clinically useful approach to classification that will facilitate research into etiological factors and inform intervention approaches that are tailored to the unique developmental profiles of each child and family.

THE PROBLEM WITH SYMPTOM-BASED APPROACHES

Symptom-based approaches to diagnostic classification (in comparison to the developmental approach that forms the basis of ICDL-DMIC system) have strived for reliability among clinicians in making a diagnosis. Lists of symptoms that are readily observable are used in the belief that they facilitate reliable judgments. The symptom-based approach, however, has not demonstrated clinical validity, including predicting clinical course or informing clinical practice, to the degree hoped for. For many diagnoses, the reliability among practicing clinicians making the diagnosis has been disappointing. Allen Frances, M.D., Chair of the DSM-IV American Psychiatric Association (APA) Task Force, recently commented in an article in *The New Yorker* magazine that the reliability hoped for was not realized and that the reliability among practicing clinicians was very poor (Spievel, 2005). In moving towards DSM-V, the APA Task Force is shifting towards a dimensional, rather than categorical, approach.

The most significant weakness in the symptom-based approach has been the confusion it has brought regarding the boundaries between disorders and the usefulness of the diagnostic categories for planning optimal treatment approaches. The degree to which many conditions evidence comorbidity with other conditions illustrates the problems with a symptom-based approach that is not sufficiently grounded in an understanding of etiological factors or the developmental pathways leading to disordered functioning. For example, often the symptom-based approaches have designated diagnostic categories, including boundaries between conditions, based simply on the consensus of experts, including decisions about how many of the symptoms are necessary for the diagnosis (e.g., three out of five, rather than two out of five).

Yet there are insufficient studies documenting what it means if the patient meets only two out of five (i.e., there is no data supporting a clear line between two versus three of the criteria). Therefore, most evidence points to a dimensional approach where symptoms or disorders may be expressed in varying degrees (i.e., shades of gray) rather than clear "you have it or you don't." DSM-V anticipates heading in this direction.

The length of time symptoms need to be manifested for a disorder to be diagnosed is another example of over-specificity. Many criteria state that the symptoms must be present for at least X number of weeks. Again, there is insufficient data on the implications of a patient evidencing it two days less than the indicated two weeks.

Most importantly, studies of prognosis and predictive validity are hampered by not controlling for the appropriateness of the treatment program the patient is receiving. For example, most children with autism are believed to continue to evidence the symptoms of the disorder five to eight years in the future. But how many of these children were in inappropriate or inadequate treatment programs? Prognosis with an optimal treatment program is not yet definitively known, due to the lack of comparative clinical trials of the most promising approaches and lack of a sufficient number of long-term naturalistic studies (Committee on Educational Interventions for Children with Autism, 2001).

Reliability studies are also fraught with problems. Criteria that are easy to agree on are not necessarily the criteria that are meaningful for clinical planning or research on etiological factors and developmental pathways. In general, there is a healthy tension between the goal of capturing the true complexity of multifaceted clinical phenomena and developing criteria that can be reliably judged and employed in research. It is vital to embrace this healthy tension and pursue a step-wise approach where complexity and clinical usefulness is a cornerstone for efforts at increasingly systematic operational definitions and research on reliability and clinical validity. A scientifically-based system is one that recognizes a step-wise progression that begins with accurate recognition and description of complex clinical phenomena and builds gradually through a series of steps toward empirical validation. Oversimplification or favoring what is measurable over what is meaningful does not serve the creation of a scientifically-based system.

At present, it is important to acknowledge that we do not yet have an empirically validated diagnostic system for mental health, developmental, and learning disorders of infancy and early childhood. We do have emerging data and a great deal of clinical experience. Therefore, an accurate statement of the field is that it is currently operating on expert consensus with supportive, but incomplete, data.

Because of these and related considerations, as indicated above, there is a general movement towards more dimensional approaches to classification. Furthermore, dimensional approaches recognize that many difficulties exist in terms of degrees of challenge, rather than with clear boundaries. Dimensional approaches recognize the multiple components which may contribute to a disorder.

MULTIDIMENSIONAL CLASSIFICATION BASED ON THE DIR MODEL

As indicated, dimensional approaches tend to be based on an implicit understanding that most mental health and developmental disorders are based on complex dynamic, developmental processes. We have formulated a developmental, biopsychosocial model to describe these processes that contribute to mental health, development, regulatory-sensory processing, language, and learning disorders in infancy and early childhood–the Developmental, Individual-Difference, Relationship-Based (DIR) approach. The DIR approach focuses on (**D**) Developmental capacities - the level of emotional, social, and intellectual functioning (technically called functional emotional developmental capacities). It also focuses on biologically-based (**I**) Individual processing differences in the way an infant or young child reacts to and comprehends different sensations, such as auditory, visuospatial, or tactile, as well as the way in which the child plans, sequences, and executes actions. It also focuses on the (**R**) Relationships, including child/caregiver/family and other relationship patterns. (This model is described more fully in Appendix 1 of this manual.) A diagnostic classification system for infancy and early childhood mental health, developmental, language, and learning disorders based on our dynamic, developmental model facilitates understanding of these disorders and, most importantly, guide intervention and treatment planning.

A vital feature of a dynamic, developmental approach is that it emphasizes the multiple relationships between different areas of development. Infants and young children with a specific type of problem often have challenges in many related areas of functioning. For example, a preschooler with an impulse control problem will often have challenges in terms of caregiver/child interaction patterns and different aspects of sensory processing, language, and cognition. Similarly, children with language problems may often also evidence contributions from challenges in motor planning and sequencing and other aspects of sensory processing.

Thus, a comprehensive approach to infancy and early childhood requires a multidimensional and multidisciplinary focus which includes a number of axes. It should be highlighted, however, that a dynamic, developmental, multi-axial approach that includes all the relevant dimensions of human development is especially vital for a diagnostic system for infants, young children, and their families. During infancy and early childhood, not only is the brain and mind growing more rapidly than it ever will again, but it is literally forming the relationships between its different components. Attending to these interrelated components is vital in classifying disorders as the basis for meaningful intervention planning and research.

A CLINICALLY MEANINGFUL APPROACH

It is very important to make sure that what is considered expert consensus represents the most meaningful diagnostic classification approach possible. This means that it is necessary to have an approach that is based on clinically meaningful categorizations that recognize dimensional processes and the full range of human functioning (i.e., the depths of human feelings and relationships) and also takes into account what is known about developmental pathways, etiology, and response to optimal interventions.

Recognizing these important goals enables us to climb the steps of science without skipping over important ones. If we sacrifice meaningful categorization for quick reliability, we wind up with a system fraught with problems. Agreement does not suggest clinical validity. Therefore, the next goal is to improve our conceptual framework by deepening and broadening it. We can then use it as the basis for future studies that enable the field of infant and early childhood mental health and development to progress in a more integrated manner which recognizes the interactive and interrelated components of development and human functioning.

Clinical Judgment and the Diagnostic Process in Infancy and Early Childhood

The diagnostic process for infants, young children, and their families requires clinical experience and judgment. As indicated, clinical science must progress in an orderly sequence, beginning with observations and descriptions that capture the true complexity and subtlety of the phenomena being dealt with, and then gradually progressing to more and more refined operational criteria that can be reliably measured and employed for studies of predictive validity, etiology, and intervention efficacy.

As will be seen in the body of this manual, the ICDL workgroups were extremely cautious in the way they approached the complex, clinical phenomena that characterize infant and early childhood disorders. Premature attempts at specificity are avoided and rich clinical descriptions are emphasized.

UNIQUE FEATURES OF THE ICDL-DMIC

The ICDL-DMIC has a number of unique features that operationalize the perspective outlined above. For example, each of the disorders classified under the heading "Interactive Disorders" is described in terms of its clinical phenomena, presenting symptoms, developmental pathways, and therapeutic implications. In addition, each disorder is described along a number of axes, which attempts to capture and emphasize an important component of, and/or contributor to, the disorder. These include the infant's or young child's level of emotional and social functioning, child-caregiver and family interaction patterns, motor planning and processing differences (regulatory sensory processing profile), language functioning, visuospatial capacities, and unique stressors that may be affecting the child and his or her family.

The goal of the DMIC is to present both a rich, detailed clinical picture of each infant or young child and his or her family and, at the same time, provide a framework for systematically organizing these rich descriptions into clinically meaningful categories. It is this balance—comprehensiveness and systematization—that guided the ICDL work groups in creating this manual. The goal is to provide a diagnostic system for infancy and early childhood mental health and developmental learning disorders that provides the basis for understanding the nature of the child's challenges and for formulating comprehensive and effective intervention approaches.

Another goal is to provide a diagnostic system that is useful for research into etiology, early developmental pathways, and intervention outcomes. Only a diagnostic system that describes the full complexity of disordered functioning and characterizes different subtypes can provide a basis for basic research on underlying etiologies and developmental pathways (see, for example, the section on the different subtypes for Neurodevelopmental Disorders of Relating and Communicating–200).

OVERVIEW OF THE ICDL-DMIC MULTI-AXIAL SYSTEM

The approach presented in the following sections reflects ICDL's developmental framework for classifying the full range of infant and early childhood mental health, developmental, and learning disorders. We will consider three broad categories of mental health disorders:

1. **Interactive Disorders**, involving symptom patterns such as anxiety, depression, and disruptive behaviors;
2. **Regulatory-Sensory Processing Disorders**, involving symptom patterns such as inattention, overreactivity, sensory seeking; and
3. **Neurodevelopmental Disorders of Relating and Communicating**, involving symptom patterns, such as self-absorption, perseveration, and dysfunctional communication (e.g., ASD patterns).

These categories include the kinds of problems that are currently conceptualized in DSM-IV-R, but not in a sufficiently developmental or comprehensive manner.

Interactive Disorders refer to challenges where a primary contribution to the difficulty stems from the infant or child-caregiver interaction patterns and related family and environmental patterns. Regulatory-Sensory Processing Disorders refer to those challenges where differences in the child's constitutional and maturational variations, in terms of sensory over- or underreactivity, visuospatial, auditory and language processing, or motor planning and sequencing difficulties are a primary contributor to the child's challenges. Neurodevelopmental Disorders of Relating and Communicating refer to developmental disorders, including autism spectrum disorders, where there are significant difficulties with the fundamental capacities to relate, communicate, and think.

Neurodevelopmental Disorders of Relating and Communicating often include regulatory-sensory processing difficulties and interactive difficulties. If, however, basic relating, communicating, and thinking are disrupted, the problems would be classified under this category. Regulatory-Sensory Processing Disorders may also involve interactive difficulties. However, if constitutional-maturational variations are a significant contribution, the problems are classified in this category. Interactive Disorders may involve constitutional and maturational variations as well as infant-caregiver interactions. However, in Interactive Disorders, the constitutional-maturational variations are not in the clinical (i.e., disordered) range and the major contributor to the problems stems from the caregiver-child interaction and related family and environmental patterns.

The only exception to the principles stated above relates to disorders involving trauma. These are classified under Interactive Disorders. Reactions to trauma may involve regulatory-sensory processing changes, such as sensory over-responsiveness; responses to trauma may also often involve anxiety or depression. When a clear trauma can be identified and is clinically thought to be responsible for the symptoms, priority is given to the diagnosis of traumatic stress disorder.

In addition, a new feature of our diagnostic manual is the inclusion of Language Disorders and Learning Challenges.

Language Disorders include challenges in communication in the context of a developmental framework that considers all components of language (e.g., gestures, motor, sensory, social, etc.). These can constitute a primary disorder when not part of another major disorder, such as Neurodevelopmental Disorders of Relating and Communicating. Language capacities also have their own profile (see Axis IV) because of the significance of language in development, as well as its impact on overall development.

Learning Challenges are included in this classification in order to identify the early pathways associated with later learning differences and challenges at school age. The goal is to optimize early interventions which may head off or ameliorate these challenges later. These include learning difficulties in reading and reading comprehension, math, and written expression, as well as organizational capacities (i.e., executive functioning).

A child may evidence a Language Disorder or Learning Challenge in addition to Interactive or Regulatory-Sensory Processing Disorders. However, if a child evidences Neurodevelopmental Disorders of Relating and Communicating, her language or learning problems would be subsumed under the broad umbrella of that neurodevelopmental disorder.

ICDL Multi-Axial Classification Approach

The approach to classifying infant and early childhood disorders should always include a comprehensive evaluation, a clinical formulation, and recommendations for a comprehensive intervention program. Appendix I specifies the approach to comprehensive assessment and evaluation and Appendix II, the framework for planning a comprehensive intervention program.

In order to organize the information from a comprehensive evaluation and to capture the unique qualities of each infant and young child and his or her family, it is essential to construct a comprehensive view of each child that includes presenting problems and functioning captured by Axis I, Primary Diagnosis, as well as other relevant capacities that are necessary to understand the child and his family and plan an appropriate intervention program. These include a functional emotional developmental profile, a regulatory-sensory processing profile, a language profile, a visuospatial profile, caregiver-infant and family patterns, stressors, and other medical or neurological diagnoses. These profiles form the basis of a multi-axial diagnosis. Axes II through VII are accompanied by clinical ratings or descriptions where the clinician may indicate the relative degree to which a particular capacity has been mastered. Each is briefly described below and is summarized in Figure 1. More detailed criteria are contained in following sections.

Figure 1: Diagram of Multi-Axial Approach

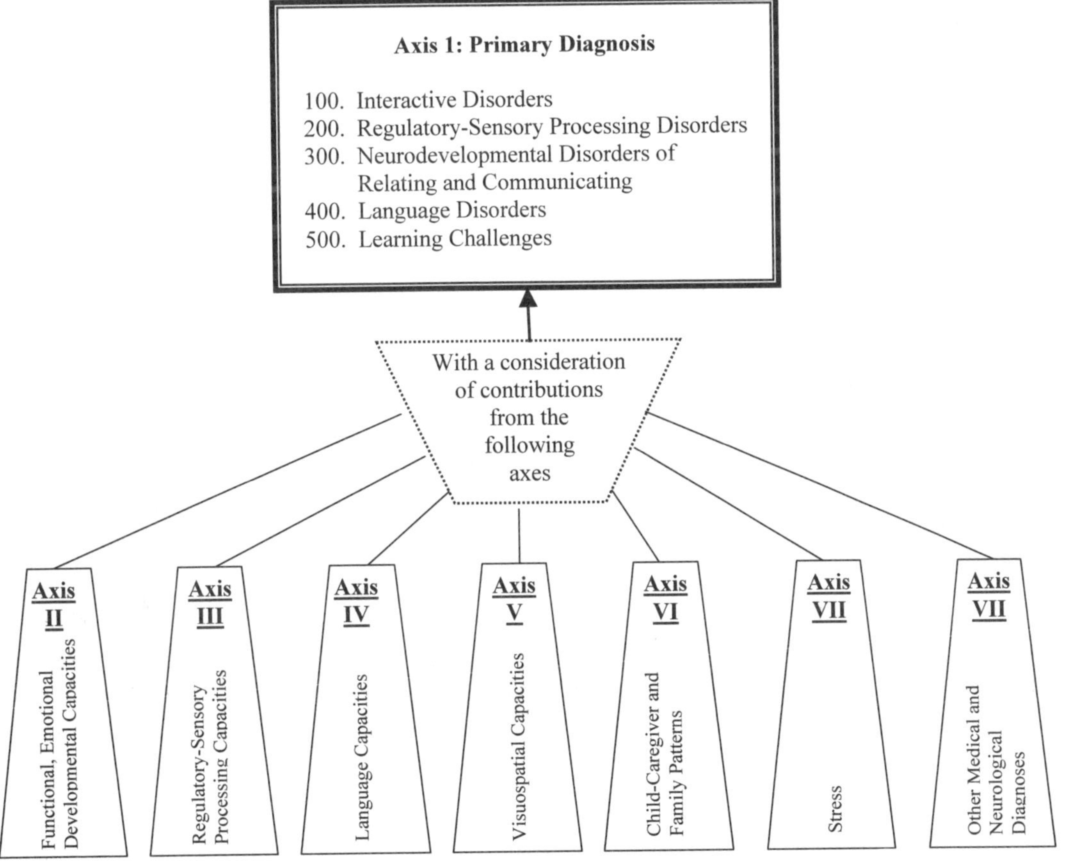

- **Axis I–Primary Diagnosis:** The broad diagnostic category—Interactive Disorder, Regulatory-Sensory Processing Disorder, Neurodevelopmental Disorder of Relating and Communicating, Language Disorder, and/or Learning Challenges—and the specific type of disorder within the category.

- **Axis II–Functional Emotional Developmental Capacities:** The relative mastery of each of the functional emotional developmental capacities, including shared attention and regulation, engagement and relating, two-way intentional, affective signaling and communication, long chains of co-regulated emotional signaling and shared social problem solving, creating symbols or ideas, building bridges between ideas- logical thinking.

- **Axis III–Regulatory-Sensory Processing Capacities:** The regulatory-sensory processing capacities, in terms of sensory modulation, sensory discrimination, and sensory-based motor abilities, including postural control and motor planning.

- **Axis IV–Language Capacities:** Includes gestural and verbal communication (comprehension and production) at each developmental level.

- **Axis V–Visuospatial Capacities:** The progressive development of visuospatial aspects of body awareness and sense thinking, location of the body in space, relation of objects to the self and other objects and people, conservation of space, visual logical thinking, and representational thought.

- **Axis VI–Child-Caregiver and Family Patterns:** Characteristics of infant or child-caregiver interaction patterns and family or environmental patterns.

- **Axis VII–Stress:** Stressors related to situations, conditions or events in the family's or child's life which can impact the child's emotional functioning and development when appropriate protective factors or adequate resiliency are not evident.

- **Axis VIII–Other Medical and Neurological Diagnoses**.

While the multi-axial approach summarizes the child's functioning, it does not replace the narrative developmental formulation that describes in more detail each of the factors outlined in these axes.

As may be apparent, different disciplines may have different degrees of familiarity with the concepts embodied in these axes. For example, occupational therapists may be quite familiar with the content of the regulatory-sensory processing axis, but less familiar with the axis describing functional emotional developmental levels. Mental health professionals may be more familiar with the functional emotional developmental levels axis and the family and interactive patterns axis and less familiar with the regulatory-sensory processing or language axes. The visuospatial processing axis may be relatively unfamiliar to many experienced clinicians. Clearly, a team approach with different professionals collaborating may be very helpful in formulating a comprehensive diagnostic profile that includes attention to all the axes outlined above.

In addition, individual clinicians using this system may find that they can comfortably use some of the axes but not others. Use of the full system may be viewed as a goal to strive for. As that goal is being pursued, we hope the use of the axes one is familiar with, coupled with an awareness of the importance of the other dimensions functioning and the possible need for consultation with colleagues is very helpful. The long-term goal is to have more and more clinicians working with infants and young children with emotional, developmental, language, and/or learning challenges to have opportunities for additional training and experience that would permit the full use of this system.[1]

SELECTING A PRIMARY DIAGNOSIS

Most infant and early childhood disorders are characterized by multiple elements or dimensions, for example, interactive and family patterns, and regulatory-sensory processing patterns. These disorders include anxiety, and mood disorders, disruptive behavior, elective mutism, as well as sleep, eating, and elimination disorders. A multi-axial approach allows a systematic description of each of the contributing elements. However, the primary diagnosis is made based on a clinical judgment regarding the predominant contributing factor. Before concluding on a primary diagnosis, all the axes must be fully evaluated in order to determine the various dimensions contributing to the presenting problems. Once all this information is considered, clinical reasoning guides the experienced clinician in selecting the predominant pattern.

The decision process would first consider the most comprehensive disorder where multiple elements of development are derailed. For example, Neurodevelopmental Disorders of Relating and Communicating includes Regulatory-Sensory Processing Disorders, Language Disorder, and emotional constrictions. When relating and communicating are not significantly derailed then the Regulatory-Sensory Processing Disorders are considered next to see if the presenting behavioral patterns are coupled with motor and/or regulatory-sensory processing challenges. When a regulatory-sensory processing contribution is significant, it takes precedence over the interactive elements in the designation of the primary diagnosis.

When the primary diagnosis is an Interactive Disorder, more than one type of Interactive Disorder may be identified. Since there is so much overlap in the symptoms of the various Interactive Disorders, the clinician must consider when the symptom is part of a broader disorder such as anxiety, mood or disruptive behavior, and when it is itself the primary disorder. In other words, clinical reasoning must determine if the multiple symptoms are significant enough to constitute an additional diagnosis or are part of the

[1] To that end, the Interdisciplinary Council on Developmental and Learning Disorders (ICDL) offers a variety of training programs and is increasing the availability and comprehensiveness of these programs, including plans for a graduate degree program in the near future (see http://www.icdl.com and http://www.floortime.org for further information)

primary problem. For example, if a child with Anxiety Disorder also has sleep problems, but the sleep problem is intermittent or a temporary disruption of a developmental capacity already mastered, along with possible other disruptions in eating or toileting, then an additional diagnosis would not be necessary. However, if the sleep problem is very intense or of longer duration, and also meets the description of the primary disorder, then it could be considered a second primary diagnosis. Similarly, if a child manifests disruptive or oppositional behavior, Anxiety Disorder or Disruptive Behavior Problem could be considered and the differentiating consideration would be whether the child has a pattern of impulse control problems in various situations or emotional states. If not, then Anxiety Disorder may be the only primary diagnosis selected. More than one diagnosis is permitted under this system. In addition, as indicated earlier, we emphasize a Language Disorder or Learning Challenge can be used as a second primary diagnosis when a child evidences a significant difficulty in either of these areas of functioning.

CLINICAL THRESHOLDS FOR DIAGNOSIS

Deciding when a behavioral or emotional pattern constitutes a disorder rather than a disruption or variation within the normal range presents the clinician with a challenge. This can be especially difficult during the first five years when development is proceeding rapidly and has so much variation influenced by individual differences. It is also a challenge when so many of the same symptoms can relate to different disorders given the limited number of symptoms in the infant's and young child's repertoire.

As indicated above, the attempts to define specific criteria for disorders in order to reach reliability do not always have solid evidence. In addition, many of the current classification approaches go beyond the available research in their specificity by requiring a specific number of criteria for a diagnosis. Yet, there are insufficient studies documenting what it means if the patient meets only two out of five (i.e., there is no data supporting a clear line between two versus three of the criteria).

Similarly, there's insufficient data on how long a symptom should be evidenced, as if two days less than the indicated two weeks is scientifically based. Criteria that are easy to agree upon are not necessarily the criteria that are meaningful for clinical planning or research on etiological factors and developmental pathways. We do not yet have a scientifically-based diagnostic system for mental health, developmental, and learning challenges, but we do have emerging data and a great deal of clinical experience.

Since we are currently operating on expert consensus with supportive, but incomplete, data, this classification system utilizes functional or operational considerations to make the clinical judgment of whether the presenting problems cross the clinical threshold to be considered a disorder. The following hierarchy should be considered:

- Is the child functioning within his or her age-expected functional developmental capacities? What is the range of the child's comprehension and expression of emotions with gestures and/or words or play, in comparison to age expectations?

This could be evaluated using Axis II–Functional Emotional Developmental Capacities, as well as other clinical information and assessments.

- How well is the child functioning within the family structure on a daily basis including routines of sleep, meals, play, relating to family, caregivers and sibling interactions? Is the environment stable? Is the child stable?

- Is the child adapting to daycare or preschool adequately and able to enjoy these environments and learning experiences?

- Is the child participating in expected social interactions, developing friendships, and able to play with peers?

- What are the child's emerging attitudes and feelings towards himself or herself and others (e.g., angry, depressed, suspicious, etc.) in comparison to what's expected for his or her age (e.g., some degree of negativism is expected during the preschool years)?

The child may present significant challenges in any one of these areas which may be sufficient to warrant a diagnosis—for example, difficulties in relating and communicating. In some cases, more than one area may be involved but the problem may not be spilling over significantly to preschool or peer play, such as a disorder of emotional range and stability where constrictions are significant and family interactions cannot support healthier emotional development. Sometimes the threshold is not crossed until the preschool brings the problem to the attention of the family—the problem may not be perceived or evidenced at home, yet is significantly impeding the child's adaptation at school. The greater the number of areas of functioning that are involved, the more likely a diagnosis is indicated.

Furthermore, in addition to the detailed descriptions of the primary diagnosis to guide clinical judgment, Axes II through VII require a clinical formulation indicating the degree to which impairment is evident. The more severe the impairment or delay of the expected developmental capacities, the greater the evidence for the disorder(s). Clinical judgment relies on evaluating the functional or operating areas and each of the dimensions in this multi-axial system to determine if the clinical threshold for a diagnosis has been crossed.

Even when the clinical threshold is not crossed, the diagnostic process and evaluation provides the parents with a better understanding of their child's profile of strengths and vulnerabilities and allow anticipatory guidance to better support the development of the child and family in the future.

In the sections that follow, each broad group of disorders is described and selected therapeutic implications are considered.

Making a Diagnosis: Case Illustration Using the ICDL-DMIC Multi-Axial Approach

In the prior section, we briefly described the primary diagnoses that need to be considered and the different axes that need to be taken into account. In order to illustrate how to decide which primary diagnosis is most appropriate and utilize the different axes, this section presents a case study that illustrates how a trained DIR clinician approaches a differential diagnosis in a complex case and uses the multi-axial evaluation to organize a comprehensive treatment plan.[1]

Making a proper diagnosis, particularly when many competing diagnoses are possible, is important. An appropriate diagnosis can lead to the best intervention plan to help the child move forward and make consistent progress. However, as indicated earlier in this manual, a diagnosis, even a multi-axial one, is only a summary of the detailed developmental profile captured in a narrative description of the child. As the illustration below demonstrates, however, the narrative description can be systematized by the recommended multi-axial diagnostic approach described in this manual and summarized into meaningful categories.

There are also brief case vignettes following the discussion of some of the primary diagnostic categories. These are intended only to illustrate that category, not the use of the entire profile, as is the goal of the following case study.

CASE ILLUSTRATION

Case History

Charlie first came in at age 3½. His parents told me that he had already been diagnosed with a number of different labels and they were completely confused. One of his presenting problems was that he wasn't playing with peers at his preschool and tended to either play alone or avoid the other children. During one evaluation, he was therefore labeled Social Anxiety Disorder.

This little boy also had difficulty with language. He could speak, but wasn't always able to understand complex instructions that would be appropriate for a 3 to 3½ year old, like a two- or three-step suggestions (e.g., "Please get the teddy bear and the truck and bring them to me"). If asked why he wanted to go outside, he would often look confused. Sometimes he could answer a question, such as "Where is the car going?" and other times he would ignore the question and just push his car forward. These challenges had led to a diagnosis of Language Disorder.

Occasionally, his parents reported, Charlie would jump around the room in a seemingly aimless way, particularly if he got excited. At those times, he would flap his hands a

[1] The DIR Institute provides an interdisciplinary educational program and DIR® Certificate Program for clinicians to conduct assessment and intervention using the DIR approach. See www.icdl.com for further information. It may be useful to review this case again after reading the entire manual.

bit and walk on his toes. Other times, he would seem to get mesmerized by a fan or by looking toward a light. However, his parents could usually draw him away from those occupations by touching him or getting in front of him. Nonetheless, they were concerned about these patterns.

In one evaluation, the diagnostician put together Charlie's social problems with peers, language challenges, and his tendency to become a little bit aimless, jump up and down and flap his hands (what the clinician called "self-stimulatory behavior"), and made a diagnosis of an autism spectrum disorder. She also used the term, PDD-NOS (Pervasive Developmental Disorder, Not Otherwise Specified). This is a diagnostic label usually reserved for a child who has features of autism, but who might not meet all the criteria necessary for that disorder. PDD-NOS, however, does place a child on the autism spectrum.

During an evaluation with an occupational therapist, the parents reported that their son was very reactive to certain types of sensations. In loud, noisy rooms, for example, with a lot of music or with children speaking loudly, he would cover his ears and seemed to get over-stimulated. Also, Charlie had difficulty chewing and even swallowing some very chewy kinds of foods. The occupational therapist felt that he had a sensory integration problem, as well as low muscle tone in parts of his body. She also diagnosed him with planning difficulties (dyspraxia).

Charlie's parents felt confused by the myriad diagnoses and the many different intervention recommendations they received as a result of them. For the PDD and autism spectrum disorder a special needs school with an autism program was recommended. For the language problems, an intensive speech therapy program was recommended to help him reach age-expected language levels. Occupational therapy was recommended to work on Charlie's muscle tone and sensory modulation and sensory integration challenges. For the Social Anxiety Disorder, the clinician recommended a consideration of medication, even though Charlie was only 3½, to reduce his anxiety. The parents were concerned because the medication suggested was an SSRI-type in the categories of Paxil, Prozac, etc., and they had read in the newspapers recently that that might be associated with negative side effects.

Formulation of the Primary Diagnosis: Axis I

It was clear from this background that we needed to do a fresh and complete evaluation to get a picture of what was going on with Charlie. In that way, we could formulate a proper diagnosis and intervention plan. We used a multi-axial approach to formulate the diagnosis, using a consideration of the Axes II - VII, along with the Axis I considerations, to observe and describe Charlie in many areas of functioning.

The Parents' Report

We began by helping the parents talk more about their current concerns, and where they thought Charlie had vulnerabilities and strengths. Since his vulnerabilities had been described when we took the history, we explored what they thought were Charlie's strengths.

For example, even though he was anxious at school and avoided the other children, at home with his parents he could be very warm and intimate, crawl up into their laps and want to cuddle. He loved sitting late at night with his father, looking at pictures in a book. He also had a very close relationship with his mother. Charlie and his mother would roll trucks on the floor during the daytime in fun games and she reported that he liked to come into the kitchen when she was cooking. Sometimes he would get out a little toy pot and pretend to stir and cook with her. They felt that he was a very loving little fellow.

The parents pointed out that, at times, Charlie could be very creative in his pretend play. When mother played with trucks with him, for example, sometimes the trucks would go and visit daddy's office. If she asked him why the truck was going there, though, he often couldn't answer. Sometimes, he just changed the subject and had the truck bang into daddy's "office," as though he got a little anxious with a question he couldn't answer. Mother felt Charlie had little creative flairs where he would invent something new in the play from time to time. She also felt his strength was that he could tell her when he wanted. If he wanted some juice or to watch a favorite video, he would ask, "Mommy, can I watch the Barney tape?" or "Can I watch this or that?" If she said "No," he would sometimes get upset, but she also thought it was a strength that he wouldn't throw a major tantrum. He might stomp around a bit or whimper, but then he would recover after a few minutes.

In terms of his developmental history, the parents reported that Charlie progressed as expected and was looking at them as a little baby. He was able to smile by 3 or 4 months and seemed happy. He was able to be purposeful in terms of reaching for and interacting with them, and he made sounds and babbled back-and-forth with them before the end of his first year.

Charlie was a little delayed in rolling over, crawling, and walking. He didn't walk until about 15 months, which concerned them. Even now, they reported, he was not as well coordinated as the other children, and this fit in with what the occupational therapist had said to them about low muscle tone and difficulty with motor planning and sequencing. The parents also noted that it became very clear in his second year of life that he was very sensory responsive to things like loud noises and certain kinds of touch - he only liked soft, cotton garments and didn't like rough or even synthetic garments. He got fussy when things were near his skin that he found uncomfortable.

Charlie's parents reported that he began using words a little bit late, using two words together closer to age 2. He had some single words around 18 months, but wasn't progressing like other children in terms of understanding "why" questions or even complex "where" questions. However, he seemed to be making progress.

Charlie had no unusual medical disorders. He had shown some eczema as a baby and they had eliminated milk products to help with that problem. They still kept milk and dairy products away because of his tendency toward eczema. That seemed to be helpful.

Clinician's Observations – Functional Emotional Developmental Capacities – Axis II

We began our observation of Charlie by assessing his functional emotional developmental levels. We looked at the areas of shared attention, engagement, two-way purposeful communication, shared social problem solving, the creative use of ideas, and the logical use of ideas.

We observed Charlie very carefully as he played with his mother and father in the office. First we observed their spontaneous play and then we observed how they played together when we gave them some suggestions to help bring out Charlie's highest level of functioning.

We saw that in a one-on-one situation in a calm environment without noise and a lot of other children around, Charlie was able to focus and attend (Level 1) and interact with his mother and father, rolling cars or trucks back-and-forth. He was able to show a lot of joy and happiness and smiled warmly at his parents during the play (Level 2). He made a lot of gleeful sounds when, for example, his father blocked his truck and he had to make his vehicle into a "flying truck." He was able to be purposeful, engaging in a lot of back-and-forth, two-way communication with vocalizations back-and-forth and gesturing (Level 3). At one point, Charlie took his parents by the hand to go to the door because he wanted to go out to get a toy that he had seen (Level 4 - Shared Problem Solving). Although he couldn't explain why he wanted the door opened, eventually Charlie was able to say, "Toy, toy there" (Level 5). It required some multiple-choice help to get him to be able to answer the question, however. We got a toy from the other room and he came back in as a happy boy and used the toy, a little gas station, to fuel his cars.

Sometimes Charlie seemed to get distracted from his play themes, jumping from one idea to another. He could meet physical challenges in his play with a little bit of support and help from his parents, but he tended to get avoidant and change subjects rather quickly when the shared social problem solving aspects (Level 4) got a little bit challenging.

Charlie could be creative in his use of ideas (Level 5) and he could use his available language, expressing simple phrases or sentences to respond to his father saying, for example, "What's this?" or "Where is the car going?" "Going to school or garage?" He could use language meaningfully, for example, when he asked for some juice, "Can I have juice now?" (Level 5). He could also respond to, "Are you thirsty or hungry?" and indicate he wanted, "a lot of juice" when shown two glasses, one with a little and one with a lot. One time, he said "Going to school...play with Zoogie (a stuffed animal he loved at school)." He then took the toy car and an action figure to the play school house. Here he was showing nice potential for expanding his creative play.

When it came to connecting his ideas together (Level 6), Charlie could answer most of the "w" questions (what, where, and who), but had trouble with "why" questions. With multiple-choice help, however, he could get them. With lots of back and forth conversation he understood the "why" questions, but didn't quite have them fully mastered. He could, however, tell you how he felt when obstructed.

Charlie showed lots of good capacities in the functional emotional developmental levels when we observed him in pretend play, interacting with parents. He evidenced competencies at all the levels, with sluggishness at the sixth level of combining ideas together to elaborate in logical ways. He also needed work on expanding his imaginative play and his flexibility with shared social problem solving. The constrictions seemed to be related, in part, to his motor planning and language challenges.

Clinician's Observations: Regulatory-Sensory Processing – Axis III

As we were observing Charlie's functional emotional developmental capacities, we also looked at his sensory, motor, and visuospatial processing capacities (Axis III). For example, one time in the play, his father set up a challenge that meant Charlie had to climb over something, which was difficult for him. Rather than follow through, he just went to the other side of the room and started playing by himself with another toy. We encouraged the father to go over and join Charlie with that other toy and then to move the toy behind the barrier he wanted Charlie to climb over, offering to help him get to it. With that assistance, Charlie allowed his father to help him and he climbed over the barrier, got to the other side, and got the toy he wanted. In general with hard motor tasks, Charlie tended to avoid and give up easily. He also had a little trouble with sequencing and with putting many steps in a row together to solve a problem.

At one point, we took out some drawing paper and crayons. Charlie had difficulty holding the crayons-he tended to "fist" them. He could scribble, but not really make circles or other shapes or copy shapes his parents drew. He did seem to enjoy just scribbling with a fisted crayon and making colors.

Also, we played some "Simon Says" games to see whether or not he could do two or three things in a row. He could do one thing like, "touch your nose" or "touch your head," but had a hard time doing two or three commands in a row ("Touch your head and then your nose"). Importantly, however, when I asked him to just verbally repeat three things that I said, he could do so easily, suggesting that his challenge was more in the area of executing the sequence of actions, rather than his remembering or sequencing a series of ideas.

To check for reported over-responsiveness to sound, we suggested that father "toot" the horn on his toy truck. Sure enough, as father's toots became loud, Charlie held his ears, got a little fidgety, and began jumping around, walking on his toys and shaking his hands a little bit. He was clearly overloaded by the loud sounds. This also indicated that when he got sensory overloaded, he wasn't able to coordinate his body in a rhythmic or organized way. He needed to do the jumping and hand shaking as a way of dealing with the sensory overload.

At the end of the observation period, we had a good picture of Charlie's regulatory sensory processing challenges. He evidenced some motor planning and sequencing challenges, or dyspraxia, and some muscle tone difficulties. This contributed to making postural control, or balance, and coordination a little bit harder for him. These also made fine motor skills harder for him (e.g., holding the crayon properly). These challenges, plus his sensory over-responsivity were consistent with what we call Regulatory-Sensory Processing Disorders (Axis I - 200s).

Clinician's Observations: Language Capacities – Axis IV

During our observation of Charlie and his parents at play, we also looked at his language functioning very carefully. Typically between age 3-3½, children are learning to answer "why" questions and he was just beginning to learn to answer them. However, he was quite creative in his pretend play, as indicated earlier, and could, for example, talk about the fact that "I am mad and I'm going to bang my car into your truck," when I challenged him with, "What are you going to do now that I'm blocking your road?" He was also able to tell me who he liked at school, his favorite food, and that "Mommy plays with me a lot" and "Daddy is at work and doesn't play."

In terms of language functioning, he showed relative mastery (though he needed work to expand these capacities) of the first five levels described in our language axis (from self-regulation, engagement, and two-way communication up through using word combinations and sharing meanings). He wasn't quite as far along in the sixth stage of Early Discourse, as would be optimal, but was on the right trajectory. My impression was that with a little greater emphasis at home on shared pretend play and back-and-forth conversations, Charlie would make good progress.

Clinician's Observations: Visuospatial – Axis V

We also looked at Charlie's ability for visuospatial processing. Although his motor problems made it hard for him to copy shapes, he also didn't seem to have a very good understanding of the way visual designs were constructed. For example, when I asked him to show me how to make a shape, in spite of his otherwise functional verbal abilities, he was unable to direct my hands.

In addition, we played a little search game in the room to see if he was a systematic searcher, and whether or not he could take into account the whole room and figure out a systematic search strategy. Here Charlie showed challenges when he looked in two places and then gave up and got distracted, rather than searching in all four corners of the room. He was able to be cautious about his boundaries with me and his parents (i.e., not invading our space). At the same time, however, he found it hard to anticipate where a ball was going to end up when I rolled it in his direction. He also found it hard to build even simple structures out of blocks. Therefore, the initial impression was that visuospatial capacities required further observation and would likely require some intervention work.

Clinician's Observations: Child-Caregiver Family Patterns – Axis VI

We also explored the family patterns and family relationships. We found that there was a solid relationship between mother and father and there was no marital stress or problems. There were no siblings yet, although they were hoping to have more children.

When we watched the parents play with Charlie, we were looking for whether they were intrusive or over-stimulating, or if they were having trouble being soothing and calming. They seemed to relate to Charlie at each of his developmental levels. They were calm and regulating; they were engaging. They were interactive and were also quite creative in the way they wanted to play with him.

In terms of the family dynamics, we didn't see any real interactive reasons for Charlie's anxiety. This helped us rule out one of our Interactive Disorders (100s). Although we did see Charlie's anxiety, we didn't see an interactive anxiety-based problem.

We also looked at interactive caregiver/child interactions and family functioning. Here we saw some relative strengths. This family seemed to be supporting Charlie's development, and, in fact, it was my impression that he was doing as well as he was doing because of the strength of the way his caregivers were interacting and playing with him, and the warmth one could feel in the whole family. There were relatively strong family patterns that were helping this child negotiate and navigate development and make consistent progress, even though there were some constitutional-maturational variations resulting in the regulatory-sensory processing and language challenges.

Clinician's Observations: Stress – Axis VII

During the course of the clinical session, we looked for stressors in Charlie's life as possible contributing factors. In this family, there were no unusual stresses, no recent illnesses, grandparents passing away, moves from one house to another, or job changes for the parents. The only stress for this little guy was trying to cope with preschool and the noise and activity level in the classroom.

Clinician's Observations: Other Medical and Neurological Diagnoses – Axis VIII

Finally, we looked for other medical or neurological diagnoses that might have contributed to Charlie's challenges. According to parent reports and medical records, other than a history of some allergies and eczema, he had been pretty healthy. There was no history of seizures or metabolic disorders. Charlie had regular pediatric evaluations and there were no physical contributions to his challenges, other than the ones we described in terms of the uneven maturation of his central nervous system.

Diagnostic Impressions – Summary of Observations

When we put together the history, the review of his current functioning, the challenges, and the observations just made in the clinical setting, we were able to come to a picture that helped us see Charlie in terms of his unique developmental profile. This allowed us to consider a proper diagnosis and plan an appropriate intervention plan tailored to his individual needs.

Although by history we knew that Charlie had been given a number of diagnoses—including Social Anxiety Disorder, PDD-NOS, Autism Spectrum Disorder, Language Disorder, and Sensory Integration Disorder—we now wanted to see this child's functioning as a whole. The key to making a proper diagnosis is not to give a separate label to each component, but to see how all these different pieces fit into one pattern.

First, it was important to see if it was possible to rule out some of the diagnoses that were given. The most severe one, and the one that was greatly worrisome to the parents, was the Autism Spectrum Disorder and the PDD-NOS diagnoses.

Using the information gleaned from our observations along the axes during the clinical sessions, we saw some of the behaviors that are usually associated with these disorders, but we also saw some strengths that were not usually associated with them. When Charlie got overloaded, he showed some tendency to hand flap and to jump up and down. He was avoiding other children at school, but he appeared to have a very nice capacity for warm intimacy. He was able to signal with his emotions and get into reciprocal back-and-forth emotional signaling. He was also able to use his emerging ideas very creatively (based on his affect or emotions). His ideas were driven by his wishes, needs, desires, or feelings. He wasn't scripting his ideas or just using his memory. He was making progress in becoming a logical thinker.

The fact that he was avoiding other children seemed more related to the sensory overload, the immaturity in his motor system, the low muscle tone, not feeling confident in his body, and to the anxiety and confusion that he felt, than a more primary problem with relating to others.

Based on the observations primarily in Axes II, III, and VI, we felt that Charlie did not evidence either an Autism Spectrum Disorder or PDD-NOS, which in our diagnostic classification system would have fallen into the Neurodevelopmental Disorders of Relating and Communicating (300s).

Next we looked at the possibility of Interactive Disorders (100s). Since Charlie was anxious at school, and we could see him get anxious whenever the task was hard, what would be the best way to characterize the anxiety? Would these anxiety patterns fit into an Axis I primary diagnosis of 101. Anxiety Disorder?

Again, when we observed Charlie in session through the course of the complete evaluation described above, we formulated a profile of his functioning, his strengths, and areas of challenge. Charlie was a warm, related, interactive, creative, bright little boy who was sensory over-responsive, who had areas of low muscle tone, and some coordination problems. His anxiety was most intense in noisy, sensory-overloading environments, such as school or at times when he needed to sequence many movements in a row. Because he evidenced clear sensory over-responsivity and motor planning and sequencing problems, he clearly had regulatory-sensory processing differences that were related to his challenges. When they are present to a significant degree, Regulatory-Sensory Processing Disorders take precedence over Interactive Disorders.

As we described earlier, Charlie had many of the developmental foundations for language and was functioning close to age expectations in his language capacities (Axis IV), having mastered the earlier stages. The impression was that he would continue to make progress with appropriate interactions at home. Therefore, while there were some language challenges, Language Disorder as a primary Axis I diagnosis was not indicated.

Although some of Charlie's challenges might have some impact on his ability to learn as he went to school, we felt that a comprehensive intervention program aimed at his regulatory-sensory processing challenges would work on challenges related to Axis I: 500. Learning Challenges. In such an instance, it is not necessary to use a second primary diagnosis.

Diagnosis

Our diagnostic impression, therefore, was of a primary diagnosis of a 200. Regulatory-Sensory Processing Disorder. We used the 201. Over-Responsive, Fearful, Anxious Pattern (this captures his sensory over-responsivity, secondary anxiety, and avoidance of peers and other activities at school) as his primary Axis I diagnosis. We also used 205. Inattentive, Disorganized Pattern. This described his motor planning and sequencing challenges and low muscle tone, evidenced in his difficulties in carrying out multi-step actions. His other challenges, particularly in visuospatial capacities are described in Axis V. Charlie's language challenges are described in Axis IV.

Intervention Plan

Formulating the diagnosis led us to recommend and plan an intervention program that would deal with each of these areas in a supportive and comprehensive manner.

We began with the home program, recommending that his parents do Floortime with him every day. Because he was functioning well, we recommended each parent do at least two 20-minute sessions with him. At other times, we suggested that they just enjoy the interaction with their son, as they had been doing. We recommended minimizing screen time (TV, videos, computer games) to 30 minutes or less a day. In the Floortime, we recommended that they play as they had in the office, making Charlie's pretend dramas more complex and throwing in the occasional "why" question to help him think more logically. In the beginning, they could help him answer the questions with multiple choice help. In this way, we would help Charlie get more practice in receiving complex information and thinking. We suggested that the parents try out complex directions once in a while, so he would have to sequence more actions in a row and do that as part of the pretend play to help him also practice his language skills. If progress was not sufficient, we would add in speech therapy. The home program was aimed at strengthening the Axis II Functional Emotional Developmental Capacities and helping Charlie master the higher levels of thinking and interacting.

As part of the comprehensive intervention program we designed for Charlie, we an occupational therapy treatment program to work on his primary diagnosis of Regulatory-Sensory Processing Disorder. The program would need to address his sensory modulation challenges, motor planning and sequencing difficulties, and his muscle tone problems. As a result, Charlie started attending one occupational therapy session a week with a qualified OT, and played twice a day in an active enjoyable home program. This involved games and play at home or in the park to help Charlie overcome challenges related to his primary diagnosis. At least twice a day for 20 minutes each, we suggested a physical workout involving some running, jumping, spinning, perceptual motor games (e.g., throwing, catching, kicking big Nerf balls, balance and coordination games, walking over balance beams, etc. as well as some search games–treasure hunts where he would learn to more systematically use his visual abilities to search around the room).

We incorporated Floortime into these OT activities, where climbing, swinging and obstacle courses turned into adventures searching for jungle animals on a Safari, climbing mountains, spaceships to the moon, adding pretend to elaborate movements, problem solving, language and reasoning.

To help Charlie with the social anxiety he was feeling (related to his challenges in Axis III), we wanted to get him more comfortable with his peers, taking into consideration his sensory over-responsivity. We wanted to help him tolerate wider ranges of unexpected and background sounds coming from larger groups. The first suggestion was that Charlie should work up to having four peer play dates a week. The parents had been avoiding that because "he wasn't enjoying his friends." However, the principle is that if the child finds it hard to do something, he requires more practice, not less, in doing that activity. The goal at first in the peer play dates was simply to create games where he and his friend would have to interact together. If they were playing nicely doing some pretend play, or just running after each other, or being silly together, that was fine - we wouldn't interfere. But if they were moving in their own directions or getting into parallel play, we'd create a little problem solving game or drama where they had to do something together so that they would resume communication and interaction between the two of them. Initially, we recommended that the parents select peers that weren't too noisy or rambunctious and wouldn't frighten or overwhelm him.

In terms of his school program, we recommended that the educators and aides create an area in a corner of the room where Charlie could have his own little fort or tent area, which would be a little bit away from the other kids when needed, especially during free play. In this way he could avoid the sensory overload and not get banged into. Also, it would be less likely that he would be quite caught in the middle of the room and get overwhelmed, either visually, by sound, or by touch. We encouraged one of the aides at school to get him and another little friend on a one-on-one "play date at school" where they could all play in the tent or small fort. Gradually, they could add another child and then another. Pretty soon, Charlie was playing with two other children in the preschool setting. This was done very gradually so he wouldn't feel overloaded.

Also, we worked with him to say, "Too loud, too loud" when it was getting too noisy. He got so he could run up to the teacher and go, "Too loud" and she could see if he needed a little break. If so, one of the aides could take him for a little walk outside or take him to a place where he wouldn't get so overloaded.

We also shortened his school day a little bit. Parents, teachers, and aides noticed that Charlie got most overloaded between 11:00 a.m. and 12:00 p.m. That was when he seemed to start jumping around and hand flapping. Therefore, we shortened his school day to between 9:00 a.m. and 11:00 a.m. That seemed to work a little better for him. We thought we could gradually expand it once he got a little more used to a wide range of sounds and more involved playing with peers.

At home, we suggested that the parents and helpers work with him on using his gestures and words to indicate when something was uncomfortable or overloading. For example, when the noise level got loud, rather than jumping, flapping, and getting uncomfortable, he could jump over to his mother and father (or helper) and say, "Too loud," using his words, as well as holding his ears. We also developed some games that he could play with music, making it louder and softer. We also had father play a lot of "modulation games," where they would do things like singing, clapping, walking, etc., soft, loud, medium loud, and loudest, sometimes using drums and other instruments, so he could be in control of some of his sound world. He was also helped to identify other unexpected sounds in the environment. He gradually learned to adapt to a wider range of surprise sounds without getting so anxious or so scared by them.

These strategies together resulted in a good rate of progress. Charlie has done very well. Interestingly, a year and a half later his language skills are age-appropriate. He's a bright little guy who is enjoying friendships. He still doesn't like big, noisy environments and finds the school yard difficult, but he enjoys one-on-one play and small groups. He is very creative in his play and enjoys superhero dramas where he too can run and leap over all kinds of obstacles in hot pursuit of the robbers. Charlie's visuospatial skills are getting better and better as his parents continue to do lots of treasure hunt games, and games involving throwing, catching, tracking, and using both his visual and motor system in space. He now better understands how space works in a larger environment as he works with his body in space. As his motor and visuospatial skills develop, he can enjoy many more activities with his friends, including playing ball, construction, moving through obstacle courses, drawing, and other kinds of games that he does as part of the occupational therapy-guided home-based play program.

Basically, Charlie is making very good progress. He and his family are seen periodically by the clinician to monitor his progress, adjust his program when needed, and anticipate next steps. We decided to start kindergarten a year later than his typical age group to let his motor system, sensory modulation, visuospatial and language skills develop. He has responded very well to this comprehensive intervention approach and is expected to make very nice progress in a regular kindergarten class.

Contributed by: Stanley I. Greenspan, M.D. and Serena Wieder, Ph.D.

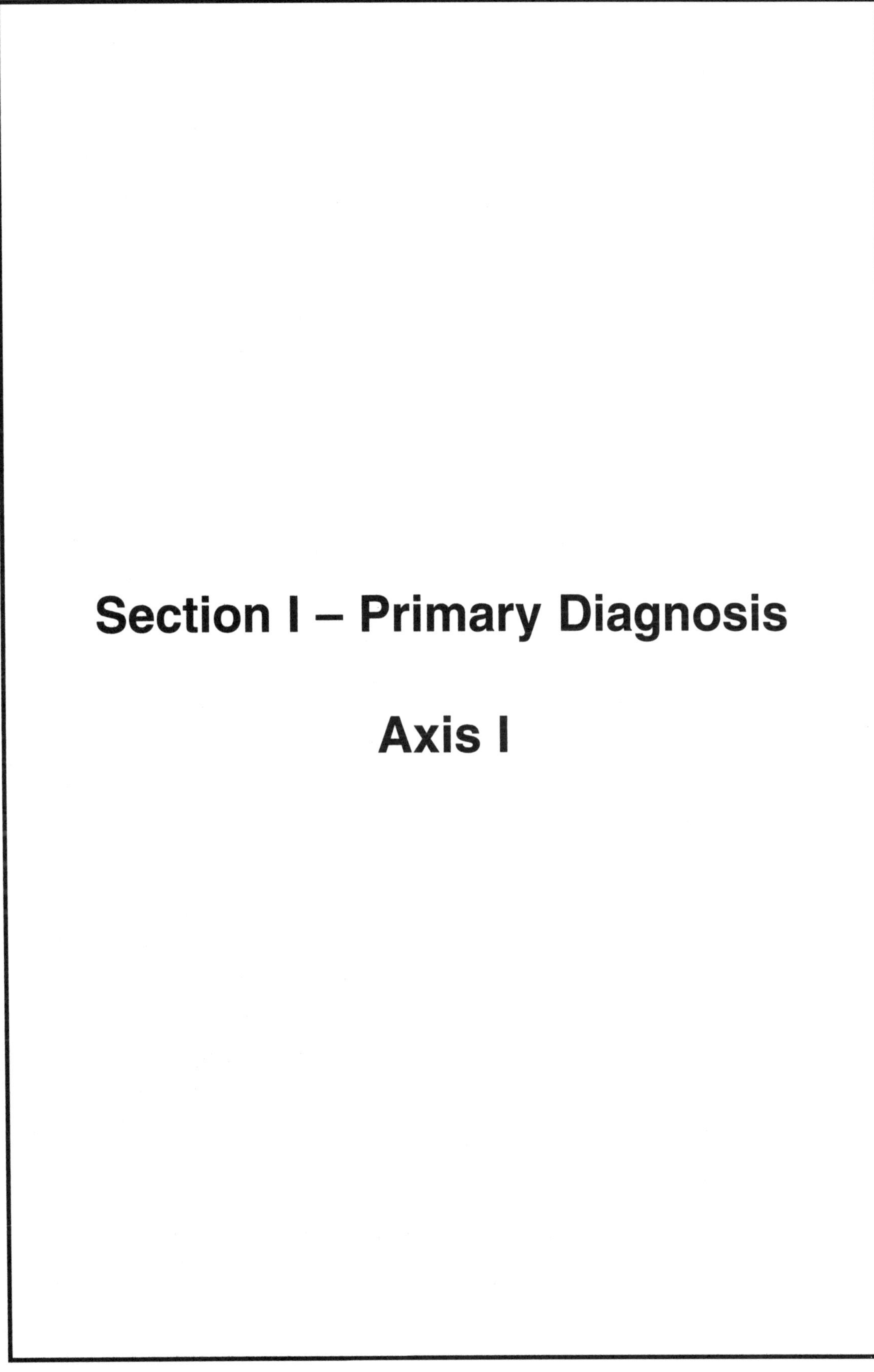

Section I – Primary Diagnosis

Axis I

Axis I: Interactive Disorders[1]

100. Interactive Disorders

101. Anxiety Disorder
102. Developmental Anxiety Disorder
103. Disorder of Emotional Range and Stability
104. Disruptive Behavior and Oppositional Disorder
105. Depression
106. Mood Dysregulation-Bipolar Patterns
107. Attentional Disorder
108. Prolonged Grief Reaction
109. Reactive Attachment Disorder
110. Traumatic Stress Disorder
111. Adjustment Disorder
112. Gender Identity Disorder
113. Elective Mutism
114. Sleep Disorder
115. Eating Disorder
116. Elimination Disorder

The descriptions of these interactive disorders includes the most salient features of the presenting picture, caregiver interactions, and regulatory-sensory processing capacities. In addition, a suggested developmental pathway, and therapeutic implications are provided for the most common disorders.

Interactive disorders are characterized by the way a child perceives and experiences his emotional world and/or by a particular maladaptive child-caregiver interaction pattern (Greenspan, 1992). The caregiver's personality, fantasies, and intentions; the child's emerging organization of experience; and the way these come together through child-caregiver interactions are important components of the basis for understanding the nature of the difficulty and for devising an effective intervention plan. As with all infant and early childhood disorders, it is important to consider the contributions not only of child-caregiver interactions but also of the child's regulatory-sensory processing profile (Axis III), and family and environmental stress factors (Axes VI and VII).

Infants and young children with interactive disorders tend to have their primary challenges with child-caregiver, family, or environmental patterns rather than their regulatory-sensory processing profile. Although each child has a unique regulatory-sensory processing profile, constitutional-maturational variations are not a major contributing fac-

1 The Work Group on Interactive Disorders includes: Serena Wieder, Ph.D., Stanley Greenspan, M.D., Lois Black, Ph.D., Griffin Doyle, Ph.D., Barbara Dunbar, Ph.D., Barbara Kalmanson, Ph.D., Lori Jeanne Peloquin, Ph.D., Ricki Robinson, M.D., MPH., Ruby Salazar, LCSW, Rick Solomon, M.D., Rosemary White, OTR, Molly Romer Witten, Ph.D.

tor in interactive disorders, as they are in the category of Regulatory-Sensory Processing Disorders, which we describe in the next section.

In cases where a thorough Developmental, Individual-Difference, Relationship-Based (DIR) assessment of a child and family reveals that the child's presenting pattern and developmental lags stem primarily from some difficulty in interaction patterns, then an interactive primary diagnosis is selected. The evaluating clinician must also consider the interaction patterns characteristic of each of the six developmental levels and determine which patterns have been negotiated successfully and which are absent or constricted. These are captured in Axis II.

As discussed above, many symptoms can arise from disorders of interaction. Regardless of the symptom, the goal of treatment is not only to alleviate it, but also to facilitate the child's progress toward an age-appropriate developmental level and toward an age-appropriate degree of stability and range of thematic experience.

Symptoms that can reflect an interactive disorder include anxiety, fears, behavior control problems, and sleeping and eating difficulties. The same symptoms can be reflective of any number of diagnoses. This is understandable in light of the limited number of behaviors or limited expression of feelings infants and young children are capable of. This category also includes transient situational adjustment reactions, such as a child's response to his mother's return to work. It also includes certain reactions to trauma in which the response does not involve multiple aspects of development.

DISCUSSION AND ILLUSTRATION OF AXIS I: INTERACTIVE DISORDERS

Consider a withdrawn 4-year-old who never formed relationships well. As a baby, she tended to disengage, particularly when confronted with anger or other intense feelings; her parents never knew quite how to woo her back. Under the pressure of competition from other children, she becomes angry and withdraws. Another 4-year-old, in contrast, engaged well from infancy, learned two-way gestural communication, and learned to symbolize his emotions; however, he has difficulty clearly distinguishing between aggressive feelings and warm, loving feelings. Whenever he feels aggressive, he becomes frightened and anticipates that others will reject him; he copes with these feelings by becoming aloof and withdrawn. The behavior or presenting patterns of these two children may appear identical, but the underlying interactive disorders that give rise to their difficulties are very different.

The first child displays an aloof, cautious manner upon entering the evaluating clinician's playroom. She may not warm up at all, or may warm up only very slowly. Whenever the situation does not feel quite right to her, or the play or conversation suggests any emotion, she withdraws anew. The clinician has the strong impression that this child never mastered the very early developmental task of engagement and intimacy. Once treatment begins, this understanding guides the therapist not to wait passively for the child to begin talking about her feelings; hanging back would simply replay the child's early experiences of disengagement. Instead, the therapist tries to empathize with the child's uncertainty about how to be close and tries to explore associated fears.

When the second child comes into the playroom, he will likely be warm and engaged, use interactive gestures, and play out themes such as aggression and love, showing that he can represent emotional experience. However, the clinician begins to see that he confuses aggressive and loving themes in his play, and that as these themes become increasingly merged and chaotic, the child cuts his play off at a critical point. This child clearly negotiated the interaction patterns of early development well, but had difficulty negotiating complex symbolized feelings in the context of an ongoing relationship. The therapist needs to discover what it is about the child's key relationships that prevented him from learning that aggressive and loving feelings can be part of the same relationship.

It is important to highlight how critical multiple observations of interactions with the child are, including those with the evaluator. This is especially important when symbolic play representing the child's experience was not observed during the prior interactions and can then be elicited by the evaluator for those children capable of dynamic play.

101. Anxiety Disorder

Infants and young children may evidence persistent levels of anxiety and fear which impede age-expected range of emotions and functioning. Anxiety can take the form of specific fears or verbalized worries, obsessions or preoccupations, excessive tantrums, distress and agitation, and avoidance behaviors. When considering any form of anxiety, several perspectives need to be considered.

First, is the anxiety primarily related to a Regulatory-Sensory Processing Disorder (see 200. Regulatory-Sensory Processing Disorders)? Second, is the anxiety primarily related to expected developmental transitions or tasks the child is having difficulty mastering? Or third, is the anxiety primarily related to infant-caregiver interactions. The primary source of the anxiety may not always be clear.

The clinician should first consider the regulatory and sensory processing contributions, then the developmental aspects, and finally the interactive components described below. Using the various axes in this multidimensional system helps identify the primary and contributing factors, as well as the degree to which the child's functioning is impaired. When a known trauma has occurred, Traumatic Stress Disorder (see 110. Traumatic Stress Disorder) takes precedence.

Presenting Pattern

Depending on the age of the child, the expression of anxiety takes different forms. Infants and very young children who cannot yet communicate or elaborate verbally show anxiety of a more generalized nature in which symptoms—such as excessive fearfulness, tantrums, agitation, avoidance, panic reactions, and worries—are in evidence on a persistent basis, even when the child is not threatened by separation from a primary caregiver. The older child may talk about his fears but not respond to reassurances, or may have a freeze, fight, or flight reaction. In some cases the child may even have a counterphobic reaction where they do just what they are afraid of to alleviate the anxiety they cannot control and "get it over with!" The child is clearly distressed and fearful and cannot carry on usual routines and activities without significant disruptions during the day or night.

We also observe, even in very young infants (3 to 4 months of age), hypervigilant behavior. The child appears frightened, overly reactive, and overly focused, as though there was imminent danger. Infants who are abused may show this reaction quite early in their development, although it can manifest itself at any time.

Most typically, anxiety is manifested in a moderate level of apprehensiveness and fear in relationship to many age-expected experiences, such as playing with peers, going into a new social setting, attending a birthday party, performing in school, or trying new foods. These behaviors may be accompanied by whining, crying, withdrawal, and refusal. Not infrequently, difficulties with sleeping or eating, and in older children difficulties with toilet training and comfortable patterns of elimination can arise from the child's anxiety even when they are not the source of the anxiety. It should be noted, however, that difficulties with sleeping, eating, toilet training, and elimination can also be related to Regulatory-Sensory Processing Disorders (see 200. Regulatory-Sensory Processing Disorders), depending on whether the primary contributing factors lie in infant-caregiver interactions or constitutional-maturational variations. When it appears that both factors are playing a major role, the primary diagnosis should be of a Regulatory-Sensory Processing Disorder (see 200. Regulatory-Sensory Processing Disorders). Regardless of the primary diagnosis, the child's developmental profile always reflects the relative contributions of constitutional-maturational variations, child-caregiver interactions, and family and environmental factors.

An interactive disorder is considered when the anxieties and fears are related to the primary caregiver(s) not sufficiently providing regulating, comforting relationship patterns. For example, the caregiver may be unable to use various strategies, such as helping the child anticipate what might be anxiety-producing through problem-solving conversations, practice in pretend play, preparing the child for what will occur, and planning strategies to use to help the child become less anxious. The caregiver may not be able to soothe, negotiate, and reassure the child sufficiently if the anxiety increases.

Often, the caregiver is also anxious and distressed. The caregiver's anxiety may stem, in part, from anticipating the child's anxiety and feeling ill equipped to help or feeling annoyed or overly worried. The caregiver may also be bringing his or her own anxieties to the situation at hand, such as social inhibition, or a specific phobia such as fearing dogs, or over-identifying with the child who reminds her of similar experiences in her childhood. In either case, the interaction between the child and caregiver increases the anxiety and distress.

Developmental Pathway

A particular type of infant-caregiver interaction combined with a particular regulatory-sensory processing profile (within the normative range of individual differences, but not at the level of a disorder) often results in the child evidencing excessive anxiety. Individuals prone to anxiety tend to be over-responsive to sensations like sound and touch, and to experience and express affect intensely. In a child at risk for anxiety patterns, the caregiver does not shut down, but instead over-reacts to the child's emotional communications. As a consequence, the child feels overwhelmed and disregulated. Instead of experiencing a loss or rupture in the relationship (as the depressed child might), the anxious child constantly feels overwhelmed and experiences dysphoric or unpleasant affects associated with being overwhelmed.

For example, when the toddler shows strong emotions, such as crying to be held or fed, the caregiver reacts as though this routine communication were a major catastrophe. The caregiver may vocalize loudly, speed up the affective rhythm of interaction, and intrude into the child's physical space by quickly picking him up before he gestures his wishes.

Therapeutic Implications

The child prone to anxiety requires long chains of especially soothing, reciprocal emotional interactions, rather than this type of over-reactive response. As the child progresses into the symbolic realm, he may internalize expectations of being overwhelmed. He is often unable to use affects as a symbolic signal of the need to use various coping strategies, because he is constantly experiencing affects as overwhelming. An unsettling feeling that for another person might serve as a signal (e.g., "I'd better do something about this aggressive partner I have") is for the anxiety-prone person the first step in an escalating feeling of anxiety, sometimes leading to panic. As the child grows up, he tends to continue to experience difficulty in relationships because, based on the earlier patterns, he expects to be intruded on or overwhelmed. Especially soothing relationships in therapy and in life can be very helpful. Along with verbal awareness of his affective and interactional patterns as well as symbolic elaboration in play and conversation, the anxiety-prone individual needs to experience new ways of engaging in interactive, affective exchanges and signaling.

102. Developmental Anxiety Disorder

Development itself can induce significant anxiety in some children who have difficulty negotiating the expected emotional milestones and making developmental transitions. As development launches children into new experiences and uncharted emotional territory, some apprehension or mild anxiety is expected with emerging emotional awareness, until the child begins to feel safe and later develops regulating interactions around emotional understanding of his or her experience. For example, recognizing a stranger and realizing this person is not someone you know reflects this awareness. With repeated interactions, which are sensitive and responsive to the infant, he or she begins to experience the new person as safe and enjoyable, and is able to adapt. Similarly, as the infant or toddler recognizes the experience of separation, sensitive caregiver interactions help the child adapt and make use of additional solutions, such as a transition object (a teddy bear or blanket) to feel secure.

As the child continues to develop, other emerging emotional experiences may challenge his sense of security and competence. For example, fears of bodily injury, what is real or not (monsters or ghosts), aggression, and related worries may emerge. With supportive interactions, the child develops an understanding of these experiences through regulating interactions, conversations, and symbolic play. She learns to take charge of her own security through words and play, using good judgment and seeking support when needed.

In some cases, however, the anxiety is very intense and highly disruptive. For example, the child may be extremely fearful of separation from his primary caregiver and venturing out into new situations. Overt behaviors include desperate clinging, crying, and tantrums. In addition, the child may be overly anxious even anticipating the separation. He may not function as usual, even when separation is not involved, and avoid expectably interesting age-appropriate experiences with toys, peers, or new physical settings. In other cases, anxiety persists way beyond the developmental stage and may generalize to other fears as well.

As an interactive disorder, the child's individual differences and/or the caregiver's experience may underlie the anxiety. Multiple dynamics can contribute to the intensity of the anxiety or prolong it. Caregivers who find it difficult to provide adequate support to their child to master new developmental tasks may have or have had similar anxieties themselves.

The child may be at risk or vulnerable due to other health matters in the past. The caregiver may have conflicts or fears related to the child growing up, or is reminded of her separation challenges in the past as well. In some cases, the child's anxiety masks other problems related to the parental relationship or other environmental stressors. The child may sense some threat or danger related to the caregiver and want to stay with her. Or, the child may be more over-responsive to the unexpected impact of touch and sounds in a new busy environment and become anxious without the security of a protective caregiver nearby. When the child presents with dominant regulatory-sensory based challenges, the anxiety related to separation and other fears should be considered under a primary diagnosis of Regulatory-Sensory Processing Disorder (see 200. Regulatory-Sensory Process Disorders).

While stranger and separation anxieties are very familiar, other developmental anxieties are identified less frequently. For example, the toddler becomes aware her body can get hurt, usually after she has mastered some motor autonomy in being able to walk, run, and climb. This awareness is not yet discriminated, in that the child does not yet "know" if it is a big deal or little deal as each bodily insult may be experienced as a potential catastrophe with attendant kisses and band-aids for the boo-boos. With developmental maturation and adequate sensory-motor capacities, these concerns typically resolve within the next year or two, as seen when the child seeks help if really hurt, takes appropriate risks during physical activities, and copes with doctor visits or medical procedures. When the expected developmental anxiety does not resolve, and the child continues to be excessively anxious, avoids physical risks, tends to panic, and is fearful of bodily injury, even in the absence of experiencing real injury or trauma, a diagnosis of Developmental Anxiety Disorder (see 102. Developmental Anxiety Disorder) can be used.

Caregiver interactions play a critical role here as well. On the one hand, if caregivers are also anxious about bodily injury because of their experiences, trauma, or fears, they may find it hard to provide the reassurance and supportive experiences their children need to master body competence. On the other hand, if they are embarrassed or ashamed of their child's fears or timidity, they may transmit these feelings or even shame their children. These interactions can exacerbate the child's anxiety and need to be carefully examined to understand the caregiver's experiences.

As development moves forward, additional emotional milestones can generate anxiety, including negative affects such as jealousy, competition, fighting, retaliation, and other forms of aggression. As children become aware of these affects, they may always insist on only being the "good guy," only claim positive feelings, deny negative motives and feelings, have frightening dreams, and avoid conflict or competition lest they lose. Anxiety is often palpable as the child shows alarm, fear, impulsivity, and even panic in the face of threats related to aggression. The child may even become aggressive towards others.

Typically, these heightened emotions are accompanied by the development of symbolic solutions as the child begins the process of differentiating reality and fantasy. When children begin to report dreams and worries about ghosts and monsters, they are beginning to imagine the first symbols of danger and vulnerability. Those who can, counter their fears with symbolic solutions of magical power (wands, wizards, and witches), employ symbolic play with action figures, or dress up drama to "fight back" and outwit their or their playmates imagined "enemy." Some children become the enemy or bad guy just to be sure they are in charge of the danger. Eventually, children can explore both the "good guy and bad guy" sides and abstract the reasons for their fighting. These symbolic experiences lay the foundation for higher level abstract thinking and personal standards.

When the child is not prepared to deal with the broader range of affects, anxiety can increase significantly. This is indicated when the child keeps safe by avoiding all negative emotions, protesting vehemently, getting angry, or throwing objects if approached with these themes by other children. The anxiety can escalate into panic as the child experiences himself in danger, or can drive the child into avoidance of experiences that make him uncomfortable, or even trigger regressions as the child tries to escape into the safety of dependency. Other children move into these new emotions more slowly, may temper their anxiety through over-reliance on magical solutions, may attempt to control the environment, and are unable to move forward into logical reasoning and building the boundary between reality and fantasy.

As with the other developmentally-based anxieties, caregiver interactions can have a crucial impact on the child's emotional development. Here, too, the caregiver's comfort or discomfort with certain emotions can support or impede the child. If the caregiver is only loving when the child is "good" and rejecting of anger, jealousy, meanness, and aggression, the child may not get the support to experience the full range of emotions safely and learn that both positive and negative feelings can be part of relationships. If the child does not have the opportunity and encouragement to experiment and practice with feelings in safe symbolic ways, the developmental process can be derailed.

Anxiety Disorder and Developmental Anxiety Disorder can have similar presenting patterns (see 101. Anxiety Disorders and 102. Developmental Anxiety Disorder). Reserve developmental anxiety for difficulties related to specific transitions into more complex emotions as development unfolds and progresses. It is not used when the anxiety is linked to known specific frightening experiences, abuse, trauma, or Regulatory-Sensory Processing Disorders.

Presenting Pattern

Children with developmental anxieties present with similar patterns as children with other anxieties and trauma reactions. Some children cling, cry, lash out, hit, bite, or tantrum, often in panic proportions. Others may just appear very apprehensive and subdued, if not alarmed, and withdraw from their usual interests and refuse activities. The verbal child may protest or express more worries and fears, show mood shifts, and avoid or withdraw from anxiety-inducing situations. In some cases, the child is afraid to go to sleep or wakes up frequently, reporting frightening dreams or nightmares, or is unable to report feelings but perhaps appears sweaty or anxious. Eating can also be disrupted, with changes in appetite and choices of foods or even difficulty holding food down. All children with this challenge evidence more intense or prolonged reactions than expected at developmental crossroads, and are not readily soothed or reassured.

The anxiety can also be readily transmitted back-and-forth from child to caregiver and caregiver to child. In some cases, the child's development may have been proceeding smoothly until the anxiety becomes obvious. In others, it is preceded by struggles to master earlier developmental transitions. The anxiety may also be a very intense but transient experience, as the child is actually trying to move forward developmentally and his anxious, disorganized, and even regressive behavior can be the step taken backwards before moving forward.

Developmental Pathway

The child may not have experienced affective signaling and/or symbolic capacities to regulate, communicate, and comprehend the emerging emotions, or may not be employing them effectively to deal with the expanding range of emotions development inevitably presents. Both individual differences in the child that contribute to greater vulnerability negotiating the steps in emotional development, and caregiver child interactions around these steps can result in developmental anxiety. The caregiver may not realize what the emotional developmental tasks at hand are and why they may be challenging the child. They may not be sufficiently aware of how their emotional experiences in their past influence their present caregiving and have unresolved conflicts or fears in similar areas that intrude into the child's emotional experience.

A number of regulatory-sensory processing vulnerabilities can also contribute to the excessive anxiety evidenced around developmental challenges. These include over-responsiveness in auditory, tactile, or vestibular-proprioceptive capacities, poor visuospatial processing, and motor planning problems. Any one or all of these can make navigating new emotional territory more challenging, especially as expectations increase for the child to interpret and respond to the environment appropriately and not be derailed by unexpected sensory intrusions.

Therapeutic Implications

It is important for the caregiver to understand the child's widening range of emotions in development and related typical anxieties. The caregiver may need support to comprehend and integrate new emotions and themes in co-regulated affective interactions and symbolic play and conversations. The caregivers are also developing, and may need to examine how their past and experience of certain emotional themes may be influencing their children. Guiding parents to more sensitive co-regulated affective exchanges and using symbolic solutions in pretend play and conversations provide the children the safety to experiment and master new emotional experiences.

103. Disorder of Emotional Range and Stability

Infants and young children tend to show a gradual increase in their emotional range and stability as they develop from early infancy into the preschool years. For example, a 2- to 3-month-old infant tends to shift emotional states rapidly and evidences a few global emotions, such as joy, delight, distress, rage, and so forth. In contrast, a 16-month-old toddler may evidence warmth and security, pleasure and delight, curiosity, excitement, caution, fear, annoyance, assertiveness, rage, sadness, and so forth. The adaptive toddler, however, experiences and expresses these emotions in a relatively stable manner in relationship to expectable experiences; for example, happiness and pleasure come in when mommy or daddy comes to the door with a big smile and a readiness to get down on the floor and play. Anger and frustration may predominate when a favorite toy is put back on the shelf because it is bedtime.

Although difficulties with age-expected emotional range and stability may be subtle and less obvious than states of anxiety, these kinds of difficulties can have long-term consequences and are important to recognize. The child's capacity to experience the full range and stability of age-expected emotions is an important foundation of his future social and intellectual development.

To determine if a child has difficulty with age-appropriate emotional range and stability, a clinician must have a roadmap of expected emotional development in infants and young children, observed in their relationships and interactions with family and friends, as well as in pretend play themes. These would start with emotions related to dependency, pleasure, security, separation, disappointment, bodily competence, injury, surprise, joy, and satisfaction. More negative emotions emerge as the child encounters the reality around him in relation to others. He may feel anger, jealousy, sibling rivalry, competition, aggression, and a wish for control and power over others. These "negative" emotions can challenge the caregiver-child interactions if the relationship does not embrace the full range of human feelings. As the child masters reality testing and reaches higher emotional developmental levels, emotions expand to friendship, loyalty, justice, and morality.

While the rudiments of most emotions are present from infancy, emotions get more and more differentiated as the child develops in the first five years of life and is able to describe more complex feelings and the reasons for these feelings, including ambivalence and conflicting emotions. A 2-year-old may first bop his baby sister and then hug and kiss her. At 3, he may pout and grab her toy. At 4 years, he may protest verbally that mommy never spends time with him and the baby always comes first, but also acknowledges his love for the baby. Between 5 and 6, he may be protective and helpful, but can also talk about his jealousy.

It is the lack of differentiation, range, and stability of emotions that characterizes this disorder. In contrast to children with developmental anxieties, these children present with constrictions and a very narrow range of affects or interests, but not the full blown intensity of anxiety reactions.

Presenting Pattern

Many infants and toddlers do not evidence the increasing range and stability of emotions just described. As toddlers and preschoolers, they may persist in evidencing only a few global emotional states, such as joy and rage, depending on the circumstances. The lack of stability may be seen in rapid fluctuations from one emotional state to another or variations in the intensity of the same set of emotions, with little or no capacity to tolerate frustration in an age-expected way resulting in disrupted functioning. Or, they may even confuse or reverse emotions inappropriately. Questions about feelings are hard to answer and the connection between thoughts, feelings and behavior are fleeting and little reflection is available. Interests tend to be limited as the child selects and focuses on just a few areas such as construction, vehicles, or transformer toys, and seems uninterested in the emotional drama that could accompany these ideas. Play with other children may also be affected as the child has fewer emotionally based ideas and is less interested in the symbolic play of others.

Developmental Pathway

Sensory under-responsivity and low muscle tone, or a mixed pattern of under-responsivity and over-responsivity, as well as over-responsivity to sensations alone, can contribute because they make emotional regulation more difficult. The key contribution, however, is from caregiver-child interaction patterns that do not optimally foster a broad range of feelings at each functional emotional developmental level. Clearly, sensory modulation challenges can make it more difficult to negotiate the functional emotional developmental capacities in a stable, regulated manner and vice versa (see Axis II for a description of the functional emotional developmental capacities). Consider the following example.

The child may be under-responsive to his own bodily sensations of emotion, e.g., not feeling the tightening of his muscles as he gets angry, or feeling the scowls in his face as he gets frustrated with a task, or the pit in his stomach as he becomes fearful. When coupled with interactions that suppress the safe expression of a full range of emotions or only find certain emotions acceptable, the child has fewer opportunities to explore and navigate his emotional world. Parents may deny the child's feelings, e.g., "Don't feel mad; don't feel sad." Or, "There is nothing to be afraid of!" or "You have to always be nice." Others are conflicted about recognizing or expressing their own emotions and avoid the same in their children, sharing only happy times. The child may learn to accommodate his parents' comfort level.

Therapeutic Implications

Reading the more subtle cues of an under-responsive child helps the caregiver tune the child into his emotional experience safely with lots of empathy and sensitive exploration. Helping the over-responsive child be more regulated is also essential. It is helpful to encourage lots of co-regulated affect signaling and symbolic dramatic play as well as elaborate conversations about emotional themes related to favorite interests. Parents also need to explore their own discomfort or conflicts about feelings and the meaning it has had in their lives in order to broaden their emotional range.

104. Disruptive Behavior and Oppositional Disorder

Disruptive behaviors are a common challenge in infancy and early childhood. As a toddler begins to walk, problems with impulse control often first emerge. For example, a toddler may hit, bite, or scratch instead of using interactive gestures and emotional signals to convey intentions. During the preschool years, children may display a combination of attentional and disruptive behavior challenges. The preschooler may evidence a high activity level, show poor frustration tolerance, react to frustration with pushing, hitting, or throwing objects, being oppositional, and rapidly shift from one activity to another. Often, when assessing the child's relative mastery of functional emotional developmental capacities, we observe that while the child has some mastery of each level, he shows constrictions at each level. These constrictions can especially impede self-regulation and social problem-solving where disruptive behavior derails symbolic solutions using language, negotiations, and pretend play to express needs and feelings, resolve conflicts, be flexible, and delay gratification.

In addition, when the child behaves disruptively, we often observe a caregiver interaction pattern characterized by a lack of regulating and limit setting as caregiver responses to the infant's signals. The caregiver may read and respond to the infant's signal of pleasure and joy or fear with a variety of appropriate reciprocal gestures (smiles beget smiles, fear begets comfort, and so forth), but when the same toddler begins to show annoyance and anger, the caregiver may evidence, often due to momentary anxiety, a lack of response or an exaggerated response. Sometimes caregivers appear almost "stone-faced" at the moment of truth, as the child is getting increasingly angry and beginning to get ready to push or bite. Other times, the caregiver may move in too quickly in an overly punitive manner. Not infrequently, one caregiver "freezes" while the other is overly punitive. The result is that the child does not receive sensitive reciprocal regulating and limit-setting responses.

In some cases, disruptive behavior can be more extreme with even young children acting very aggressively. They might hurt others, set fires, destroy property, or torture animals with little remorse. They may become aggressive in a caregiving environment that is overly punitive or unavailable and be relatively unable to successfully master the organizational levels dealing with engagement, empathy, co-regulated emotional signaling, and limit-setting. If the immediate environment doesn't provide warmth and nurturing, as well as firm, consistent limits, or if limits are imposed abusively, the tendency toward seeking sensation can take on an enraged quality, with indiscriminate, aggressive acting out.[2]

The child with disruptive behavioral patterns who also evidences clearly dominant regulatory-sensory processing challenges should be considered under that dimension. When disruptive behavior appears more response to the environment or specific frustrations, rather than the specific sources of anxiety, this diagnosis should be considered.

Developmental Pathway

The pathways include the way the child reacts to and comprehends different sensations and plans actions (an expression of his or her biological patterns), the ways in which his or her caregiving environment interacts with these individual differences, and the levels or stages of emotional and intellectual organization that are negotiated through these interactions.

For example, infants and toddlers who are under-responsive to touch and sound and, therefore, sensory-seeking or crave sensation and are physically very active often become aggressive in a caregiving environment that is overly punitive or unavailable. They are relatively unable to successfully master the organizational levels dealing with engagement, empathy, co-regulated emotional signaling, and limit-setting.

Children who are over-responsive to sensations such as touch and sound may easily become overloaded in noisy or busy environments, such as a preschool or a shopping mall. A sudden, unexpected touch from another child can easily be misperceived as hostile or aggressive by the tactilely over-responsive child. He may then push or hit as a response. Infants and toddlers who are sensory over-responsive to sensations such as touch and sound (an expression of a different biological pattern than the under-respon-

[2] Among children deprived of nurturing affection in the early years of life, including those in institutional care, two tendencies have been observed. One group of children became withdrawn, depressed, or apathetic. Some stopped developing physically, failed to gain weight, and even became quite ill and did not survive. Those in the other group sought out sensation, becoming aggressive, promiscuous, and indifferent to others, relating to them only to fill their own concrete needs (Spitz, 1945). Other researchers found a higher than expected degree of subtle difficulties in the functioning of the nervous system among antisocial children and adults, with problems in perception, information processing, and motor functioning (Bowlby, 1944; Lewis, 1992; Yeager & Lewis, 2000)

sive child), likely become aggressive if the caregiving environment is too intrusive or overwhelming. While such a pattern is related to a very different underlying processing challenge, in comparison to the sensory-seeking child, it nonetheless can manifest itself with aggressive behavior.

Therapeutic Implications

For each developmental pathway leading to disruptive behavior or aggression, we have been able to identify specific family, environmental, educational, therapeutic, and social-community patterns that can facilitate adaptive development and help children overcome their challenges.

As a child is beginning to use facial expressions, gestures, and body postures that will lead to a push or a hit, the caregiver would ideally respond with a hand gesture and vocal tone indicating, "What's going on?" or "What do you want?" and then a series of interactive gestures that help the child express the desire for this or that toy or to be helped to a quieter room. If the child escalates further and is almost about to hit, ideally the caregiver would respond with limit-setting hand gestures, indicating, "stop" and with vocal tones and facial expressions showing serious concern and firmness. If the child escalates even further, the caregiver may need to use firm, consistent, but gentle limit-setting actions, such as holding and comforting and perhaps removing the child from the action he is having trouble handling. The limit-setting action conveys to the child that the parent can help him control his behavior and that he can't engage in his desired activity until he calms down. Whenever possible, pre-empting severe disruptions by providing adequate transitions or cues to help the child anticipate frustration or disappointment, can help the child self-regulate and engage in some problem-solving discussions. Once the child is upset, the goal of the caregiver is to soothe the child, so he realizes he can calm down, and perhaps to find an alternative activity that can be mutually satisfying. The child experiences the removal from the original desired but difficult activity as a limit-setting consequence that, together with the soothing care, help him to internalize limits in the future.

Clearly, this type of optimal interaction is difficult for caregivers, who themselves may have anxieties or conflicts around disruptive behavior or aggression. When a caregiver-infant interaction pattern combines the elements that support inattentiveness (only short bursts of interaction) and disruptive behavior (difficulties with limit setting), the infant or young child may evidence both features.

Ongoing relationships help the aggressive child develop empathy and a desire to use his abilities for constructive interactions. Very firm limits, lovingly applied, are also crucial in teaching him to control his assertiveness. Practice in labeling feelings and pretend play help him develop a richer inner life. Parents can encourage safe and constructive physical activities such as sports. They can also involve him in communication that enables him to ponder, give names to his feelings, consider their consequences, and most important, develop compassion for others. A child with these kinds of supportive early relations has a chance of becoming a bold, imaginative leader.

Adaptive interactions begin with early nurturing and reciprocal affective interactions. The key is long chains of back-and-forth signaling that help the toddler feel secure and regulate his sensory craving behavior. In other words, lots of physical activities with back-and-forth emotional signaling and regulation are helpful. The caregiver is active and slows down the action through regulated affective interactions (e.g., "Let's see if our trucks can go slow and kiss rather than crash"). Intrusive, punitive caregiver affective patterns or caregiver withdrawal intensify the maladaptive patterns.

Importantly, each type of underlying processing contribution requires a very different interactive approach in order to help the child. Therapeutic implications for each are described below.

1. Children who are over-responsive to sensations require a great deal of soothing and regulation and, over time, need to learn how to self-calm and remove themselves from situations where they are overloaded. While they need to learn to describe their feelings rather than act them out, the feelings that they eventually describe are very different from the ones a sensory-seeking child describes. The sensory over-responsive child is likely to describe fear and panic and being overwhelmed, whereas a sensory-seeking child is likely to describe his pleasure in activity and the need for activity as a way of feeling whole and together.

2. Many children with aggressive behavior who are either sensory-seeking or sensory over-responsive, also may evidence motor planning and sequencing challenges as well. This additional processing challenge tends to intensify the likelihood of aggressive and/or antisocial behavior because children with planning and sequencing challenges have a hard time constructing a larger pattern of behavior that includes a pattern of internal limit setting. In other words, it's harder for these children to sequence together a pattern where they experiment with assertiveness and create for themselves a proper boundary between constructive assertiveness and destructive aggression. As their ability to construct larger patterns improves, they are able to sequence together the steps that involve assertive exploration and appropriate limit setting. Also, children with motor planning and sequencing challenges are more likely to feel confused, humiliated, or have other negative feelings about themselves, which may contribute to angry feelings.

3. In a similar way, children with auditory processing challenges or visuospatial processing challenges may also have difficulty operating within a complex social or academic setting. They may have difficulty with the basics of following verbal directions or understanding where they are in physical space. They may also have difficulty in seeing the forest for the trees and easily get lost in the "trees" (those with visuospatial processing problems). These additional challenges contribute to feelings of anxiety, embarrassment and humiliation and, in many circumstances, increase both aggressive and depressive feelings, both of which can fuel aggressive actions in children.

In general, we have found that the more processing challenges there are, the greater the likelihood of aggressive behavior if certain challenging environmental conditions are also present. As indicated earlier, the environmental conditions that contribute to aggressive behavior often include the lack of sufficient nurturing; regulating affective interactions; firm, persistent, but gentle limit setting; and support for imaginative and reflective thinking, especially with regard to the world of feelings. A comprehensive program needs to involve the family and the educational system, as well as, if indicated, specific therapies to strengthen underlying processing capacities or work on understanding feelings.

105. Depression

In healthy development, infants and young children gradually expand their capacities for emotional expression and experiencing a wide range of feelings. This gradually expanding capacity is part of the infant-caregiver relationship pattern. Adaptive interactive patterns enable the infant to successfully negotiate each of the functional emotional developmental capacities, and thereby experience, by the time they are toddlers, a large range of emotions from joy, pleasure, and enthusiasm to transient sadness and fear. They are also able to enjoy assertiveness and exploration, as well as a growing curiosity.

Presenting Pattern

Infants and young children can begin showing a consistent mood pattern, rather than the range of emotional states expected for their age and developmental stage. For example, some toddlers and preschoolers display a persistently sad or depressed affect. They may indicate they are sad or well up with tears when asked about feelings or even when seeing someone else feeling sad or crying. They appear to show little pleasure or interest in their usually enjoyable activities and do not initiate fun activities. Sometimes they may have difficulty showing or verbalizing expectable feelings of sadness in situations that would ordinarily elicit sad feelings, or insist they are happy even as they cry or look very sad. As they become symbolic, they may play out and talk about depressive themes. Preschoolers may, for example, enact in play and/or verbalize persistent feelings of being bad, and slightly older children may even talk about wishing they were not alive or present themes of dying in their play (which is not part of a bereavement or trauma situation).

Infants and young children may also evidence persistent agitation and irritability, with nothing pleasing them, or in contrast, may move very little, show little energy, and turn down activities they may have once enjoyed. Other children have sleep or eating difficulties (with weight loss or gains), which are common symptoms related to various sources of stress.

The severity of the mood disorder may be reflected in the intensity of just a few of the behaviors described above, or the increasing number of challenges, the longer the child feels depressed. Infant-caregiver interaction patterns often play a major role in the child's difficulties in regulating mood. The child may experience the loss of love or support when the parent cannot accept his or her full range of behavior and feelings. For example, the parent may be very loving in response to compliance and being good, but pull away when the child is angry or aggressive. The parent may not be able to respond to the child when his own conflicts are triggered and he is ambivalent or unpredictable to the child.

The depression becomes apparent over time when the child experiences some loss or conflict with others and is unable to rely on an internalized, nurturing image to soothe and comfort. Such difficulties can, if left unaddressed, persist into adulthood. See the case example below.

Developmental Pathway

Sensory over-responsiveness, stronger verbal processing capacities, and weaker visuospatial processing capacities characterize the pattern we have observed in many individuals prone to depression. In a child at risk for depressive patterns, the caregiver tends to shut down when the child's affect is becoming intense (i.e., the caregiver finds it hard to maintain a pattern of co-regulated affective interaction at these moments of heightened affect). The child experiences a loss or rupture in the relationship, sometimes only for a few seconds. This very brief sense of loss becomes associated with strong affect. As expectations are formed, due to better pattern construction, the child expects loss and/or emptiness when he has strong feelings. As he becomes more symbolic, this pattern can be experienced in terms of images of loss and, later on, "I must have caused the loss by being bad or angry or demanding." Instead of an internal security blanket of warm, soothing, comforting images and expectations, the child experiences loss and sadness.

Therapeutic Implications

One aspect of therapeutic work with the child (or adult) with depressive tendencies is working on the flow of interaction, helping the caregiver maintain co-regulated, affective interactions, pulling the child in with extra enthusiasm, as needed, rather than temporarily withdrawing or freezing and, at the same time, helping the caregiver understand what might have happened to bring on these tendencies. The goal is to help the child become able to experience, express, and explore a broad range of affects, including feelings of anger, entitlement, and fear of loss. Helping the child learn to visualize the nurturing parent can help alleviate the sense of loss and encourage self-soothing and adaptive responses.

To illustrate how infant-caregiver interaction patterns, as well as the child's regulatory-sensory processing profile and the caregiver's personality, can contribute to this type of challenge, consider the example of a bright, talented, and precociously verbal 4-year-old who became depressed when she experienced competitive situations at preschool.

When a child became competitive with her during playtime, she felt the other child was unfair and had a feeling of loss; she then got depressed and didn't play with or talk to the other children for the rest of the morning. This sequence occurred routinely when she experienced competition. She could describe a feeling of "being all alone" during these moments. Her therapist asked her if she could bring to mind an image of her mother and picture her nurturing her at these times. She said, "I can't picture my Mommy." She was unable to create a nurturing internal image. Her therapist later learned that she had a mother who had consistently responded to her strong feelings not by nurturing her, but instead by shutting down and becoming "stone-faced".

A clue to this pattern was the child's reaction to her therapist's periodic temporary loss of empathy and relatedness. If, for example, the therapist looked out the window for a second, the child would immediately look quite sad. Instead of trying to pull the therapist back in, she would look down and her voice would go into more of a monotone, as though she were giving up.

It wasn't sufficient, however, just to verbally point out this pattern. It was also necessary to create a different type of affective interaction and rhythm. The therapist needed to pull her back in with animated affective gestures and literally challenge her with his affective gestures to take the initiative. He did this with very distinct expectant looks, which communicated, "Can you keep the affective rhythm going, or are you going to intensify my momentary lapse with an even bigger one?" Eventually, therapist and patient were able to explore this pattern in play and with words.

Initially, this patient didn't have the basis for recreating a multi-sensory, affective experience of nurturing in her own imagination. She didn't have the internal affective image or feelings to get her through a tough time. Instead, she would get depressed because she had no internal, representational security blanket to fall back on. The security blanket was absent at the level of two-way, presymbolic affective communication and at the level of symbolization. As she learned to initiate affective interactions at times of loss, she also gradually became able to imagine and symbolize an internal security blanket made up of images. She could feel and picture her mother or friends in nurturing interactions.

This patient was also much stronger in her verbal processing capacities than her visuospatial processing, a pattern we have observed in many individuals prone to depression. Because of these processing patterns, she took a long time to progress to the level of feeling and picturing nurturing interactions. She began by describing them and gradually progressed to picturing and feeling them.

As her explorations broadened, she was able to deal with many additional conflicts. For example, she was very competitive with her stone-faced mother and had sought out her father as an ally in the family triangle. Only after she was able to construct internal, nurturing images, however, was she able to explore her own competitiveness, triangular relationship, and other conflicts.

106. Mood Dysregulation: A Unique Type of Interactive and Mixed Regulatory-Sensory Processing Disorder Characterized by Bipolar Patterns

In recent years, there has been growing interest in early identification and treatment of bipolar-type mood dysregulation in children (Geller, Zimmerman, Williams, Bolhafner, & Craney, 2001; Egland, Blumenthal, Nee, & Sharp, 1987; Lish, Dime-Meenan, Whybrow, Arlen-Price, & Hirschfeld, 1994; Cytryn & McKnew, 1974; Carlson & Weintraub, 1993; Radke-Yarrow, Nottelmann, Martinez, Fox, & Belmont, 1992). In children, manic or hypomanic states often cause aggressive behavior or agitation rather than the frantic, grandiose thinking commonly seen in adults.

Diagnosing bipolar patterns in children is therefore difficult (Harrington, Fudge, Rutter, & Pickles, 1991; Strober, Morrell, Burroughs, Lampert, & Freeman, 1988). We do not have a clear understanding of the antecedent variables leading to bipolar disorder in children, although a host of neuropsychological vulnerabilities or deficits have been suggested, including problems in the areas of language, motor development, perception, executive functioning, and social functioning (Sigurdsson, Fombonne, Sayal, & Checley, 1999; Castillo, Kwock, Courvorise, & Hooper, 2000). Furthermore, a comprehensive intervention program that addresses family interactions and educational issues, as well as biochemical treatments, has not been formulated.

Presenting Pattern and Developmental Pathway

We propose a novel hypothesis: bipolar patterns in children can be understood as arising from a unique configuration of antecedents involving sensory processing and motor functioning, early child-caregiver interaction patterns, and early states of personality organization. Specifically, we suggest that children at risk for developing bipolar-type mood dysregulation share the following characteristics (Greenspan & Glovinsky, 2002):

1. An unusual processing pattern in which over-responsivity to sound, touch, or both coexists with a craving for sensory stimulation, particularly movement (most over-responsive children are more fearful and cautious). Sensory craving is usually associated with high activity and aggressive, agitated, or impulsive behavior. Therefore, when they are overloaded with stimuli, children with this unusual combination of processing differences cannot self-regulate by withdrawing, as a cautious child might. Instead, they become agitated, aggressive, and impulsive, thereby overloading themselves even more.

2. An early pattern of interaction, continuing into childhood, characterized by a lack of fully co-regulated reciprocal affective exchanges. In particular, caregivers are unable to interact with the infant or child in ways that help her up-regulate and down-regulate her moods to modulate states of despondency and agitation.

3. A personality organization in which the fifth and sixth functional emotional levels of development have not been mastered. Emotions either are not addressed at

the symbolic level, instead remaining at the level of behavior or somatic experience, or are represented as global, polarized affect states rather than in integrated form.

Therapeutic Implications

The DIR assessment of a child and family determines whether or not the child has this combination of characteristics. A comprehensive, developmentally-based intervention program must address all three issues. A program can be designed to head off the interactive experiences that intensify the child's sensory processing difficulties, and the child can be helped to understand her particular processing challenges and to prepare herself for situations in which these will likely pose a problem.

A child with constrictions at the early, presymbolic level of two-way affective interaction can be helped to master the capacity for long sequences of co-regulated affective exchanges, necessary for a more stable mood. For example, when she begins to show more agitation in her voice and movement, the therapist might deliberately shift to a more soothing, comforting tone to down-regulate the intensity of affect. When she becomes more apathetic and self-absorbed, the therapist might employ a more energetic rhythm of preverbal and verbal exchange, speaking faster and using more animated hand gestures to up-regulate the child's mood. The therapist might also explore, with a verbal child, how she feels during these shifts of affective rhythm and intensity. During such discussions, the child can be helped to symbolize and reflect on the feelings she is experiencing.

A child who can use words to describe actions but who cannot symbolize emotions can be helped to advance through the levels of development described in Axis II: first, to begin using words to describe feelings as concrete entities, which are close to and demand action ("I'm mad," "I'm hungry") and second, to use affects as a signal of internal experience ("I feel mad," "I feel hungry"), thus making possible reflection and problem-solving.

A developmentally-based treatment program for a child with patterns suggesting a bipolar disorder might involve several components, including individual psychotherapy for the child, perhaps twice a week; weekly sessions with her parents to help them create a family environment that facilitates her development; and work with the school to help staff understand and adapt to her. It might also include specialized educational programs to strengthen processing weaknesses and facilitate social and emotional growth in the school setting.

By ensuring that the parents fully understand their child's developmental profile and therapeutic goals, the therapist can increase the likelihood that they support the long-term, comprehensive approach that is necessary to help a child with bipolar patterns. Having very specific goals that are easily understood, but that nonetheless embrace complex psychological processes (e.g., the child begins naming, and later reflecting upon, intense feelings) helps the parents to participate effectively and to monitor their child's progress. The therapist also needs to help the parents work through whatever conflicts may previously have precluded a commitment to long-term therapy.

107. Attentional Disorder

Infants and young children may evidence challenges in sustaining attention, one of the most complicated mental health disorders. It is complicated because while certain shared symptoms, such as inattentiveness, characterize a large number of children who receive this diagnosis, there may very well be many different patterns (i.e., many different pathways) leading to these symptoms, and many different reasons for inattentiveness. A comprehensive approach to understanding attentional problems needs to look at the different and combined processing patterns as well as the different developmental organizations and interactive patterns.

In this section, we focus on challenges with attention that stem primarily from interactive difficulties and the developmental pathways that contribute to these challenges. Attention needs to be given to the relevant developmental tasks at hand to explore whether developmental anxieties (fears) or social challenges in/or the environment may be disrupting the child's attention and can be addressed or modified.

Later we focus on attention difficulties as a Regulatory-Sensory Processing Disorder (see 205). In both the interactive and regulatory-sensory processing attention problems, the same developmental pathways are involved and interactions can be more challenging. Using the multi-axial system helps the clinician determine which contribution is most dominant and which primary diagnosis to use. Based on this complete profile, the clinician will determine which developmental pathway is contributing to the symptom choice. Do the dominant features of the interactive challenges make it the primary disorder? Or, are the developmental pathways associated with regulatory problems of greater significance, thereby making the regulatory-sensory processing challenges the primary disorder?

Presenting Pattern

Variations in attention can be expected in early development. Difficulties sustaining attention can be observed as early as 2 to 4 months when the infant becomes more capable of turning and focusing to look and listen and coo responsively. By 8 to 12 months, the infant may attend only fleetingly, rather than in the sustained manner needed for two way interactions such as peek-a-boo or pat-a-cake, or enjoying a shape sorter together. In the second year of life, the toddler might just move from toy to toy and appear highly distracted even when playing with an object of choice. Later, the young child may always be on the move, always changing topics, unable to stick with a conversation or a game. Another pattern involves spurts or intermittent stop-and-go interactions. Or, the child may be too self-absorbed or over-focused on special interests and find it hard to shift his attention to others, even when called.

Variations in attention can also be related to the functions at hand so that young children may be attentive to books, videos, or other forms of entertainment, but less so when expected to attend to and participate more actively in what others choose or where there is less interest and less interaction available as in circle time. Often, the tolerance or expectations of the environment affect perceptions of the problem, e.g., a child playing alone for long periods might be considered an asset rather than self-absorbed, or changing activities every few minutes at pre-school or at home may be considered necessary because assumed attention is very short in young children. Despite all these variations, attention difficulties are readily identified, and determining the primary contributions based on the child's individual profile is the next step.

Developmental Pathway

Motor and regulatory-sensory processing patterns and child-caregiver and family interactive patterns (and often combinations of both) can be significant contributors to attentional challenges. First, consider interactive patterns.

As in anxiety and depression, we have observed a pattern of reciprocal affective interchanges characteristic of attentional difficulties. Typically, co-regulated reciprocal affective interactions with caregivers are established from about 9 to 24 months. When we observe an infant-caregiver interaction pattern characterized by short bursts of back-and-forth communication or signaling, rather than long chains of back-and-forth communication, a problem is evident. Some caregivers respond to the child's short bursts of interaction by becoming fragmented with the child. They jump from one thing to another with him rather than trying to sustain a long chain of interaction. They also frequently give up entirely and let the child play alone.

Other caregivers attempt to over-control the child, which can tend to lead the child to be rigid. Such a child seems to focus, but it is not true, shared attention. There is no real back-and-forth problem-solving. Over-control also mobilizes catastrophic affects that can lead to even shorter interactions. The child's constitutional-maturational variations as well as the caregiver's characteristics contribute to this type of interactive pattern. In addition, the caregiver's attentional capacities should be explored.

The absence of consistent opportunities for communication and interaction with adults can lead a child to become more self-absorbed or preoccupied with her own interests and seemingly inattentive to others. The critical factor, however, is that these children can be readily wooed into interaction and focus when engaged in a wide range of conditions, e.g., in quiet environments, in the class, in a small group, etc.

In some cases what appears as poor attention may also be related to anxiety and avoidance patterns, and other interactive disorders should be considered. Chaotic families or very self-absorbed ones can certainly contribute, and one may also see symptoms of anxiety and/or depression in children in such settings.

In most cases, when regulation, interaction, and engagement are available, poor attention usually relates to Regulatory-Sensory Processing Disorders (see 200. Regulatory-Sensory Processing Disorders) or developmental disorders described later.

In considering the interactive patterns of children with attentional problems, there appear to be two reasons for the short bursts of interaction. One, they bring unique biological patterns into the interaction. The other is the interactions that stem from these or intensify them, as described above. Now let's look at the regulatory-sensory processing differences that may contribute to the developmental pathways of attentional problems.

As a group, children with attentional challenges tend to have one or a number of processing differences most frequently with motor planning and sequencing. Six regulatory-sensory processing and modulation patterns, as well as some combinations, are associated with problems with attention. These are described below.

1. **Motor Planning and Sequencing:** It is hard for children to engage in long action sequences (i.e., a number of actions in a row). In their spontaneous play, they'll tend to do two actions in a row, such as take the car and put it into the house. They do not do eight or ten actions in a row, such as take the car, put it in the house, then take it out of the house and go to the pretend schoolhouse, then go to the store, etc. We see children who, even as toddlers, can sequence four or more actions in a row (e.g., moving trucks different places) and children who can only do one or two sequences. When a child has biologically-based motor planning and sequencing challenges and perhaps other processing challenges as well, it's harder for him to engage in long chains of back-and-forth interaction. If he's a one- or two-step action sequencer, the adult interacting with him is going to have to work with him much harder to sustain an interaction than with a child who ordinarily is a four or five-step action sequencer. When older, children with motor planning problems may have a hard time with such basic skills as learning to tie their shoes, learning a complicated sequence of dance steps, mastering the steps involved in new sports, as well as in following directions that involve motor performance. Therefore, motor-based schoolwork can be very challenging. Children with this problem can have difficulty with a range of basic academic and social tasks that often are associated with a lack of attentiveness. For example, they are inattentive and have difficulty complying with a range of school activities, including such basics as standing in line and marching in an orderly way to the library or lunchroom; organizing their backpacks with the proper homework assignments; carrying out the steps in doing the homework; and returning the homework the next day. Children with this challenge may understand all the concepts involved in the homework, but receive a low grade because they either don't take the homework home or don't hand it in the next day. Because of their difficulty with sequencing, they may also have difficulty in handling complex social interactions as involved in negotiating different relationships at a party or on a soccer field. In addition, sequencing ideas in an essay or an oral argument may also be problematic.

2. **Under-Response to Basic Sensations:** Such children often have challenges in registering basic sensations, such as touch and sound. Therefore, they tend to retreat into their own fantasies. A typical 4-year-old with this pattern would be

described by his parents as "tuning out" all the time and engaging in pretend play on his own. His teacher would describe him as "tuning out" as well, and that she has to work very hard to get and maintain his attention.

3. **Sensory-Seeking:** These children may be under-responsive to sensations such as touch and sound, as is the previous group. They tend to be physically active and seek out sensory input, sometimes, to compensate for their under-responsivity. They tend to differ from the previous group in another important way—they are often under-responsive to the sensation of movement and, therefore, crave it, which tends to contribute to their activity levels. They are also less likely to have low muscle tone, which the previous group often does evidence. This also contributes to their ability to seek out sensation, in comparison to the previous group, who would tire quickly from too much activity. The sensory-seeking group also tends to have difficulty with registering sensory input and, therefore, is often inattentive when someone is trying to talk with them or challenge them to focus on an academic task. Because they also tend to seek sensations, however, they frequently fidget, touch everything nearby, and attempt to create loud noises and movement for themselves and others. Therefore, they often evidence high activity levels and move rapidly from object to object. They may also, in their zest for new sensations, evidence a great deal of risk-taking and aggression. The aggression can become especially prominent if children don't receive sufficient nurturing interactions, limit setting, and practice in creative (imaginative) thinking and reflective problem-solving.

4. **Over-Responsive to Sensation:** Children with this pattern tend to over-respond to basic sensations, such as touch and sound. In a noisy classroom, they tend to be distracted easily by the sounds around them, such as another child chewing or the sound of the boiler or air-conditioner or a noise outside. Rather than retreating into their own fantasy worlds and having a hard time registering sensations, these children register too many sensations and jump from one thing to another. They have a hard time sustaining their attention. They may also evidence some reactive aggression and impulsivity when they are overloaded with sensation. In this group, it is often the sensory overload, rather than a fundamental difficulty with anger, that is associated with this type of behavior.

5. **Auditory-Verbal Processing Challenges:** Children with this pattern evidence inattentiveness secondary to processing or comprehending auditory, verbal experiences (i.e., language). They may show difficulties with following directions, understanding the sequence or steps in solving a problem, or their ability to comply or carry out any number of social or academic tasks. Their confusion and lack of sustained direction often leads to, or appears to be, inattentiveness. This pattern may be especially difficult to diagnose if the auditory processing and language challenges are subtle.

6. **Visuospatial Processing Challenges:** This pattern relates to difficulties in processing or comprehending visuospatial experiences. Visuospatial experiences have to do with understanding spatial relationships, such as where the park is in relationship to one's own house, or how the different rooms in a new house are laid out or how to find a hidden object, or, at a more advanced level, how to be able to picture different visual designs from different angles, such as figuring out the mirror image of a pattern of blocks. Advanced concepts in mathematics and science also depend a great deal on visuospatial thinking, as does the more general ability to "see the forest for the trees." Children who have difficulties with visuospatial processing often have a hard time understanding the larger patterns within which they are operating and, therefore, can easily get "lost in the trees." They may be quite gifted verbally and have excellent verbal memories, but nonetheless, have difficulties with complex patterns that require a great deal of sequencing or difficulties with the ability to put all the pieces together into a larger whole. Such children can easily evidence distractibility and inattentiveness when the tasks are oriented towards "big picture" thinking, or require the manipulation of objects or concepts in spatial contexts.

7. **Combinations and Severity:** Many children evidence combinations of the above underlying processing difficulties. The more severe the interactive patterns described earlier and the processing differences, often, the greater the attentional difficulties.[3]

Therapeutic Implications

A comprehensive approach to understanding attentional problems needs to look at the different subtypes that relate to these different and combined processing patterns as well as the different developmental organizations and interactive patterns described above. When a child has biologically based motor planning and sequencing challenges and perhaps other processing challenges as well, it's harder for him to engage in long chains of back-and-forth interaction, and this may intensify family challenges. At the same time, family challenges can intensify the processing challenges.

To the degree the caregiver can engage the child in longer and longer chains of reciprocal interaction through mobilizing the child's interest and affect, the more the child can learn to extend his reciprocal interactions in spite of his processing problems. In other words, practice with long chains of back-and-forth, affective interactions can help the child learn to compensate for his processing challenges. This is the key to the type of co-regulated reciprocal interaction pattern that may help the child learn to sustain his attention. Even more importantly, long interactive sequences also help the child strengthen his planning and sequencing abilities, as well as other processing abilities. When a child is engaged in long, back-and-forth interactions, he is practicing and strengthening all his processing skills because they are being used in a more complex and challenging

[3] It is important to note that neuropsychological and educational batteries do not always test for all these processing challenges. For example, they do not test for over- or under-responsivity to sensations such as touch and sound. They do, however, pick up auditory-verbal processing challenges and certain types of sequencing challenges.

manner. The key is to mobilize the child's affect and challenge him to use each processing ability as part of long sequences of co-regulated, affective exchanges. For example, a caregiver entices a toddler to search in both of her hands for a much-desired toy. The caregiver is able to challenge the child into ten circles of back-and-forth signaling during the search game. Such a simple, everyday search game, however, affords the child an opportunity to strengthen a number of processing capacities.

First, he is planning a ten-step action sequence rather than only a one- or two-step sequence. Second, he is practicing a visuospatial problem-solving capacity (i.e., searching for a hidden object). Third, he is processing sounds and words as the caregiver suggests he look in this "hand" or that "hand." Fourth, he is practicing motor skills and patience as he is challenged to open up the caregiver's hand, finger by finger.

Some caregivers, however, respond to the child's short bursts of interaction by becoming fragmented with the child. They jump from one thing to another with him rather than try to sustain a long chain of interaction. They also frequently give up entirely and let the child play alone.

Other caregivers attempt to over-control the child, which can tend to lead the child to be rigid. Such a child seems to focus, but it is not true, shared attention. There is no real back-and-forth problem-solving. Over-control also mobilizes catastrophic affects that can lead to even shorter bursts of co-regulated problem-solving interactions.

In attempting to mobilize the child into longer chains of co-regulated interactions, it is important to recognize that because the child may be used to short bursts, it is quite challenging. Initially, the key is to join the child in his rhythm. If he is more active, one tries to move with him, even as he moves around the room. If he is slower-moving and seems to be more absent-minded, one gets into a slow-moving rhythm with him.

It is also very important to pay attention to his natural interests and harness his positive affect. There is no better way to harness affect than to pay attention to what a child naturally enjoys. Does he enjoy, for example, a high-pitched voice or a low-pitched voice? Does he enjoy movement or sitting still? Does he enjoy one toy versus another? If he prefers physical objects to a person, you can join in with those physical objects, i.e., place the toy on your head and create a problem for the child to solve. By doing that, he is drawn into interaction. The caregiver and the toy become one and the same.

By harnessing his pleasure, enthusiasm, and interest, the child's affect is heightened. Once there is a heightened state of pleasurable affect and you are in rhythm with him, the key is to extend that interaction a few more reciprocal interchanges, as in the example of enticing the child to search for the toy. As you sustain the child's pleasure and the rhythm, it is usually possible to extend the reciprocal interaction to a few more circles of communication, and then a few more, and then a few more.

It is important not to get caught up in repetitive actions (i.e., opening and closing the door, or putting the car in and out of the garage). It is best to move to more creative and innovative actions as one keeps the rhythm going and extends the circles of communication.

Try appealing to all of the child's senses simultaneously—sound, sight, touch, smell, and movement in space as well. The key is finding the right level of sensation. If the child is over-responsive, you have to be soothing (in the over-responsive pathway). If the child is under-responsive, you have to energize up in an animated and interesting way for that sensory pathway. For example, for a child who is over-responsive to sound, use soothing vocalizations. If a child is under-responsive to sound, use highly energized vocalizations. For a child who is easily overloaded by visual complexity, keep the visual challenge simple. For a child who requires visual complexity, lots of colors and patterns are preferable. A child who prefers robust movement in space may enjoy roughhousing or other activities that involve lots of movement. A child who is initially more stationary, although he may learn to enjoy more movement, has to be approached more gradually and enticed into greater movement. For the child who has trouble with auditory processing, start with simple vocalizations or words, building up to more complicated ones including, as the child gets older, games that have directions in them where the child can win by following gradually more complex directions. Because each of these processing areas is now part of ongoing back-and-forth interactions, the child is learning to attend, interact, and use his senses more adaptively, all at the same time.

As you tune into the child's rhythms, find pleasurable affects, join those pleasurable activities, extend circles of communication, and harness all the sensory processing and motor planning capacities of the child simultaneously, you help that child learn to focus and attend and at the same time strengthen his or her underlying processing capacities.

In addition, many children require specific therapeutic or educational approaches, including special technologies to help them strengthen their underlying processing capacities. For example, some children require occupational therapy or speech therapy.

If we can begin such a program during the toddler years, we can work to increase a child's capacity for co-regulated reciprocal interactions during the stage at which the child is just learning how to sustain attention and engage in shared social problem-solving. By using co-regulated interactions, the child can be helped to become a dynamic attender and a problem solver. At the same time, he can strengthen his underlying processing capacities, which makes it easier for him to sustain this capacity to focus and attend and problem solve in the future. Even for older children, such a program can be helpful.

Not infrequently, children with attentional difficulties also have difficulties modulating their activity level. They can become very active, intruding into other people's space, or under-responsive, lost in their own worlds. These patterns are often in evidence in the early infant-caregiver interactions with toddlers on the move all the time, or self-absorbed and relatively inactive. The co-regulating interactive partner, however, can modulate the child's activity. For the child who is too active, the partner joins the activity, but then slows it down. With the slightly older child, modulation games can be played where, for example, they create a copycat game with rules like: go fast, slow, super slow, slow motion; or play the drums: hard, soft, super soft. The child who vocalizes loudly and seems to intrude into other people's space with his loud voice can also be assisted by the counter-regulatory interactive partner who helps him modulate with imitating soft sounds and whisper sounds, as well as loud ones.

The interactive partner may have more influence on the child's behavior than we are accustomed to assuming. For example, the pattern of response she institutes can increase the frequency of the child's behavior, including his activity level. It can influence the rigidity or emotional sensitivity of the behavior. The more variable or unpredictable a pattern of response (or reinforcement), the harder it is to extinguish behavior under its influence (i.e., the more rigid it is). While sustaining behavior has a positive advantage for the stability of certain behaviors, there are also negative consequences. These behaviors remain less sensitive to changing environmental contingencies, and therefore are more fixed and rigid.

Consider the following examples. A caregiver is preoccupied and responds to the child's gestures or other behaviors based on the number of behaviors the child initiates, but does so in a somewhat unpredictable manner (this is called a random ratio pattern of response or reinforcement). Such a pattern of response leads to very high activity levels because the child gets more responses or reinforcements if he initiates lots of behaviors. In contrast, what if the pattern of response to the child is based on how much time has passed (e.g., a self-absorbed caregiver only tunes into the child periodically)? Such a pattern where the caregiver responds one time after five seconds and the next time after eight seconds, etc., leads to very low activity levels. The activity can get so low that the child looks more and more self-absorbed. These patterns of response can exert a potent influence on behavior (Ferster & Skinner, 1957). Ironically, this type of potent caregiver influence can be subtle and it may appear that only biological factors are controlling the child's behavior. Often, however, both biological and experientially-based factors are working together.[4]

In summary, we have suggested that problems with attention can have a number of different developmental pathways. Each of these combines unique processing profiles with different types of early infant-caregiver (and later) interaction patterns.

4 There is a large literature on operant learning theory that looks at the impact of different response patterns on behavior (i.e., schedules of reinforcement). This literature may be helpful as an added conceptual framework (Greenspan, 1975).

108. Prolonged Grief Reaction

The loss of a parent or primary caregiver is so profound it always requires clinical attention.

Presenting Pattern

Reactions can take many forms and may progress over time. Most often, when infants and young children experience the loss of a primary caregiver, they evidence an initial grief reaction characterized by the child searching and protesting the caregiver's absence. The child may also withdraw, become more passive and self-absorbed, and avoid expected or pleasurable activities. Fear, anxiety, and agitation following the loss may give way to despondency and self-absorption, depending on the length of the loss. In other cases, the child may hardly seem to be reacting, especially if they take on the role of comforting or distracting the other grieving members of the family by "entertaining" or becoming more demanding of the caregiver and insisting they be cared for.

Reactions can also take the form of increased separation anxiety and some children cannot tolerate separation from the remaining caregiver and are very clingy. Some express their anger and aggression at the remaining parent who is still there, with or without the idealization of the missing parent. In some cases, children appear to carry on in one environment but not another such as at pre-school or daycare versus at home. Many evidence sleep and eating disruptions, weight loss, weight gains, become ill, have a variety of somatic complaints, reduced frustration tolerance, or other regressions in recently mastered developmental tasks such as toileting, dressing, and other forms of feeling "helpless." The persistence and/or multiplicity of these symptoms move expected grief reactions to the level of a disorder.

Comprehending the permanence of the loss is developmental in nature, but it is important not to underestimate the impact of the loss on infants and toddlers or children with significant developmental delays who may have many of the reactions described above, which other caregivers may not always link to the loss and grief or don't expect the child to remember. For the verbal child, it is not unusual for the child to express that she expects the return of the parent or imagines they are living elsewhere and they will be able to reunite at some point. Similarly, some children show marked distress at reminders of their missing caregiver, while others seek reminders that are positive reflections of their experiences and they want nothing changed or moved.

Whatever the reaction of the child to the loss of a parent or primary caregiver and however they try to comprehend its meaning, it is important to help the child, given the overwhelming significance of the loss and the child's limited resources to understand the reason or the finality of the loss. The age of the child and the emerging developmental profile of the child determines, in part, how long a period of loss is necessary for it to be considered a prolonged grief reaction or disorder.[5] An important factor is the availability

[5] Bowlby described and the Robertsons filmed very young children evidencing such a grief reaction when separated from their primary caregivers during a hospitalization. (These famous films are available at the New York University film library (Bowlby & Robertson, 1953)

of a nurturing substitute caregiver who provides extra security and emotional warmth, the opportunity to express feelings, and, in preschoolers, the opportunity to play out emerging worries and fears as well as feelings of loss. Such a caregiver can be especially helpful in enabling the child to cope with grief.

Developmental Pathway

Disruption of the child's functioning is likely to take the form of any vulnerability in the child's constitutional maturational patterns before the loss. Children who are over-responsive may become more irritable and fussy, with increased reactivity to the environment. Under-responsive children may become more withdrawn and self-absorbed and less responsive to attempts to arouse and engage them. Many children have mixed patterns and may show many fluctuations in unpredictable ways—sad and withdrawn one hour and frustrated and aggressive the next. If regulation was fragile to begin with, more difficulties are to be expected. But, even when the child's functioning is good, some short- or long-term dysregulation can be expected.

Therapeutic Implications

Where the loss of a caregiver is permanent, due to the death of a parent or permanent separation from a parent, it is essential to have a nurturing substitute caregiver available to help the child reestablish a sense of security. Guidance to other caregivers on how to talk about the loss from a developmental perspective and to recognize grief reactions is essential. In addition to daily comfort, daily stability in routines and playtime, increasing symbolic play, increasing talk time, not making abrupt moves if possible, and psychotherapy or counseling for the child and surviving family may be necessary. Even during relatively brief separations from a primary caregiver, such as a hospitalization or other reasons during which for some reason the caregiver cannot be present, the availability of another nurturing caregiver is extremely helpful.

When grief reactions are not dealt with and/or a child is exposed to multiple losses, as may happen in neglectful families and in multiple foster care placements, we may also see the gradual setting in of a coping strategy characterized by impersonal relationship patterns, aggressive behavior, or both.

109. Reactive Attachment Disorder

Forming an attachment or, more broadly, an emotionally trusting relationship, is a well-established critical dimension of healthy emotional development. We can observe, however, many compromises in forming or sustaining healthy relationship patterns.

Presenting Pattern

Attachment problems include a wide range of challenges, from infants and young children who are not able to engage in any type of intimacy, do not seek or respond to comfort, and may be either very despondent, withdrawn or self-absorbed, to those who are diffusely aggressive, impersonal and promiscuous in their relationships. Others show more subtle variations in degrees and qualities of intimacy, empathy, and the capacities for negotiating and sustaining relationships.

When extreme, disruptions in early attachment patterns can be associated with compromises in growth and weight gain (failure to thrive), as well as language, cognitive, and social difficulties. The most severe versions of these reactions are seen in children who grow up in orphanages that do not provide sufficient nurturing care and in children who experience extensive neglect or abuse within their families. If attachment problems have significantly disrupted the fundamental capacities of relating, communicating, and thinking, the child may appear like a child with neurodevelopmental disorders of relating and communicating, such as autism, with little capacity for shared attention, social reciprocity, or social problem-solving and require the same type of treatment program as children with derailed development.

In many cases, however, attachment and relationship problems in infancy and early childhood are not extreme. There are many subtle variations within which the early relationship lacks emotional depth, range, and optimal levels of trust and security. In looking at the more subtle attachment and relationship problems of infants and young children, the clinician should employ a framework that considers the implications of infant-caregiver relationships in light of the infant's capacity to successfully master each of the functional emotional developmental capacities. The attachment relationship needs to be viewed from the perspective of the full range and stability of age-expected feelings and progression through each of the functional emotional developmental capacities (Axis II). These levels may be difficult to negotiate with parents who have often experienced severe deprivation themselves as seen in multi-problem families, and then are unable to form intimate attachments with their own infants. The interactions may also be embedded with anxiety, despair or ambivalence and other compromises in the parent's experience or current relationships.

The clinician also needs to consider the contributions of the child's regulatory-sensory processing profile. For example, infants who are very responsive to sensations such as touch and sound may evidence far more insecurity in their early relationship patterns than other infants. On the other hand, challenges in forming relationships can lead to challenges in sensory modulation, sensory processing, and motor planning, which can appear to have a biological origin, even when they are secondary to interactive challenges. Infants who are born with very competent nervous systems, including good muscle tone and abilities to focus, attend, and respond to visual and auditory sensations, can lose these competencies during the first 2 to 3 months of life if their environments are either very chaotic or non-nurturing (Greenspan et al., 1987). Infants can develop low muscle tone, under-responsivity to touch and sound, as well as difficulties in auditory and visuospatial processing or sensory hypersensitivity and patterns of avoidance (in the more chaotic, over-stimulating environments). Even when these patterns are secondary to interactive difficulties, they may be indistinguishable from infants who are born with these processing challenges such as infants with extreme regulatory or neurodevelopmental difficulties in relating and communicating.

Developmental Pathway

Two major pathways and their variations need to be considered. One pathway includes the interaction between the environment and the child. When the environment is neglectful, abusive or otherwise stressful, it may not be able to provide the nurturing interactions necessary to form relationships which can support each functional developmental level (see Axis II). In some cases the environmental stress may be related to external factors such as poverty, family disruption, or illness. In other cases, the parents may not have the personal emotional and relationship capacities to help their child form a secure relationship and maintain it.

Understanding the child's unique individual profile and the contribution of the child's challenges highlights the other major pathway. For example, the infant may be more sensory over- or under-responsive or have challenges in the way he or she processes auditory and visuospatial information and plans motor actions. These variations can challenge the parent's competency and derail the development of a secure and trusting relationship as the infant and parent struggle to regulate and enjoy their interactions.

Therapeutic Implications

In working with the infants in multi-risk families who suffered severe emotional deprivation, as well as infants and young children who evidenced or developed processing differences, we were able to identify pathways to helping the infants and young children as well as the parents. Multi-risk families, however, require a great deal more family support and outreach as part of a comprehensive program. Establishing the safety and survival of the family and developing a therapeutic relationship with each is essential (Greenspan et al., 1987).

The therapeutic implications for promoting the relationship include tailoring nurturing interactions to the child's individual processing differences and working with individual processing differences at each of six early levels of affective organization, including the level that deals with co-regulated affective signaling, which can be exceedingly challenging for these children to master. Co-regulated, affective interactions tailored to the child's processing differences often enable the child to negotiate intimacy on his own terms (e.g., resolving approach-avoidance interactions more and engaging in more finely tuned regulation through affect signaling). Caregivers who work through their conflicts as well via affective signaling, coupled with verbal explorations of their perceptions, feelings, memories, and meaning of the child, as well as understanding the uniqueness of their child's tendencies, often show progress.

Understanding the child's sensory over- or under-responsivity and the way she processes auditory and visuospatial information and plans motor actions provide therapeutic implications for facilitating relationships for even the most challenging children—for example, strategies for not overwhelming the over-responsive infant or calming the overstimulated infant supports engaging and affective signaling. Similarly, learning to engage the under-responsive child and woo her into rhythmic interactions improves affect cuing and enjoyable two-way interactions, and opens the door for the child to form symbols and use language creatively and meaningfully, form peer relationships, and relate to others with a high degree of empathy and reflectiveness.

110. Traumatic Stress Disorder

The term "Traumatic Stress Disorder," rather than "Post Traumatic Stress Disorder" is used because infants and young children often respond to severe trauma or stress immediately. The reaction may then continue, depending on factors discussed below.

Presenting Pattern

Infants and young children may be exposed to a range of traumatic stresses that can disrupt their emotional, social, language, and intellectual development. Children experiencing or witnessing serious unexpected events that threaten them or others, such as accidents, animal attacks, fires, war, natural disasters, or overwhelmingly frightening interpersonal events such as abuse or a parent being killed, are some examples.

Such children may experience a disruption in a number of basic capacities. Most common are disruptions in sleep, eating, elimination, attention, impulse control, and mood patterns. Physiological disruption is common and reflects the enormous impact of the traumatic stress on the young child's autonomic functions and regulation of basic states such as startle responses, increased heart rate, heavy breathing, shaking or sweating. Other children become sick and needy. The child may also find it difficult to focus and may be so on guard, anxious, or avoidant she is unable to participate in and enjoy typical routines or social activities.

New fears not present before the trauma may also emerge as the child becomes more worried about other things and displaces fears of recurrence of the traumatic event. These fears may be accompanied by nightmares. Others ask continuous questions about the event, repeating questions they already know the answer to. Children who play symbolically may re-enact the trauma in their play over and over again, unable to change the story.

The clinician should consider this diagnosis whenever a known single event or series of discrete events are associated with an immediate or delayed disruption in the child's age-expected range of emotional and social or related language and cognitive capacities. The child's reactions may be tempered by the parent's ability to help the child feel safe again as quickly as possible, but may surface later on. The clinician needs to look for any disruption in ongoing mastery of the functional emotional developmental capacities in relationship to a traumatic event. For example, in evaluating regulation and shared attention, difficulties with concentration and/or over-vigilance may make it difficult for the child to attend and engage in the aftermath of insecurity following the trauma. Engagement may be disrupted as the child may either feel distrustful or angry for the failure to protect him or becomes more clingy, frightened, or sad. The child may also become less communicative and helpless, unable to sustain the longer back-and-forth problem-solving interactions he had before. If he is able to play symbolically, the child may reenact some form of the trauma as the victim or the perpetrator, or may become avoidant and constricted, unable to use symbolic play or language to deal with his feelings. Reality testing can get derailed as the child resorts to denial, confuses what is real or not real, or regresses to magical thinking.

Developmental Pathway

The child's basic regulatory and developmental patterns often interact with the stress. Infants and toddlers who are under-responsive to touch and sound and sensory-seeking or crave sensation and are physically very active, often become aggressive and/or antisocial following the trauma, especially if they also suddenly lose the caregiver's protective security provided through engagement, empathy, co-regulated emotional signaling, and limit-setting. Children who are under-responsive but not sensory-seeking may shut down further and appear more lethargic or depressed and difficult to arouse.

Children who are over-responsive to sensations such as touch and sound may easily become hypervigilant or overloaded. The sensory over-responsive child is also likely to describe fear and panic and "being overwhelmed." Even a sudden, unexpected touch from another child can easily be misperceived as threatening or aggressive. He may then push or hit when others become too intrusive or overwhelming. Caregiver-child interaction patterns that are soothing and regulating, foster initiative and social responsiveness, and the elaboration of emotions and ideas in play and words often help children deal with stress. Where these patterns are compromised, stress can be more difficult.

Therapeutic Implications

Re-establishing the security of the child is paramount and this includes securing the basic safety of the family who can then try to quickly restore the safety of their children. Healing or working through the trauma requires increased nurturing and reciprocal affective interactions, as well as regulation and calm soothing with gradual support for the child's initiative. Pretend play following the child's lead so he or she can explore feelings at his or her own pace is very helpful. Parents or other caregivers can involve the child in soothing communication that enables him to ponder, give names to his feelings, and be assured all is being done to help him feel safe again. The goal of the caregiver is to help the child calm his fears, so he realizes he can calm down, and to reassure him how he is protected, and gradually to help him express and explore feelings, including fears. Children who are more sensitive to sensations require a great deal of soothing and regulation.

Any prior regulatory-sensory processing challenges, whether in auditory processing, visuospatial processing challenges, or motor planning can become exacerbated and disrupt the functioning of the child who may, for example, have difficulty following directions, feel lost or confused in space, or not be able to sequence problem-solving interactions. These experiences can contribute to further anxiety, insecurity, and may increase aggressive or depressive feelings.

Clearly, this optimal interaction may be difficult for caregivers, who themselves have just experienced the trauma and are very anxious. Other ongoing relationships may be needed to help the family and child feel secure and deal with fears. It is essential for caregivers or their substitutes to provide stable environmental conditions with sufficient nurturing, regulating affective interactions, and firm but gentle limit-setting if needed. It is also important to provide many opportunities for play and conversation to help the child work through the trauma and strengthen overall developmental capacities.

111. Adjustment Disorder

Infants and young children, like older children and adults, evidence temporary challenges in response to expectable situations that they have difficulty adapting or adjusting to. Experiences such as a change of caregiver, starting school, conflicts with peers, temporary illness of a parent, birth of a sibling, separation and divorce, or moving from one house to another may trigger an adjustment reaction. What is unique, however, about the infant's or young child's adjustment reaction is the types of behaviors and interactions that vary from their prior adaptation.

Presenting Pattern

In addition to easy-to-observe temporary shifts in sleeping, eating, minor regressions in language and behavior, mood shifts, poor frustration tolerance, increased anxiety or fears, oppositional behaviors, or impulse control patterns, one must also look for subtle changes in the child's ongoing mastery of each of the functional emotional developmental capacities described in Axis II. Does the child who was fully engaged withdraw even a little? Does the child begin to object to going to pre-school or leaving the house? Does symbolic play get restricted to earthquakes or battles?

In choosing this diagnosis, it is critical to identify the source of the challenge (e.g., a parent's absence on a business trip), the changes in behavior and mood relative to prior functioning, and the way in which the challenge is disrupting the child's mastery of functional emotional developmental capacities (e.g., his typical optimism and happiness). Having these pieces of information enables the available caregiver to provide extra stability, security, and opportunities for the child to communicate, through gesture, play, or verbalization of his concerns.

Developmental Pathway

Adjustment reactions can have a number of different developmental pathways related to the child's unique processing profiles and prior adaptation. A temporary disruption can relate to the most recently mastered developmental task such as separation or toilet training. A child-caregiver interaction pattern characterized by a caregiver over-responding to a child's expectable feelings can be associated with a tendency to become fearful with a temporary challenge. A regression can occur in the area the child struggled in the past, such as falling asleep related to over-responsiveness to sound or difficulties self-calming. The under-responsive child might withdraw or become more self-absorbed. Symptoms can also relate to the processing system that is less developed, e.g., not listening or following directions (weaker auditory processing) or losing and not finding favorite toys (weaker visuospatial processing). It is often possible to understand the family dynamic or sensory based reasons for the adjustment reaction by examining the child's earlier adaptations and profile.

Therapeutic Implications

Understanding the source of the trouble and its effects on the child also enables parents and caregivers to lessen the nature of the challenge. For example, a father who is away on a business trip can call more frequently and make sure his toddler can hear his voice on the speakerphone. Mother can provide the child with a picture of daddy or a "Daddy and Me" photo album to look at while they are talking, and she can then engage him in playing with a daddy doll. In general, increasing caregiver availability, security, interactive opportunities, and times for symbolic play provide a basis for helping the child cope with new concerns. When persistent measures to support the child do not alleviate concerns, other primary diagnoses should be considered.

112. Gender Identity Disorder

In infants and young children, gender is beginning to form. One can see gender-specific behaviors throughout infancy and early childhood. These become more pronounced in the latter part of the second year and into the third and fourth years of life. Children's difficulties with their own biological gender are most frequently identified when a preschooler insists on dressing up as the opposite gender, not simply as part of playful exploration and experimentation but as a persistent pattern. In play, there may be a strong preference for opposite-gender roles, dolls, and so on. There may also be a strong preference for opposite-gender playmates as well as for activities associated with the opposite gender. Verbal preschool children may express a clear dislike for their own anatomy and a wish to change their genitals. This reaction can be particularly strong and associated with a great deal of anxiety as the preschool child becomes more aware of the anatomical differences between boys and girls. The patterns of preference for the opposite gender and dislike of or anger at one's own gender can begin in early childhood. If not addressed, they can persist and intensify as the child develops. These patterns can emerge at older ages as well.

Often, there may be unique constitutional-maturation variations as well as caregiver-child interactions and family patterns contributing to a child's gender identity difficulties, for example, a parent's wish for a child of the opposite sex or parental conflicts. Underlying concerns with separation from the primary caregiver, conflicts over aggression and assertiveness, conflicts identifying with the same gendered parent or the absence of a positive relationship may contribute to the child's difficulties (Coates, Friedman, & Wolfe, 1991).

Developmental Pathway

Children tend to be more over-responsive to sounds, lights, and touch, as well as more challenged by difficulties with sensory modulation, motor planning and sequencing, and visuospatial processing. This combination, coupled with caregiver conflicts and the developmental tasks at hand, may undermine the security and physical and emotional competence of the child who then seeks change of gender. Since gender conflicts also emerge at the time the child is expected to expand his emotional range and become more able to experience increasing negative emotions such as anger, jealousy, retaliation and fears of aggression, the child may seek to avoid or flee from his own gender which may mask the anxieties related to these feelings.

Therapeutic Implications

A comprehensive intervention program that works with the child-caregiver relationship patterns, family relationships, and the child's constitutional-maturational variations is often required. It is important not to overlook the importance of treating the over-responsiveness and modulation challenges, and strengthening sensory-motor and visuospatial processing to increase the child's competence and coping with his body and the expectations of the environment. Creativity through art, music, and movement are also opportune ways for greater symbolic expression and working with the child.

113. Elective Mutism

Elective mutism refers to a continuing difficulty in talking in social situations coupled with an ability to comprehend language and to speak in other settings such as home. While this pattern is reported to be found in less than one percent of children, it is nonetheless challenging for parents, educators, and the child.

Presenting Pattern

Children with elective mutism tend to be anxious and are often very reactive to changes in or new environments, especially ones with lots of people, noise, etc. where sounds and movements can be surprising and unpredictable. The inability to speak is often associated with a subjective state of overwhelming fear and vigilance. Often the child attempts to retreat in a selective manner. In play or conversation with a child with elective mutism, one often observes content having to do with fear, worry, and danger. One may also see patterns of avoidance, e.g., seemingly safe non-emotional scenes such as very friendly tea parties. Relationships are often characterized by an anxious dependent pattern with a reluctance to take initiative and be assertive. While the child appears most anxious and becomes selectively mute and over-vigilant in selected settings, constrictions of the functional emotional developmental capacities are evident even where the child is comfortable speaking. Unresolved developmental anxieties related to fears of body damage, aggression, and other negative emotions are evident with constricted capacities to symbolize and express feelings safely in play or conversation. Although related to anxiety disorders, the highly specific symptom of elective mutism warrants a separate disorder.

Developmental Pathway

The somatic state is one of tension and anxiety and, as indicated earlier, over-reactivity to sensation. The child with elective mutism is also described in the section on

Regulatory-Sensory Processing Disorders (see 200. Regulatory-Sensory Processing Disorders, Sensory Modulation Challenges [Type I]—over-responsive). Often, early infant-caregiver interaction patterns do not optimally support the child's initiative and self-regulation. Over-anxious caregiver response patterns, dysregulating ones or those that undermine initiative should be looked for.

Therapeutic Implications

Often the anxiety level can be reduced by, for example, inviting a child from school to the child's home to increase confidence, familiarity, and experience with speaking to that child in a calm and secure setting. If this is followed by having that child, who is now familiar, play with the child with elective mutism in a little tent in a corner of the room, one may begin hearing some vocalizations and words. Eventually a third child can be added to the group, and so forth and so on, until the child becomes comfortable speaking in the middle of the classroom. In other cases, someone the child is comfortable speaking with can go with the child to the new or stressful environment. Caregivers should be helped to provide regulating and initiative-supporting reciprocal affective exchanges. These themes should also be supported in pretend play, reality-based problem-solving conversations, and in overall family patterns.

114-116. Sleep, Eating and Elimination Behavior Disorders - Introduction

Difficulties with sleeping or eating, and in older children, difficulties with toilet training and comfortable patterns of elimination, are very common in infancy and early childhood. In some cases, they initially appear to be the only challenge the child experiences. Often, these difficulties arise in response to various interactive challenges, including trauma, anxiety, and adjustment reactions to transitions, illness, and psychosocial stress. The choice of the symptoms is often determined by the underlying sensory-motor vulnerability in combination with the developmental anxiety and/or interactive patterns. Difficulties with sleeping, eating, toilet training, and elimination can also be related to Regulatory-Sensory Processing Disorders (see 200. Regulatory-Sensory Processing Disorder).

The clinician needs to determine whether the primary contributing factors lie in infant-caregiver interactions or constitutional-maturational variations. When it appears that both factors are playing a major role, the primary diagnosis should be of a Regulatory-Sensory Processing Disorder. When it appears infant-caregiver interactions play a major role, then the primary diagnosis should be an interactive disorder. Regardless of the primary diagnosis, the child's developmental profile always reflects the relative contributions of constitutional-maturational variations, child-caregiver interactions, and family and environmental factors. Axis II (Functional Emotional Developmental Capacities) highlights the relative strengths and weaknesses of the dyad and their adaptive areas of emotional interactions.

114. Sleep Disorders

Establishing sleep-wake cycles is one of the first tasks of infancy and most children establish sleep-wake routines within the first few months or year of life. Many factors may contribute to challenges. Disruptions in sleep patterns can naturally occur with illness, changes in location, transitions in development, and other stress, but usually get re-established with the resumption of security and soothing relationships. In some cases, healthy sleep routines were not established early on or there were inconsistent times or settings for sleep, or when infants do not learn to fall asleep on their own and are used to being held, fed, or lying in physical proximity of the parent. Some infants rely on nursing or sucking a bottle to initiate sleep. Parents do not always learn other techniques for helping the child calm and fall asleep independently. Other infants do not change their patterns even after maturation appears to have resolved fussy and irritable periods during infancy but sleep rhythms still do not get established. In still other cases, the environment is too chaotic to sustain routines and security with resulting disorganized sleep patterns.

Another factor to consider pertains to the culture of the family. Complaints of a sleep disorder can be subject to the perceptions and feelings of caregivers who may have varying tolerance for irregular or disrupted sleep patterns or have similar patterns themselves. In other cases, parents come from cultures where sleeping with a child is acceptable or desired and all children share this experience. What presents as a sleep disturbance for one parent, therefore, may not be a problem for another.

Since sleep disorders are such a common pathway for conveying distress, they can signify any of the primary interactive disorders described earlier, or they can be rooted in constitutionally-based Regulatory-Sensory Processing Disorders associated with other regulatory challenges described below. When the sleep disorder is highly disruptive of the child's and/or family's functioning, even when it is part of another primary interactive disorder, it can be used as a secondary primary diagnosis to highlight the attention it needs to help stabilize the family. For example, when sleep disruptions are frequent and coupled with severe anxiety related to emotional developmental challenges, a secondary sleep disorder can be considered.

Presenting Pattern

Infants and young children may have difficulty settling into sleep when they first go to bed, or wake up and cannot fall asleep again on their own. Some of these infants may even wake frequently throughout the night and are restless sensitive sleepers. Others may be hard to arouse and sleep too much. Sleep disruption can also occur when children awaken from a scary dream or nightmare as they become more symbolic and are not sure what is real or not.

It is often the interactions between caregivers and children that become the determining factor of a sleep disorder. Relationships are often characterized by neediness, negativism, and impulsivity, with different parts of this pattern dominating in different children and families. Some parents are puzzled when they hear their child can fall asleep with others but not with them, and are left feeling very inadequate. Others blame each other for not being able to get the baby to sleep and marital conflict may also fuel the maintenance of the sleep disorder.

Developmental Pathway

Infant-caregiver interactive patterns combine with underlying sensory and motor patterns including over-responsivity and/or under-responsivity related to poor arousal as contributing factors. Particular infant-caregiver interaction patterns to look for include over-responding to the infant's cues and undermining initiative; difficulty creating rhythmic, soothing interactions; insufficient interactive opportunities during the waking hours; and intrusive, frightening interactions.

Therapeutic Implications

Parents can benefit from guidance on how to establish sleep routines and respond to the individual needs of their children. This may involve altering the environment and recognizing overstimulating patterns or reactivity to touch, sounds, movement and possible contributions from the foods the child eats or breast milk (mother's diet). With toddlers and young children, the guidance may address finding other ways to increase intimacy and playful interactions and then use routines and gentle, but clear limits to guide the child to sleep.

When separation challenges have already derailed the child sleeping in his own room, a transition plan can be put in place, again coupled with increased interactions and play during the day. This also supports the child's emotional development as he learns to symbolize in play and conversations his expanding range of emotions and any attendant anxieties.

However, it is difficult to embark on a constructive approach to intervene when parents become too distressed (exhausted) or angry about the persistence of the problem and have "already tried everything!" Exploring the dynamics of a sleep problem in a family is essential for clearing the way to effective intervention. The more supportive and empathetic the family, the better it is able to help the child embark on a constructive intervention approach, and the more likely the family relationship patterns are characterized by comfort, security and shared pleasure.

115. Eating Disorders

Eating disorders, like sleep disorders, can be symptomatic of many of the interactive disorders as well as a regulatory disorder with sensory hypersensitivities and oral motor difficulties described below. When related to an interactive pattern, eating disorders may reflect the residual anxiety of resolved biological problems, such as gastrointestinal difficulties, reflux, or other illnesses with resulting anxiety and lack of pleasure around eating.

It is often the interactions between caregivers and children that become the determining factor of an eating disorder. For example, eating can become an over-relied source of comfort and self-soothing in the absence of appropriate nurturance. Refusal can become an expression of fear, anger, or rejection in the absence of symbolic expression.

Presenting Pattern

The eating disorder may involve poor or irregular intake, food refusal, vomiting, or restricted and insatiable eating. Since eating is so essential for survival, it is not a challenge that can be overlooked for long. Since the health and weight of the baby is often seen as a reflection of "good" parenting, it can become an enormous source of worry, stress, and feared inadequacy to the caregiver. The interaction between the two can result in vacillations between neediness, negativism, and anxiety with different parts of this pattern dominating in different children and families. Even simpler feeding challenges can undermine the confidence of infant and caregiver when coincidental with family disruptions, transitions, or difficult resuming or establishing more organized eating patterns.

Developmental Pathway

Two pathways are involved. The infant's underlying sensory-motor vulnerability can include both hypersensitivities to food textures, tastes, and smells or under-reactivity to tastes and smells reducing the awareness and enjoyment of eating. In addition, infants may have reduced muscle tone and oral motor difficulties which make feeding or eating challenging, e.g., difficulties getting food off the spoon, moving food to be chewed and swallowed, lip closure, etc. When these sensory-motor vulnerabilities combine with infant-caregiver interactive patterns related to conflict, anxiety, and fears an eating disorder can develop.

Therapeutic Implications

The infant's underlying sensory and oral motor difficulties need to be understood and treated, with guidance to restore the caregiver's confidence in being able to feed and nurture her child. Exploring the dynamics of eating for the child is also essential. A parent's insecurity as a competent nurturer can also contribute or confound the child's challenges. Contributing family stress, marital discord, a complicated family history, or parent eating disorder needs to be addressed therapeutically. The more supportive and empathetic the family; the better it is able to help the child embark on a constructive intervention approach that includes fostering both security and initiative as well as mastery of the functional emotional developmental milestones, and the more likely the family relationship patterns will be characterized by comfort, security and shared pleasure.

116. Elimination Disorders

Elimination disorders include functional encopresis and enuresis. There is a primary type where expected urinary or bowel control has not been reached beyond the variations of developmental expectations, and a secondary type where it has been reached, but is subsequently lost. In both types of elimination disorders, as well as in children who withhold their stool or urine, the child often experiences a range of affective states. Fear, shame, and embarrassment over the "accident" are readily observed. However, at a deeper subjective level, the child often feels unsure about his or her body. There is a pervasive sense of insecurity about bodily functioning with significant anxiety over "not being in control" of unexpected urges. Some children defend against the bodily signals to eliminate and may hide or deny their bodily needs. These children may compensate by trying to control everyone else. They may experience the demands of their body coming too unpredictably and become anxious. Some children are not sufficiently aware they need to go until too late; they have poor sensory registration of their bodies' signals coupled with reduced muscle tone leaving them confused and embarrassed.

For others, mastery of toileting implies too high expectations to be a "big boy!" or, persistent wishes to still be "baby." This conflict may be the child's or the parent's, and usually becomes intertwined as caregiver and child struggle with fears of loss and separation, changes in alliances, (e.g., babies belong to mom but big boys go to daddy!), fears of incompetence, or other conflicts.

The child's mental content in play and conversation tends to mirror the affective patterns described above. Play themes are often characterized by avoidance of strong affect, explosive bursts of affective content, and vacillations between the two. The child often verbalizes a wish to "do better" and please his caregivers, coupled with negativism and intermittent impulsivity. In the content of the child's play, one sees shame, embarrassment, avoidance, impulsivity, and fragmentation. An examination of functional developmental capacities can help identify the constrictions contributing to these problems and the specific dynamic formulation which may be relevant.

Developmental Pathway

Underlying sensory-motor vulnerabilities combined with interactive challenges contribute to elimination difficulties. For example, the child may have low muscle tone and poor motor planning, as well as sensory under-reactivity, making it difficult to sense and then execute motor control over basic bodily functions. Others may be too sensitive to or fearful of the flushing. Some limit their toileting to a specific bathroom in their home or cannot orient themselves visually and spatially in unfamiliar settings. But, somatic states also tend to express the particular type of affects and physical challenge the child is evidencing (e.g., discomfort). For some children, withholding can become a way to express anger or retaliation in the absence of more symbolic use of words or play to communicate their feelings. Relationships are often characterized by vacillations between neediness, negativism, and impulsivity with different parts of this pattern dominating in different children and families.

Therapeutic Implications

It is important to help the child deal with his sense of uncertainty and insecurity, so that he or she can arrive at a realistic picture of how the body functions. It is also important to help the child work through fears of anger or assertiveness, as well as help the caregiver and family (as a whole) provide an emotional climate that supports both security and initiative. Often, caregiver-child interaction patterns are compromised in fostering assertiveness and initiative in a secure and regulated manner at both the level of affective gestures and symbols. Sensory and motor processing can also be supported to facilitate the child's sense of competence in his body through related and other sensory-motor and visuospatial activities. It is important to help the parents deal with their feelings regarding this basic body function, what it means to them and how they feel, and what allows them to implement an effective approach to support the child. The more supportive and empathetic the family, and the better it is able to help the child embark on a constructive intervention approach, the more likely the family relationship patterns will be characterized by comfort, security, and shared pleasure.

Axis I: Regulatory-Sensory Processing Disorders[1]

200. Regulatory-Sensory Processing Disorder

Sensory Modulation Challenges (Type I)

201. Over-Responsive, Fearful, Anxious Pattern
202. Over-Responsive, Negative, and Stubborn Pattern
203. Under-Responsive, Self-Absorbed Pattern
    - 203.1 Self-Absorbed and Difficult to Engage Type
    - 203.2 Self-Absorbed and Creative Type
204. Active, Sensory Seeking Pattern

Sensory Discrimination Challenges (Type II) and Sensory-Based Motor Challenges (Type III)

205. Inattentive, Disorganized Pattern
    - 205.1 With Sensory Discrimination Challenges
    - 205.2 With Postural Control Challenges
    - 205.3 With Dyspraxia
    - 205.4 With Combinations of 205.1-205.3
206. Compromised School and/or Academic Performance Pattern
    - 206.1 With Sensory Discrimination Challenges
    - 206.2 With Postural Control Challenges
    - 206.3 With Dyspraxia
    - 206.4 With Combinations of 206.1-206.3

Contributing Sensory Discrimination and Sensory-Based Motor Challenges

207. Mixed Regulatory-Sensory Processing Patterns
    - 207.1 Attentional Problems
    - 207.2 Disruptive Behavioral Problems
    - 207.3 Sleep Problems
    - 207.4 Eating Problems
    - 207.5 Elimination Problems
    - 207.6 Elective Mutism
    - 207.7 Mood Dysregulation, including Bipolar Patterns
    - 207.8 Other Emotional and Behavioral Problems Related to Mixed Regulatory-Sensory Processing Difficulties
    - 207.9 Mixed Regulatory-Sensory Processing Difficulties where Behavioral or Emotional Problems Are Not Yet in Evidence

[1] Work Group Members include: Lucy J. Miller, Ph.D., OTR, Marie Anzalone, Sc.D., OTR, Sharon A. Cermak, Ed.D., OTR/L, Shelly J. Lane, Ph.D., OTR, Beth Osten, M.S., OTR/L, Serena Wieder, Ph.D., Stanley I. Greenspan, M.D.

Regulatory-Sensory Processing Disorders (RSPD) should be viewed on a continuum of regulatory-sensory processing variations. All children evidence unique regulatory-sensory processing profiles. They vary in the ways they respond to different sensations (such as touch and sound), comprehend these sensations, and plan actions. Some children, however, have processing differences that are extreme enough to interfere with daily functioning at home, in school, and in interactions with peers or adults, as well as with routine functions such as self-care, sleeping, and eating. As we describe regulatory-sensory processing below, note that while we focus on the disorders end of the continuum, the same patterns can characterize children without challenges and can be very helpful in understanding individual differences and the best ways to promote healthy emotional, social, and intellectual functioning. While observations of variations in motor and sensory functioning in infants and young children have a long history (e.g., the writings of (Ayres, 1964); the concept of RSPD was first introduced in the 1980s and early 1990s when Greenspan introduced the concept of Regulatory Disorders (Greenspan et al., 1987; Greenspan, 1992). Along parallel lines, the concept of Sensory Processing Disorders has been developing since Ayres (1972). In 2004, a framework describing a new taxonomy for classifying classic patterns and subtypes of sensory processing problems was presented (Miller, Cermak, et al., 2004).(Greenspan, 1992)

Regulatory Disorders as a diagnostic entity was subsequently incorporated into the diagnostic classification system of Zero To Three: National Center for Infants, Toddlers, and Families. More recently, the Regulatory-Sensory Processing Work Group of the Interdisciplinary Council on Developmental and Learning Disorders (ICDL) has brought the two streams of thought together from the occupational therapy literature and the Developmental, Individual-Difference, Relationship-Based (DIR) model of Infant and Early Childhood Mental Health (Greenspan, 1992) and reformulated and added to the description of Regulatory-Sensory Processing Disorders, which is included in this section.

All children evidence their own unique regulatory-sensory processing patterns. These variations are always important to consider when constructing a developmental profile for a specific infant or child and her family. An RSPD, however, should be considered when the child's motor and sensory differences are contributing to challenges that interfere with age-expected emotional, social, language, cognitive (including attention), motor, or sensory functioning. RSPD gives rise to some of the same symptoms and behaviors as interactive disorders, including nightmares, withdrawal, aggressiveness, fearfulness and anxiety, sleeping and eating disturbances, and difficulty in peer relationships. However, RSPD involves clearly identifiable constitutional-maturational factors in the child.

CLINICAL EVIDENCE AND PREVALENCE OF REGULATORY-SENSORY PROCESSING DIFFERENCES

Recognition and work with regulatory-sensory processing differences have a long history. Occupational therapists have clinically assessed, treated, and researched sensory processing difficulties in children since the late 1950s. Based on both clinical experience and assessment findings, tactile defensiveness was first described by Ayres (Ayres, 1965; 1966a; 1980) as an over-responsiveness to touch sensations, particularly light or unexpected touch. Subsequently over-responsiveness to sensory input in a specific sensory system (e.g., the vestibular system) or within the whole body (i.e., sensory defensiveness) has been identified and defined (Ayres, 1972a; Parham & Mailloux, 2001). Under-responsiveness to sensation has also been clinically characterized (Knickerbocker, 1980; Royeen & Lane, 1991; Dunn, 1994).

Sensory responsiveness differences have been used to characterize populations of children with difficult temperament (Rothbart, 1981; Rothbart & Posner, 1985; Thomas & Chess, 1985); regulatory disorders (DeGangi & Greenspan, 1989; DeGangi, 1991; DeGangi, 2001; Greenspan, 1981; 1992; Williamson & Anzalone, 2001); and children with autism spectrum disorders (Greenspan & Wieder 1997; 2005). In a recent study of a representative population, a parent questionnaire on regulatory-sensory processing differences distinguished infants and young children with a number of developmental disorders, including autism and cognitive deficits, from infants and children without challenges (Greenspan, 2004). Functional problems associated with regulatory-sensory processing differences have been described to include: decreased social skills and participation in play; decreased frequency, duration or complexity of adaptive responses; impaired self-confidence and/or self-esteem; deficient adaptive or daily life skills; and diminished fine-, gross- and sensory-motor skill development (Bundy, 2002; Parham & Fazio, 1996; Parham & Mailloux, 2001). While parents may struggle with issues long before children enter school, problems related to Sensory Processing Disorder (SPD) may become more apparent once a child enters a day-care or school environment (Miller & Summers, 2001).

Empirical evidence matching the behavioral manifestations such as those identified above, with physiologic indicators of sensory processing impairments, is accumulating (Mangeot, Miller, McIntosh, 2001; McIntosh, Miller, Shyu, Hagerman, 1999; Miller, McIntosh, McGrath, et al., 1999; Schaff, Miller, Sewell, & O'Keefe, 2003). Electrodermal activity (EDA), as a marker of sympathetic nervous system activity, has recently been used to document physiologic responses during a sensory challenge protocol. The EDA of children with severe Sensory Processing Disorder and Fragile X syndrome differs significantly from the EDA of typically developing children after sensory stimulation (Miller, et al., 1999). Further, children with sensory processing impairments and no other diagnosis demonstrated significantly abnormal EDA after sensory stimulation (McIntosh, et al., 1999). Parent ratings of sensory processing impairment have been shown to correlate with EDA measures, as well (McIntosh, Miller, Shyu, & Dunn, 1999).

In addition, vagal tone has been used to measure parasympathetic nervous system functioning in children identified with sensory processing impairments (Schaaf, Miller, Sewell, & O'Keefe, 2003). Results indicate that children with sensory processing disturbances displayed significantly lower vagal tone than typically developing participants, consistent with other studies that found decreased parasympathetic functioning associated with stress vulnerability, developmental and cognitive delays, and emotional and behavioral over-reactivity.

Among children, prevalence estimates of Sensory Processing Disorder based on clinical experience have ranged from 5% to 10% for children without disabilities (Ayres, 1989; Ermer & Dunn, 1998). Estimated rates of Sensory Processing Disorder for children with disabilities such as autism, derived from reliable and valid survey results, are reported to be as high as 40%-88% (Adrien, Lenoir, P., Martineau, 1993; Dahl & Gillberg, 1989; Kientz & Dunn, 1997; Ornitx, Guthrie, & Farley, 1977; Talay-Ongan & Wood, 2000). A more recent investigation of prevalence placed the rate among the general population of kindergarten-aged children at 5% using conservative estimation procedures (Ahn, Miller, Milberger, & McIntosh, 2004).

Different views regarding an appropriate comprehensive theory or the effectiveness of particular intervention strategies must not distract attention from the compelling evidence for the existence of regulatory-sensory processing differences and their relevance to understanding a range of clinical phenomena. Studies supporting the existence of regulatory-sensory processing differences and difficulties in the general population and different clinical disorders should be separated from considerations of regulatory-sensory processing theories and intervention strategies. Research is underway to examine both of these areas of interest.

DEVELOPMENTAL PERSPECTIVES ON REGULATORY-SENSORY PROCESSING DIFFERENCES

To recognize problems as early as possible, it is important to emphasize that regulatory-sensory processing differences are evident very early in life. In a study of 8-month-old children (Doussard-Roosevelt, Walker, Portales, Greenspan, & Porges, 1990; Porges & Greenspan, 1990), we were able to show that a high percentage of the symptomatic infants had constitutional-maturational differences that contributed to their sleeping problems, eating difficulties, temper tantrums, and other symptoms (DeGangi & Greenspan, 1988). The babies were either under- or over-responsive in some sensory modality or had sensory processing, muscle tone, or motor planning difficulties, in addition to difficulties with physiological regulation. These differences seemed to contribute to a skewing of parent-infant interaction patterns, which, in turn, affected the infants' personality development (DeGangi, DiPietro, Greenspan, & Porges, 1991).

The infants' constitutional-maturational differences persisted and were evident at 18 months. The families also showed signs of distress (Portales, Porges, & Greenspan, 1990). A small group of these infants who were followed to age 4 displayed more behavioral and learning problems than a comparison group (DeGangi, Porges, Sickel, & Greenspan, 1993). Clearly, children with constitutional-maturational unevenness tend to be especially challenging. They have a harder time than other children in their relationships with caregivers; their families' functioning tends to be stressed; and they eventually may experience more behavioral and learning difficulties (Miller, Robinson, & Moulton, 2004).

One can see how a child's constitutional-maturational characteristics influence interaction patterns, and hence the child's developing organization of experience, by considering a fifteen-month-old who has difficulty processing sounds she hears. At this age, children experiment with independence and negotiate separateness and connectedness by walking or crawling away from the parent, while maintaining contact through glances and vocalizations. The child who cannot process sounds across a room, however, cannot obtain reassurance from the parent's voice. If her mother says, "Hey, that's terrific! Look how nicely you're walking!" the child, unable to decode the rhythm of mother's voice, is confused and may simply stare, instead of smiling and brightening up. To feel secure, she has to come over and cling to her mother. If the mother is unaware of her daughter's difficulty in processing sound, she may feel angry or impatient at this clingy behavior and push the child away. When we talk on the phone to a loved one far away, our ability to decode the affect in the voice allows us to feel warmth and connection. The child who lacks this ability has greater than average difficulty in developing independence.

Children with visuospatial processing impairments may have difficulty maintaining their internal representations, especially under the pressure of intense affects. If a child cannot maintain a mental image of her parents or other significant caregivers, she is likely to feel a sense of loss and may experience anxiety, fear, or depression. We hypothesize that the biologic vulnerability for depression may be mediated in part through a visuospatial vulnerability that, in turn, creates vulnerability in the stability of mental representations. The loss of internal representations leads to dysphoric affects. The dysphoria experienced in depression is, in this model, in part secondary to the processing disturbance.

DIAGNOSIS OF REGULATORY-SENSORY PROCESSING DISORDERS (RSPD)

The diagnosis of RSPD involves a distinct behavioral pattern *and* a sensory modulation, sensory-motor, sensory discrimination or attentional processing difficulty. When both a behavioral and a sensory pattern are not present, other diagnoses may be more appropriate. For example, an infant who is irritable and withdrawn after being abandoned may be evidencing an expectable type of relationship or attachment difficulty. An infant who is irritable and overly responsive to routine interpersonal experiences, in the absence of a clearly identified sensory, sensory-motor or processing difficulty, may have an anxiety or mood disorder. Sleep and eating difficulties, in the absence of identifiable sensory responsivity or sensory processing differences, are classified as disorders in their own right. Further evaluation is then needed to determine whether the cause is an interactive disorder or some other underlying problem that does not fall within our three categories.

Presenting problems that can indicate an underlying RSPD include behavior control difficulties, sleeping and feeding difficulties, fearfulness and anxiety, poor motor skills, avoidance or craving of activities involving different sensations, difficulties in speech and language development, organizational difficulties (pre-executive functioning challenges), and impaired ability to play alone or with others. Parents may also complain that a child gets upset easily, loses his temper frequently, and has difficulty recovering and/or adapting to change.

Poorly organized or modulated responses in infants and children may show themselves in the following domains:

1. The physiological or state repertoire (e.g., irregular breathing, startles, hiccups, gagging)
2. Gross motor activity (e.g., motor disorganization, jerky movements, constant movement)
3. Fine motor activity (e.g., poorly differentiated movements or sparse, jerky or limp movements)
4. Oral motor activity (e.g., picky eater, food texture sensitivities, drooling)
5. Attentional organization (e.g., "driven" behavior, inability to settle down or, at the other extreme, perseveration about a small detail)
6. Affective organization, including the predominant affective tone (e.g., sober, depressed or happy); the range of affect (e.g., broad or constricted); the degree of modulation expressed (e.g., infant shifts abruptly from being completely calm to screaming frantically); and the capacity to use and organize affects as part of relationships and interaction with others (e.g., avoidant, negativistic, clinging and demanding behavior patterns)
7. Behavioral organization (e.g., aggressive or impulsive behavior)
8. Sleep, eating or elimination patterns (e.g., unable to fall or stay asleep, eats little, or has a poor schedule, difficulty eliminating or incontinent)
9. Language (receptive and expressive) and cognitive difficulties

Many attentional, affective, motor, sensory, behavioral control and language problems that have traditionally been viewed as difficulties in their own right may in some children stem from a broader, more basic RSPD. General terms such as "overly sensitive," "difficult temperament," or "reactive" have commonly been used to describe infants and children with motor and sensory processing differences. But clinicians have tended to use such terms without specifying the sensory system or motor functions involved. There is growing evidence that constitutional and early maturational patterns contribute to the difficulties of such infants, but it is also clear that early caregiving patterns can exert considerable influence on how constitutional-maturational patterns develop and become part of the child's evolving personality. As interest in these children increases, it is important to systematize descriptions of the sensory, motor, and integrative patterns, as well as the caregiving patterns presumed to be involved.

To make the diagnosis of Regulatory-Sensory Processing Disorder in an infant or young child, the clinician must observe one or more behavioral challenges and a sensory processing challenge including sensory modulation, sensory-motor, sensory discrimination or attentional problems from the list below.

Sensory Modulation Symptoms

1. Over- or under-responsivity to loud, high-pitched, or low-pitched noises
2. Over- or under-responsivity to bright lights or new and striking visual images, such as colors, shapes, and complex fields

3. Tactile defensiveness (e.g., over-responsivity to dressing, bathing, or stroking of arms, legs, or trunk; avoidance of touching "messy" textures) or oral hyper-responsivity (e.g., avoidance of food with certain textures)
4. Under-responsivity to touch or pain
5. Gravitational insecurity—that is, over-responsivity in a child with normal postural responses (e.g., balance reactions) to the changing sensations involved in brisk horizontal or vertical movements (e.g., being tossed in the air, riding a merry-go-round, or jumping)
6. Under- or over-responsivity to odors
7. Under- or over-responsivity to temperature
8. Qualitative deficits in ability to modulate motor activity, such as extreme activity or passivity (not secondary to anxiety or interactive difficulties)

Sensory-Motor Symptoms

1. Oral-motor difficulties or poor oral coordination influenced by low muscle tone, motor planning difficulties, or oral tactile over-responsivity (e.g., chewing, sucking, blowing, taking deep breaths)
2. Poor muscle tone and muscle stability (e.g., hypotonia, hypertonia, postural fixation, or lack of smooth movement quality)
3. Qualitative deficits in fine motor planning (e.g., difficulty in sequencing the hand movements necessary to explore a novel or complex toy, difficulty climbing a jungle gym). Qualitative deficits in fine motor skills including handwriting, coloring, matching construction tasks, puzzles, eye hand coordination.
4. Qualitative deficits in gross motor planning, including movements in space, obstacle courses, automatic movements while doing another task like talking
5. Qualitative deficits in articulation capacity (e.g., for an 8 month-old, difficulty imitating distinct sounds; for a 3 year-old, difficulty pronouncing words to describe an intended or completed action)
6. Poor components of movement patterns (e.g., flexion, extension, weight shifting, rotation, and balance reactions)

Sensory Discrimination Symptoms

1. Qualitative deficits in visuospatial processing (e.g., for an 8 month-old, difficulty recognizing different facial configurations; for a 2½ year-old, difficulty knowing in which direction to turn to get to another room in a familiar house; for a 3½ year old, difficulty using visuospatial cues to recognize and categorize different shapes)
2. Qualitative deficits in aspects of auditory processing, such as difficulty distinguishing between closely related sounds
3. Qualitative deficits in aspects of tactile discrimination (e.g., unable to distinguish objects through touch)

Attentional Symptoms

1. Qualitative deficits in capacity for sustained attention, including the capacity for shifting back and forth between two objects (such as a person and a toy), not related to anxiety, interactive difficulties, or clear auditory-verbal processing, visuospatial processing, or motor planning problems

TYPES OF REGULATORY-SENSORY PROCESSING DISORDERS (RSPD)

As suggested earlier, regulatory-sensory processing is an encompassing term referring to the way the nervous system manages incoming sensory information. It is the means by which sensory information is perceived and organized from external stimuli in the environment or from internal stimuli within the body to produce an adaptive response. In this context, adaptive response is defined as an effective behavioral response. Although traditionally considered from a behavioral perspective, adaptive responses may also be considered from a physiologic perspective. From this perspective, adaptive responses include an efficient physiologic response to a sensory challenge or demand.

Also, as discussed earlier, some individuals have difficulty processing sensory information and responding to it appropriately. When the sensory and motor difficulties are severe enough that an individual's daily routines and activities are disrupted and there are related emotional and/or behavioral challenges, the condition is diagnosed as RSPD. Difficulties with motor, emotional, attentional, or daily living skills may be markers of how sensory stimuli are perceived and interpreted.

RSPD is divided up into a number of specific disorders, and also contains a category of "mixed" disorders based on the predominant characteristics of the child, including behavioral patterns and emotional inclinations, as well as motor and sensory patterns. Note that the descriptions of the different types include a discussion of caregiving patterns (therapeutic strategies) that promote better regulation and organization in the child, as well as caregiving patterns that intensify the child's difficulty. Because the daily routines of caregiving involve continual sensory, motor, and affective experiences for the infant and young child, irregular conditions in the environment, changes in routine, or handling that is not sensitive to individual differences can strongly affect infants and children with RSPD, as well as their caregivers.

There are a number of specific types of Regulatory-Sensory Processing Disorders. Each is characterized by different types of regulatory-sensory processing and behavioral patterns. While each type of disorder is identified separately, there are three broad patterns that characterize them.

1. Sensory modulation problems, such as over-responsivity, under-responsivity, and sensory-seeking (Type I)
2. Sensory discrimination problems (Type II)
3. Sensory-based motor challenges (dyspraxia and postural regulation difficulties) (Type III)

SENSORY MODULATION CHALLENGES (TYPE I)

The first group of Regulatory-Sensory Processing Disorders to be described involves challenges in *sensory modulation*. Sensory modulation challenges are characterized by an inability to grade the degree, intensity, and nature of responses to sensory input. Often the child's responses do not fit the demands of the situation. The child therefore demonstrates difficulty achieving and maintaining an optimal range of performance and adapting to challenges in daily life. (See Guide for Observations in Appendix III for suggestions on observing sensory modulation differences.)

There are three subtypes of RSPD related to sensory modulation challenges.

201. Over-Responsive, Fearful, Anxious Pattern

Children who demonstrate over-responsivity to sensory stimuli have responses to sensations that are more intense, quicker in onset or longer lasting than those of children with typical sensory responsivity under the same conditions. Their responses are particularly pronounced when the stimulus is not anticipated. Children may demonstrate over-responsivity in only one particular sensory system, for example, "auditory defensiveness" or "tactile defensiveness," or they may demonstrate over-responsivity in multiple sensory systems. Over-responsivity to sensory stimuli in multiple modalities is often referred to as sensory defensiveness. Children are usually particularly over-responsive to specific types of stimuli within a sensory domain (e.g., in the tactile domain they respond defensively to light touch but not to deep pressure), rather than to all stimuli within a domain.

Responses to sensory stimuli occur along a spectrum. Some children manage their tendency towards over-responsivity most of the time, while other children are over-responsive almost continuously. Responses may appear inconsistent because over-responsivity is highly dependent on context. While children may generally attempt to avoid particular sensory experiences, sensitivities may vary throughout the day, and from day to day. Since sensory input tends to have a cumulative effect, the child's efforts to control responses to sensory stimuli may build up and result in a sudden behavioral disruption in response to a seemingly trivial stimulus.

A child's behavioral characteristics when faced with uncomfortable stimuli can fall within a broad range. At one end of this spectrum, the child shows fearfulness and anxiety, often avoiding many sensory experiences. At the other end of the spectrum, the child shows negativity and stubbornness, or obstinacy exemplified by attempts to control the environment. This latter tendency is described as a separate type below. This range of responses is often termed the "fight, flight, fright, or freeze" response, and is attributed to sympathetic nervous system activation. Secondary behavioral characteristics include: irritability, fussiness, poor adaptability, moodiness, inconsolability and poor socialization. In general, children who are over-responsive to sensation have difficulty with transitions and unexpected changes.

Sensory over-responsivity is often seen with other sensory reaction patterns. For example, children may show over-responsiveness to tactile stimuli while seeking proprioceptive stimuli. Sensory over-responsivity also may be observed concomitantly with sensory discrimination problems and dyspraxia.

Behavioral patterns include excessive cautiousness, inhibition, and fearfulness. The child avoids sensation in an effort to control unexpected incoming sensory stimuli. In early infancy, one sees a restricted range of exploration and assertiveness, dislike of changes in routine, and a tendency to be frightened and clinging in new situations. Young children's behavior is characterized by excessive fears or worries and by shyness in new experiences, such as forming peer relationships or engaging with new adults. Occasionally, the child behaves impulsively when overloaded or frightened. He tends to become upset easily (e.g., irritable, often crying); cannot soothe himself readily (e.g., finds it difficult to return to sleep); and cannot quickly recover from frustration or disappointment, especially in environments that include multiple or intense sensory stimuli. The fearful and cautious child may have a fragmented, rather than an integrated, internal representational world, and may therefore be easily distracted by different stimuli.

Further examples include:

- Avoids group activities and often plays alone
- Excessively cautious and afraid to try new things, resulting in a restricted range of exploration
- Prefers uniformity in the environment
- Prefers repetition and the absence of change or, at most, change at a slow or predictable pace
- Difficulty with transitions and unexpected changes
- Tends to be frightened, clinging, worried or shy in new situations
- May have difficulty forming peer relationships or engaging with new adults
- Becomes upset easily and quickly
- Perfectionist and compulsive
- Can appear under-responsive ("shut-down") as coping mechanism to over-arousal

Caregiver patterns that are characterized by soothing, regulating interactions; that respect the child's sensitivities; and that do not convey that the child has bad behaviors are helpful. Supportive parents anticipate noxious environments and minimize them or prepare the child for them. Enhancing flexibility and assertiveness in fearful and cautious children involves empathy, especially for the child's sensory and affective experience; very gradual and supportive encouragement to explore new experiences; and gentle, but firm, limits. Inconsistent caregiver patterns intensify these children's difficulties, as when caregivers are overindulgent or overprotective some of the time and punitive or intrusive at other times.

202. Over-Responsive, Negative, and Stubborn Pattern

Children with this pattern tend to evidence the same physiologic responses described above for the over-responsive, fearful and anxious type. However, this type of child seeks to control the sensory environments in which they find themselves and, thus, may prefer repetition and the absence of change or, at most, change at a slow, predictable pace. Rather than being overloaded and becoming fearful, anxious, and cautious, these children attempt to control their environments so that they can minimize fear and anxiety.

Behavior patterns may appear negative, stubborn, and controlling. The child can become aggressive and impulsive in response to sensory stimulation. He often does the opposite of what is requested or expected. Infants with this pattern tend to be fussy, difficult, and resistant to transitions and changes. Preschoolers tend to be negative, angry, and stubborn, as well as compulsive and perfectionistic. However, these children can display joyful, flexible behavior in certain situations.

In contrast to the fearful or cautious child, the negative and stubborn child does not become fragmented but organizes an integrated sense of self around negative patterns. In contrast to the impulsive, sensation-seeking child (described below) the negative and stubborn child is more controlling, tends to avoid or be slow to engage in new experiences rather than to crave them, and is not generally aggressive unless provoked.

Further examples include:

- Aggressive or impulsive when overloaded by sensory stimuli
- Hit, kick or bite in response to unexpected sensory stimulation, such as being accidentally jostled in line
- Defiant (child does the opposite of what is requested or expected)
- "Difficult" and hard to soothe
- Controlling
- May be irritable, fussy, difficult, not adaptable, moody, and unsociable

Caregiver patterns that enhance flexibility involve soothing, empathetic support of slow, gradual change and avoidance of power struggles. (Caregivers can avoid power struggles by offering the child choices and opportunities for negotiation whenever possible.) Caregivers' warmth, coupled with gentle, firm guidance and limits–even in the face of negative or impulsive responses that may feel like rejection–and encouragement of symbolic representation of affects, especially dependency, anger, and annoyance, also helps children with this pattern become more flexible. In contrast, caregiver patterns that are intrusive, excessively demanding, over-stimulating, or punitive tend to intensify negative patterns.

203. Under-Responsive, Self-Absorbed Pattern

Children who are under-responsive to sensory stimuli are often quiet and passive, disregarding or not responding to stimuli of typical intensity available in their sensory environment. Alternatively, they may be so enthralled by a world of their own imagination that they have trouble engaging in the here and now. They may appear withdrawn, difficult to engage, and/or self- absorbed because they have not registered the sensory input in their environment. The term "poor registration" is often used to describe their behavior, as they do not appear to detect or "register" incoming sensory information. They may also appear apathetic and lethargic. They may seem to lack the inner drive that most children have for socialization and motor exploration when, actually, they do not notice the possibilities for action that are around them. Their under-responsivity to tactile and proprioceptive inputs may lead to poorly developed body scheme, clumsiness, or poorly modulated movement. These children may fail to respond to bumps, falls, cuts or scrapes that can present a danger, as they may not notice pain, such as injuries to the skin, and objects that are too hot or too cold.

Children who are under-responsive to sensation often do not seek greater intensity in sensory input even though they may require it for optimal environmental interaction. Children with this pattern may be overlooked or thought of as the "good baby" or "easy child" simply because they fail to make demands on people and things in the environment. These children often need high intensity and highly salient input in order to become actively involved in the environment, the task, or the interaction.

In some instances, children who are easily overloaded by sensory stimulation may appear to be under-responsive when in fact they are extremely over-responsive. The observable behavior is one that suggests withdrawal and shutdown, perhaps as a defense mechanism. Children with sensory under-responsivity also may have sensory discrimination challenges and dyspraxia.

As indicated above, there are two patterns observed. Some children tend to be self-absorbed, unaware, and disengaged, while others are self-absorbed, but very creative and overly focused on their own fantasy lives. Therefore, we describe two subtypes for the Under-Responsive Self-Absorbed Pattern.

203.1. Self-Absorbed and Difficult to Engage Type

Behavior patterns include seeming disinterest in exploring relationships or even challenging games or objects. Children may appear apathetic, easily exhausted, and withdrawn. High affective tone and saliency are required to attract their interest, attention, and emotional engagement. Infants may appear delayed or depressed, lacking in motor exploration and social overtures. In addition to continuing the above patterns, preschoolers may evidence diminished verbal dialogue. Their behavior and play may present a limited range of ideas and fantasies. Sometimes, children seek out desired sensory input, often engaging in repetitive sensory activities, such as spinning on a sit-n-spin, swinging, or jumping up and down on the bed. The child needs the intensity or repetition of these activities in order to experience them fully.

Further examples include:

- Often quiet, passive or withdrawn
- May be overlooked or thought of as "a good baby" or "an easy child" simply because of a quiet demeanor and lack of demands
- Disinterested in exploring games or objects
- Apathetic, easily exhausted
- May seem delayed or depressed
- Lacking in motor exploration and social overtures
- Difficult to engage - often fail to register others' attempts at engagement
- May have diminished verbal dialogue
- May present only a limited range of ideas and fantasies
- May engage in repetitive sensory activities, such as spinning or playing on a sit-n-spin, swinging, or jumping up and down on the bed

Caregiver patterns that provide high-energy interactive input help engage the child in activities and relationships and foster initiative. These patterns involve energized wooing and robust responses to the child's cues, however faint. In contrast, caregiver patters that are low-key, "laid back," or depressive in tone and rhythm tend to intensify these children's patterns of withdrawal.

203.2. Self-Absorbed and Creative Type

Behavioral patterns of self-absorbed children, many of whom are also creative, include a tendency for the child to tune into his own sensations, thoughts, and emotions rather than to communications from other people. Infants may become interested in objects through solitary exploration rather than in the context of interaction. Children may appear inattentive, easily distracted, or preoccupied, especially when they are not pulled into a task or interaction. Preschoolers tend to escape into fantasy when faced with external challenges, such as a demanding preschool activity or competition from a peer. They may prefer to play by themselves if others do not actively join their fantasies. In their fantasy life, they may show enormous imagination and creativity.

Further examples include:

- Highly intelligent children who are in their own world
- Out of touch with actions happening around them
- Prefer to spend time on the computer or reading or in their own fantasy world
- May be difficult to engage because they are so involved in their cognitive processing

Caregiver patterns that are helpful include a tendency to tune into the child's non-verbal and verbal communications and help the child engage in two-way communication, that is, to "open and close circles of communication." Caregivers should also encourage a good balance between fantasy and reality and help a child who is attempting to escape into fantasy stay grounded in external reality (e.g., by showing sensitivity to the child's interests and feelings; by promoting engagement and discussion of daily events, feelings, and other real-world topics; and by making fantasy play a collaborative endeavor between parent and child rather than a solitary activity). In contrast, a caregiver's self-absorption or preoccupation, as well as confusing family communications, tends to intensify the child's difficulties.

204. Active, Sensory Seeking Pattern

Children with this pattern actively seek or crave sensory stimulation and seem to have an almost insatiable desire for sensory input. They energetically engage in activities or actions that are geared toward adding more intense "feelings" of sensation to satisfy a basic need or desire for sensory input. They tend to be constantly moving, crashing, bumping, and jumping, they may have a need to touch everything and have difficulty inhibiting this behavior, they may play music or the TV at loud volumes, may fixate on visually stimulating objects or events, or may seek unusual olfactory or gustatory experiences that are more intense and last longer than those of children with typical sensory responsivity.

Atypical responses occur along a spectrum; some sensory seeking behavior is normal. Often these children prefer a higher level of arousal than adults feel is appropriate in a given environment. Sensory seeking may also be seen as a means to obtain enhanced input for individuals with reduced awareness of sensation. Sensory seeking may be done in an effort to influence (increase) their level of arousal. For children who are sensory seekers, the need for constant stimulation is difficult to fulfill and may be particularly problematic in environments where children are expected to sit quietly such as in school, in movies, and in libraries. Obtaining additional sensory stimulation, if unstructured, may increase the child's overall state of arousal and result in disorganized behavior. However, if directed, specific types of additional sensory input can have an organizing effect.

The behavioral characteristics of these children when their sensory needs are not met include demanding and insistent behavior. They may be impulsive, almost explosive, in their attempts to fill their quota for sensation. They have a tendency to "get in trouble," creating situations around themselves that others perceive as "bad" or "dangerous." Secondary behavioral characteristics that describe these children include: overly active or aggressive, impulsive, intense, demanding, hard to calm, restless, overly affectionate, and craving attention. Extreme seeking or craving of sensory input can also disrupt children's ability to maintain attention for learning. Activities of daily living are frequently disrupted. Children may have trouble in school because they are distracted as they are "driven" to attempt to obtain extra sensory stimulation instead of focusing on tasks.

Behavioral patterns involve high activity, with children seeking physical contact and stimulation, for example through deep pressure and intense movement. Frequently, the motorically disorganized child's tendency to seek contact with people or objects leads to disruptive behavior (e.g., breaking things, unprovoked hitting, intruding into other people's physical space). Behavior that begins as a result of craving sensations may be interpreted by others as aggression rather than excitability. Once others react aggressively to the child, his own behavior may become aggressive in intent.

Infants in this group are most satisfied when provided with strong sensation in the form of movement, sound, touch, or visual stimulation. They may be content only when held or rocked. Toddlers may be very active. Preschoolers often show aggressive, intrusive behavior and a daredevil, risk-taking style, as well as preoccupation with aggressive themes in pretend play. When the young child is anxious or unsure of himself, he may use counterphobic behaviors such as hitting another child first, in anticipation of possibly being hit, or repeating unacceptable behavior after being asked to stop. When older and able to verbalize and observe his own patterns, the child may describe his need for activity and stimulation as a way to feel alive, vibrant and powerful. Children who have extreme sensory needs that are not met may become demanding and insistent on getting their own way. They may be impulsive, almost explosive in their attempt to fill their quota for sensation. They have a tendency to "get in trouble" as they create situations around them that others perceive as bad or dangerous.

Further examples include:

- Energetically engage in activities or actions that are geared to adding more intense "feelings" of sensation (seeming to satisfy a basic need or desire for sensory input)
- Crave sensory input in one or more sensory channels; may look like attention-seeking behavior, but actually craving sensation. Craving may be seen as:
  - Constantly moving and crashing, bumping and jumping
  - Playing music/TV extremely loudly
  - Watching visually stimulating scenarios for hours
  - Seeking olfactory or gustatory experiences that are more intense and last longer than children with normal sensory responsivity desire
- May seem hyperactive and have difficulty sitting quietly (at school, during worship situations, at the dinner table); can disrupt other children's ability to maintain attention
- May be restless, impulsive, almost explosive (in their attempt to fill their quota for sensation), and have a difficult time controlling their aggressive or impulsive behaviors ("out of control"). This results in a tendency to "get in trouble" or create situations around them that others perceive as "bad" or "dangerous."
- Child's overall state as it appears behaviorally is one of high arousal; the child gets "wound up" with increasing amounts of stimulation
- May become demanding and insistent on getting his own way

Caregiver patterns characterized by continuous, warm relating, a great deal of nurturing, and empathy, together with clear structure and limits, enhance flexibility and adaptivity. Caregivers should understand the need for extra stimulation and give the child many opportunities to acquire more stimulation, preferably through interactive, modulated play. Encouraging the use of imagination and verbal dialogue to explore the external environment and elaborate feelings further enhances the child's flexibility. Advocacy in settings outside the home is required so that others understand the child's behavior, adapt these constructive caregiver patterns, and avoid labeling the child a "behavior problem." In contrast, caregiver patterns that lack warm, continuous engagement (e.g., frequent changing of caregivers); that over- or underestimate the child; that are overly punitive; or that vacillate between overly punitive limit-setting and insufficient limit-setting may intensify the child's difficulties.

SENSORY DISCRIMINATION CHALLENGES (TYPE II) AND SENSORY-BASED MOTOR CHALLENGES (TYPE III)

As indicated earlier, in addition to challenges related to sensory modulation, there are regulatory-sensory processing disorders related to sensory discrimination challenges and to sensory-based motor challenges (postural control problems and dyspraxia). See the Guide for Observations in Appendix III for suggestions on observing these capacities.

The two Regulatory-Sensory Processing Disorders based on challenges in these processing areas involve inattentive, disorganized behavioral patterns and school performance and academic problems. Both these disorders may involve various combinations of difficulties in sensory discrimination, as well as sensory-based motor performance (including postural control problems and dyspraxia).

First, we describe each of these Regulatory-Sensory Processing Disorders in terms of its behavioral characteristics and the caregiver patterns that worsen or improve them. Then we describe the sensory discrimination challenges and sensory-based motor challenges (including postural control problems and dyspraxia) that are associated with these two Regulatory-Sensory Processing Disorders. We are describing the processing contributors to these disorders together (rather than individually), because they share various combinations of the same contributing sensory processing and motor planning challenges.

205. Inattentive, Disorganized Pattern

205.1 With Sensory Discrimination Challenges
205.2 With Postural Control Challenges
205.3 With Dyspraxia
205.4 With Combinations of 205.1 – 205.3

Behavioral patterns that are related to sensory discrimination, motor planning and/or postural control challenges include a tendency to be inattentive and disorganized. For example, the child may have difficulty following through on tasks or school assignments. In the middle of a homework assignment or household chore, the child may wander off to some other activity, seemingly unmindful of the original goal. In the extreme, the child's behavior may appear fragmented. As others put more pressure on the child, he may become more disorganized. When these challenges continue over a period of time, the child can easily become demoralized and feel depressed and/or angry. Impulsive or defiant behavior is not uncommon, nor is passivity, avoidance, and preference for activities, such as video games, which is experienced as less demanding (in terms of sequencing and organizing complex plans of action).

When challenged to be involved in tasks that are difficult, one often sees increasing avoidance, fragmentation, and disorganization, as well as "inattentiveness." It's not unusual for parents to describe a child as "organized" and "attentive" when getting ready to go to the video arcade or out for his favorite ice cream and yet "fragmented," "inattentive," and "disorganized," when attempting a multi-step math problem. Clinicians as well as caregivers often ask whether the patterns described above are different from what is often described as attentional problems or Attention Deficit Disorder. The descriptions of the different processing challenges that contribute to this type of behavioral pattern help clinicians observe the relationship between specific regulatory-sensory processing patterns and attentional and organizational challenges.

Caregiver patterns that recognize the underlying challenges can help the child strengthen the processing areas contributing to his difficulties. In addition, while the child is working to strengthen underlying processing challenges, caregivers and educators who can help the child break down complex tasks into manageable steps and provide patient, multi-sensory support (visual, auditory, and motor cues) also tend to help the child make progress. On the other hand, caregiving patterns that characterize the child as "unmotivated," "bad," or "lazy," and pressure and punish the child, rather than help him set up doable goals that can be associated with a sense of mastery, inevitably intensify the child's challenges. The key to constructive caregiver patterns is to understand and strengthen the contributing processing differences that are described in some detail below.

206. Compromised School and/or Academic Performance Pattern

206.1. With Sensory Discrimination Challenges
206.2. With Postural Control Challenges
206.3. With Dyspraxia
206.4. With Combinations of 206.1 – 206.3

Behavioral patterns associated with motor planning and sequencing challenges (dyspraxia), postural control, and sensory discrimination difficulties may include circumscribed school performance or academic challenges. For example, difficulties with motor planning and postural control can make handwriting very difficult. Sensory discrimination difficulties may make distinguishing shapes or letters difficult. Visuospatial challenges may make lining up columns in math or in understanding concepts involving graphs or diagrams difficult. Motor planning and sequencing difficulties may also contribute to problems with sequencing ideas into sentences. If the contributing processing contributions to these types of school performance and academic challenges are not addressed, the child may become avoidant, disinterested, and/or demoralized. A sense of failure, rather than a can-do, positive attitude may follow. School itself can become viewed as a place of failure and all activities in school, or school as a whole, may be avoided.

Caregiver patterns that recognize the processing contributions to the child's school performance and academic challenges and provide supportive, step-wise help tend to improve the child's overall functioning. Caregivers who can break the challenge down into small enough steps for the child to experience a sense of mastery 70% to 80% of the time are likely to be especially helpful. Caregivers who are punitive, rejecting, or overly expectant often increase the difficulties. When a child has difficulty with a particular motor or sensory discrimination task, there is little intrinsic sense of mastery or pleasure in performing it. In comparison, when a child is naturally gifted at an activity, there is intrinsic pleasure in the activity itself. Therefore, support, guidance, incentives, and breaking the challenge down into easily-mastered steps are essential to helping the child overcome his challenges and feel a sense of pride and accomplishment.

SENSORY DISCRIMINATION AND SENSORY-BASED MOTOR CHALLENGES (INCLUDING POSTURAL CONTROL PROBLEMS AND DYSPRAXIA) THAT MAY CONTRIBUTE TO INATTENTIVE, DISORGANIZED PATTERNS AND COMPROMISED SCHOOL PERFORMANCE PATTERNS

Sensory Discrimination Challenges

Sensory discrimination is the process by which specific qualities of sensory stimuli are perceived and meaning attributed to them. Children with sensory discrimination difficulties have problems discerning the characteristics of sensory stimuli. The result is a lessened capability to interpret or give meaning to the specific qualities of stimuli, to detect similarities and differences among stimuli, and to differentiate the temporal and/or spatial qualities of stimuli. Children can perceive that stimuli are present and can modulate their responses to the stimuli, but cannot tell precisely what or where the stimulus is. Children with this challenge have difficulty interpreting the spatial and temporal qualities of sensory input and, as such, cannot use time and space information or other specific characteristics of the sensory experience to guide performance.

Sensory discrimination challenges may be seen in any sensory system, and often co-occur with dyspraxia (see below). It may be seen in children who are sensory over-responsive. In these children the more primitive protective system (over-responsivity) can override detailed (discriminative) information about attributes of objects in the environment, resulting in decreased discrimination. It also frequently occurs with sensory under-responsiveness. A child who is lethargic and unable to arouse is disinterested and has difficulty engaging with people. He may lack exploration of objects and overtures to others which over time would grow his discriminative system.

Children with poor sensory discrimination may appear awkward in both gross and fine motor abilities and/or inattentive to people and objects in their environment. They may take extra time to process the salient aspects of sensory stimuli, thus appearing "slow." They may display significant frustration with an inability to make sense out of the world. This problem may lead to lowered self-confidence, attention seeking behavior, and temper tantrums when their efforts are not met with success.

Behavioral Indicators of Sensory Discrimination Challenges by Sensory System

One way to conceptualize sensory discrimination problems is by the domain that is involved. The divergent validity of the subgroups below is yet to be empirically established; hence, they are theoretical at this point.

Visual

- The discrimination of the spatial characteristics of objects and letters (e.g., "b" and "d") and difficulty with spatially guided movement
- Appears clumsy as he moves his whole body through space or as he moves parts of his body through space for tasks such as reach and grasp
- May have trouble playing games that require discriminating objects in space such as catching, batting a ball, or throwing to a target
- May have difficulty finding his way within a building or around a community environment
- With vision occluded, may not be able to find objects when they are mixed in with others or may have difficulty rotating puzzle pieces to fit correctly in the space
- Difficulty with visual motor integration activities, such as being able to manipulate objects in space mentally, in order to complete a motor activity (e.g., putting puzzles together, putting away materials or clothes in a box)

Auditory

- Difficulty identifying and distinguishing different sounds such as: "t" and "p" as in cat and cap; "b" and "k" as in bag and back
- Processes auditory information slowly, word by word, and thus may miss content in a sentence
- May appear to "stop listening" at times and it can appear as though he is not paying attention
- May not be able to discriminate the salient features of the sounds from noise in the milieu
- May "tune out" if flooded by sounds (this may look like inattention)
- May have trouble following directions and need directions repeated

Tactile

- May have difficulty identifying precisely what is touching them
- May have difficulty identifying objects with his hands (stereognosis) or identifying what type of stimulus is touching him with vision occluded

Proprioception

- Difficulty judging timing, force and distance (e.g., may hold a pencil too tightly or loosely, not use enough force to tear the scotch tape off, or kick a ball either too hard or not hard enough)
- May have low muscle tone

Vestibular

- Difficulty sensing direction of movement with eyes closed
- Difficulty sensing displacement of body center of gravity, resulting in poor balance[2]
- Difficulty sensing speed of movements

Postural Challenges

Postural challenges refer to difficulty stabilizing the body during movement or at rest in order to meet the demands of the environment or of a given motor task. Postural problems are characterized by inappropriate muscle tension, hypo- or hypertonic muscle tone, inadequate control of movement, and/or inadequate muscle contraction to achieve movement against resistance. Postural difficulties frequently occur in the presence of vestibular, proprioceptive, and visual-motor problems, and include poor stability in the trunk, poor righting and equilibrium reactions, poor trunk rotation and/or poor ocular control.

Postural control provides a stable yet mobile base for refined movement of the head, eyes, trunk, and limbs. When postural control is good, the child is able to execute functional behaviors such as reaching, pushing, pulling, and resistance against force. The sensory input supporting postural control is typically vestibular/proprioceptive and visual in nature. The degree of postural control is affected by the arousal level of the individual, as well as the modulation and the discrimination of sensory information. An individual who is under-responsive to sensory input or who has poor discrimination may not display the necessary postural tone to respond successfully to the demands of a given task or situation. Likewise, the postural control of an individual who is over-responsive may be overly rigid, leading to difficulty performing smooth graded movements.

Motorically, children with poor postural control often do not have the body control to maintain a good standing or sitting position. In addition, they may have difficulty automatically adjusting and maintaining a body posture that enables them to perform tasks efficiently. For example, when writing at a desk, they may bend far over the paper or lay their head on their arm as they write. They may have difficulty alternately raising their head and extending their neck to look up from their paper to copy words from a chalkboard and then repositioning their head, neck and eyes back onto the paper to write.

Postural challenges can occur with or without a motor planning disorder, although it is often observed with dyspraxia, particularly in difficulty with bilateral integration activ-

2 To balance, at least two of the following three systems are required: vestibular, visual, proprioception.

ities (e.g., doing activities that require use of both sides of the body together such as riding a bike, pumping a swing, etc.) and with rhythmical activities (e.g., bouncing a ball, clapping on the beat).

Behavioral Indicators of Postural Challenges

- Poor trunk stability (often called co-contraction) at rest and/or during movement
- Tendency to fixate (often called "fix") or stabilize the trunk using flexion or extension patterns resulting in poor fluidity of movement
- Difficulty stabilizing at shoulders and hips resulting in poorly refined movements of upper and lower extremities
- Tendency to avoid weight bearing in upper extremities
- Poor righting and equilibrium reactions
- Poor trunk rotation
- Avoidance of climbing and discomfort on uneven surfaces
- Avoidance or discomfort crossing the midline of the body
- Poor ocular control, such as smooth pursuits and visual shifting (e.g., localization from near distance to far distance)
- Difficulty isolating head and eye movements (e.g., can't move eyes only to look at something to his right or left; instead his whole head must move to turn his eyes)
- May appear to have visual distractibility due to problems maintaining visual focus in busy environments or during movement

The postural problems above often lead to one of the following types of patterns:

- Tendency to avoid moving around and dislike of unexpected movement
- Tendency to be very physically active but lacking control and safety awareness

Dyspraxia

Dyspraxia is an impairment in the ability to plan, sequence and execute novel or unfamiliar actions. It is characterized by awkward and poorly coordinated motor performance, which can be observed in gross motor, fine motor and/or oral motor abilities. To be diagnosed with sensory-based dyspraxia, deficits must manifest in processing of sensory information in one or more of the following sensory domains: tactile, kinesthetic, proprioceptive, or vestibular. Visual-motor deficits usually accompany this difficulty also.

Dyspraxia is most clearly characterized by inadequate planning and poor performance of new and/or novel motor tasks. These children learn by trial and error, with decreased ability to generalize skills to other similar motor tasks. Execution of discrete motor skills (e.g., standing, walking, pincer grasp) may be adequate. However, the performance of complex tasks may be compromised, including tasks that require one or more of the following: significant sequencing, important timing aspects, rhythm of motor action, or subtle adaptation in the "moment of action."

Children with dyspraxia have difficulty knowing where their body is in space, and they have trouble judging their relationship to objects, people and space well. As a result, they may be accident-prone and tend to trip or bump into objects or others. They may break toys because of difficulty with planning. They often have poor skills in ball activities and other sports. They may have difficulty with projected action sequences that require timing (e.g., jumping over, into, and through moving ropes or throwing balls at targets, especially when both the child and the target are moving). Many children have trouble with fine motor manipulative activities such as handling small objects and handwriting. Daily activities such as using utensils and dressing are often slow to develop. Due to poor planning, children are often disorganized and may look disheveled.

Some children with dyspraxia are highly creative verbally, and may prefer fantasy games to "doing." They may try to mask their dyspraxia by acting like a "class clown" or they may be reticent to participate in new group activities. Often children with dyspraxia have difficulty with ideation (or formulating goals or ideas) for actions. Because these children are unable to generate new ideas of what to do, they may resort to rigid or inflexible strategies. They may perseverate and prefer the familiar to the novel.

Children with dyspraxia are often inactive, preferring sedentary activities such as watching TV, playing video games, reading a book, or playing fantasy games. This can result in weight problems. Self-esteem may be poor as a result of dissatisfaction with their abilities and repeated failure. Children often have low frustration tolerance. They may be perceived as manipulative and controlling. These children may have an over-reliance on language to compensate for the dyspraxia, although dyspraxia can occur with language impairments. Dyspraxia often occurs with sensory discrimination challenges. In addition, it may be accompanied by sensory under-responsivity or sensory over-responsivity

Behavioral Indicators of Dyspraxia

Ideational

- Inability to formulate a goal (or idea) for action
- The child does not have an idea of what to do and may resort to rigid or inflexible behavior
- May prefer fantasy games to "doing"

Gross Motor

- Tend to be accident-prone and trip, bump into objects or people
- Generally poor in ball activities and other sports
- Difficulty participating in team sports, especially as they become more competitive
- Performance characterized by trial and error; takes the child more time and practice to learn new skills
- May break toys because of difficulty with planning and force modulation

- Difficulty generalizing previously learned motor tasks to new situations and contexts
- Fatigue easily and have decreased endurance
- Some children may have an over-reliance on language to compensate for motor problems (e.g., talking through each new motor activity or trying to turn attention away from task)
- May be reluctant to participate in new group activities
- May prefer sedentary activities such as watching TV, playing video games, reading a book, playing fantasy games
- May try to mask their dyspraxia by acting like "class clowns"

Fine Motor

- Difficulty with fine motor manipulative activities (e.g., cutting, coloring, pasting, construction toys) and (pre) handwriting
- Daily activities such as using utensils and dressing are often slow to develop due to difficulty with planning
- Often disorganized and may be disheveled-looking
- May perseverate or prefer simpler play activities

Oral Motor

- Difficulty with articulation and sometimes with sucking, chewing, and swallowing sequences
- Prolonged/excessive drooling

207. Mixed Regulatory-Sensory Processing Patterns

It is quite common for children to display mixed regulatory-sensory processing patterns. Combinations of patterns and/or subtypes in one child are common and differences among various sensory domains in the same child may be observed. For example, it is not uncommon for a child to experience sensory over-responsivity in the tactile system and sensory-seeking in the vestibular and proprioceptive systems. In addition, atypical response patterns to sensation can vary as a function of time or day, environmental context, stress, fatigue, level of arousal and many other factors. First, we discuss mixed sensory modulation patterns. Second, we discuss mixed motor and sensory processing patterns. Finally, we outline a few of the common behavioral challenges that are often related to mixed regulatory-sensory processing patterns.

Mixed Sensory Modulation Patterns

Sensory Over-Responsivity with Sensory Seeking

It is common for children to be over-responsive in one domain (e.g., tactile) while sensory seeking in another domain (e.g., movement and proprioceptive). It appears that intense movement and proprioceptive input is used by some children as a method to self-regulate their aversion to other types of sensory input. For other children sensory seeking is a way to feel active, excited and engaged (it just feels good).

Sensory Under-Responsivity with Sensory Over-Responsivity

Some children are under-responsive to stimuli at first, but when stimuli are provided systematically they quickly meet their quota and become over-responders. This is believed to be related to a narrowed band of tolerance for sensory input. It may appear from the outside as if the child is labile, swinging from one responsiveness extreme to the other. Different sensory modalities can be differentially affected, e.g., the child may remain under-responsive to olfactory stimuli (e.g., intrusively trying to smell people and objects) but show over-responsiveness to touch.

Sensory Over-Responsivity with Sudden Sensory Under-Responsivity

Some children start out with extreme over-responsivity and suddenly appear under-responsive, appearing almost to shut down. These children are also believed to have a narrow band of normal responsiveness. Perhaps they are so over-responsive that their system may actually be shutting down as a defensive mechanism so that no additional sensory input is registered by their nervous systems. They may look extremely under-responsive, but may actually be having extreme defensive reactions to stimuli.

Mixed Motor and Sensory Processing Patterns

In addition, to mixed sensory modulation patterns, there are a number of other mixed patterns that should be mentioned. These include:

- Sensory over-responsivity with sensory discrimination difficulties
- Sensory over-responsivity with dyspraxia
- Sensory under-responsivity with dyspraxia
- Sensory discrimination challenges with dyspraxia
- Postural control challenges with sensory over-responsivity
- Postural control challenges with sensory under-responsivity
- Postural control challenges with dyspraxia

Common Behavioral Challenges Related to Mixed Regulatory-Sensory Processing Patterns

The mixed regulatory-sensory processing patterns listed above can occur with and without behavioral or emotional challenges. There are a number of well-known symptom patterns that are often related to mixed types of regulatory-sensory processing problems. A few of these are listed and briefly described below. Before describing these, however, it should be noted that the challenges listed below may be related to interactive difficulties and/or unique motor and sensory processing challenges. Where the interactive elements (i.e., caregiver-child interaction patterns) are the predominant contributor, a diagnosis under interactive disorders should be considered. Where the predominant contributor is a unique motor or sensory processing pattern, the diagnosis of RSPD should be considered. Once a diagnosis of Regulatory-Sensory Processing Disorder is considered, the clinician should determine if the challenges are related to a specific pattern, such as sensory over-responsivity, or a mixed pattern, as described above. The challenges listed below are usually related to mixed regulatory-sensory processing patterns when this dimension is the main contributing factor. As with all mental health and developmental disorders in infancy and early childhood, there are always regulatory-sensory processing and interactive dimensions. The multi-axial framework recommended in this diagnostic system takes these multiple factors into account. Therefore, even if the clinician finds it difficult to emphasize one or another feature of the complex problems listed below, the multi-axial framework, nonetheless, permits a full description of the child's functioning. The very common problems listed below are included in both the interactive and regulatory-sensory processing categories because for different children, one or the other feature often predominates. It would, therefore, be an oversimplification to list them arbitrarily in only one or the other category.

207.1. Attentional Problems

Children with problems in attending and sustaining their focus often evidence a number of regulatory-sensory processing challenges. Most evidence difficulties with motor planning and sequencing. It is difficult for them to carry out a planned series of actions to solve a problem unless there is a great deal of structure guiding them. In addition, many children with attentional problems also evidence sensory discrimination difficulties, for example, in figuring out complex visuospatial patterns and solving visuospatial problems (searching systematically for a hidden object in all parts of a room). In addition, some children with attentional problems are sensory-craving and, therefore, very active and sometimes aggressive. A small percentage of children with attentional problems are sensory over-responsive and, therefore, very distractible. They are distracted by different types of sounds or sights and easily become overloaded and more fragmented in a noisy or busy setting. Also, some children with attentional problems are sensory under-responsive and, therefore, ordinary sensations, such as the human voice, which would orient a child, don't draw their attention. Instead, they drift off into their own world. Some very bright children with this pattern wind up daydreaming a great deal. Clearly, many children with attentional problems evidence combinations of the above, such as motor planning problems and sensory under-responsivity. Environmental and caregiving patterns may contribute, as well.

207.2. Disruptive Behavioral Problems

Toddlers and preschoolers with disruptive behavior often evidence sensory craving, which leads them to be very active and, at times, aggressive, even without necessarily intending to be so. Some of these children may also have areas of sensory under-responsivity where, for example, they may be relatively insensitive to pain, making this pattern even more intense. Some children also evidence sensory discrimination challenges, such as auditory discrimination, making it harder to understand limits and guidelines. Each or any combination of these patterns can contribute to disruptive behaviors. Environmental, caregiver, and family patterns also contribute.

207.4. Sleep Problems

Many children with difficulties falling asleep or sustaining sleep evidence some degree of sensory over-responsivity. Some also evidence sensory discrimination challenges. Others evidence a great deal of sensory craving and are, therefore, very active. Often, these sensory patterns are compounded by a variety of environmental factors and caregiving practices, which may contribute to the sleep challenges. From an early age the child forms certain patterns with caregivers that reinforce sleep difficulties over time.

207.4. Eating Problems

Many children with eating difficulties evidence sensory over-responsivity, especially in their oral cavity. Some also evidence low muscle tone, including low tone in their oral-motor area, as well as motor planning and sequencing challenges. Their oral-motor functioning challenges contribute to making eating a very difficult task. Other children are under-responsive to sensation in the oral cavity, also making eating difficult because expectable sensations from food are not occurring. Environmental and caregiving patterns may further contribute.

207.5. Elimination Problems

Many children with elimination challenges evidence combinations of sensory under-responsivity, low muscle tone, and motor planning and sequencing difficulties. Some, however, are sensory craving and others are sensory over-responsive. Caregiver and environmental patterns contribute, as well. For example, the child who is unable to sense when his or her bladder is full and has a hard time regulating motor actions, is more prone to having accidents.

207.6. Elective Mutism

Children with elective mutism are often sensory over-responsive and, therefore, highly anxious. Typically, a school environment is a challenging setting because of the noise and other sensations. Although over-responsivity is the largest contributor, children with elective mutism may also have dyspraxia. Attention to these differences, coupled with increasing the level of security and the gradualness with which the child enters a new setting, like school, can be very helpful.

207.7. Mood Dysregulation, including Bipolar Patterns

Often infants and young children with fluctuating moods have an underlying challenge characterized by sensory over-responsivity coupled with sensory-seeking. Therefore, when overloaded, instead of retreating and becoming cautious, they become more agitated and impulsive. As they become symbolic, this can take the form of shifting from fearful and depressive themes to angry and power-oriented themes. See the Interactive Disorder section for a fuller description of infants and young children with mood fluctuations, including bipolar patterns.

207.8. Other Emotional and Behavioral Problems Related to Mixed Regulatory-Sensory Processing Difficulties

Children with mixed regulatory-sensory processing challenges may evidence emotional or behavioral problems or symptoms not listed above. These may include: anxiety, fearfulness, negativism, and so forth. When these challenges or problems are related to mixed regulatory-sensory processing challenges, that should be indicated in this category.

207.9. Mixed Regulatory-Sensory Processing Patterns where Behavioral or Emotional Problems Are Not Yet In Evidence

In the early years of life, many children present with mixed regulatory-sensory processing challenges, but do not yet evidence clear emotional, social, and/or behavioral problems. Their regulatory-sensory processing challenges may be noted by their parent, early childhood educators, or their primary healthcare provider. For example, they may be over-responsive to light touch and have difficulty with sequencing motor responses. The recognition of these challenges provides an ideal opportunity for preventive work and family guidance that is geared to improving functioning in these and related areas, and preventing the emergence of emotional, social, and/or behavioral problems. Many parents and educators already implement such preventive strategies intuitively. However, identifying these patterns can help systematize these efforts and broaden the number of children who are helped.

Case Illustrations of Regulatory-Sensory Processing Disorder

Mario: A Case Illustration of a Child with an Over-Responsive, Fearful, Anxious Pattern

Presenting Problems

Mario was $4^1/_2$ years of age at the time of referral. His mother had become gradually more concerned about Mario, although no specific event prompted the current request for assessment. Referral had come through the pediatrician. Mario's mother had felt for some time that he was different from other children, although as he was her only child, she was not sure if this was a problem. While he was interactive with her and his dad, Mario was quiet and stand-offish around others, even members of his extended family with whom he spent a good deal of time. Mario was difficult to engage socially, and often did not seem to be able to have fun. He had no real friends in day care, and tended to play alone. He would engage others only if he was in control of the play activities. At the time of referral Mrs. Diaz had noticed increasing difficulties with eating (very picky), clothing choice, and very limited play activities. Major concerns revolved around transition to kindergarten.

Background and History

Mario was the product of a full term pregnancy, long labor, but otherwise normal delivery. His mother experienced serious complications following his birth and was hospitalized for several days. She continued to be under close medical scrutiny and care for nearly a year following Mario's birth. She was unable to provide care for Mario for approximately his first 2 weeks of life. Mario had remained at home, being cared for by his father and his aunts. It was a stressful time for all.

From the beginning Mario was difficult to bottle feed. He seemed to have a hard time settling into someone's arms for feeding, and this was accentuated when someone other than his parents fed him. Mario's mother became the primary feeder at home, and she generally either fed him in an infant seat or sitting on her lap facing away from her. Later, Mario's daycare teacher reported similar feeding difficulties.

Transition to solids foods was difficult. Mario greatly preferred the sweeter baby foods (fruits) and rejected nearly all vegetables. He ate some cereals and meats, but was picky in terms of temperature, taste, and texture. He did not tolerate foods of mixed consistency, and would simply refuse to eat if his preferences were ignored. Becoming concerned that he would develop poorly as a result of diminished food intake, Mrs. Diaz resorted to giving him what he preferred, and what she could be certain he would eat. As he transitioned off baby food onto chewable foods this pattern continued. From age 2 and through today he eats a very limited range of foods. As a toddler, he would finger feed dry foods, noodles with no sauce, soft/well-cooked pieces of meat, and most fruits. He continued to refuse vegetables. He drank milk from a sippy cup, and a little juice. It was difficult to get him to add new foods or beverages to his limited repertoire.

Motor milestones were largely on time, although toilet training was very difficult. Mario did not seem to like the bathroom, but neither did he like being in dirty diapers or pull-ups. He would remove his pull-up immediately after it became dirty, leaving it in his room. He was finally fully trained by age 4.

Mario was not an environmental explorer as a toddler, preferring to sit and work with blocks, small animals and figures. He enjoyed swinging to some extent, although only slow controlled swinging. He climbed very little as a toddler, but recently has begun to climb more if the climbing activity was aligned with his real love: playing dress up and make-believe. Mario loves nothing better than to dress in a cape and don the weapons of a super hero. He plays out complex scenarios which often include having a home base hidden somewhere out of reach; thus he began to climb. His play themes are very complex, and Mario must direct all who participate in his elaborate plays.

Language skills had never been of particular concern. Mario's mother reported that Mario began using words and sentences roughly on time, according to her books on early development. She was unable to precisely recall when he first began talking, but was never concerned about it. The play scenarios in which he engages have always been very language rich.

An area of puzzlement for Mrs. Diaz is Mario's limited emotional expression. She described him as a child who rarely showed emotional extremes in any direction. As an infant he did not often cry from hunger, although he did fuss to have his diaper changed. He was generally content to be left in an infant seat rather than fussing to be held and carried. As he grew up, Mario rarely became excited about activities or gifts, and would walk away from a disagreement with another child rather than fight over a toy. He has never been very affectionate. She views this as emotional stability. Mario can and does become upset when he is hurt, and at those times seeks comfort from his mother.

Current Status

Mario remains very picky about food. He has developed a preference for spicy foods, and limits what he eats to certain meats, most fruits, white bread, buttered noodles, and some sweets. He drinks only orange juice and milk. Mario is equally as choosy about his clothes, preferring long sleeves regardless of the weather, pants without zippers, and shirts without buttons.

Although Mario has been in daycare since he was 9 months of age, he still does not seem connected to either his care providers or playmates. He prefers solitary play, unless he can get some of the children interested in his make-believe type of play. With this play he establishes strict rules and limits so that when one of the children chooses not to comply, the game ends.

Mario continues to be very attached to both of his parents. While he continues to show only a limited degree of overt affection, he makes frequent visual contact with his mother when they are in the same room. She reports that he looks for them to pick him up promptly from day care; the day care provider indicated that once departure time arrives, Mario looks for them each time an adult enters the room. He always seems relieved when his parents come to take him home. He gives a hug and kiss hello/goodbye on request, but generally does not offer either on his own. At day care he shows preference for a few children, and one provider. He continues to avoid conflict by simply walking away.

Mario has not formed close relationships with other adult family members. He is cared for one evening each week by an aunt, and appears very fond of his cousin in this household, but remains emotionally distant from the adults. He and his cousin play well together, but according to the aunt, Mario controls all aspects of play. If the game is not going his way, he walks away and starts something new. His mother reports that Mario talks about this cousin a great deal, and is animated in these discussions. She takes this as excitement and enjoyment over being with this cousin.

Although early developmental milestones were on time, at $4^1/_2$ years of age Mario does not ride a tricycle, pump on a swing, or slide. He does not seem to enjoy games with balls or any other outside activities that involve tools. He has become good at climbing up a ladder to get into a clubhouse, and generally incorporates this into his make-believe plots. He tends to develop make-believe scenarios that involve good guys and bad guys, and weapons of some sort.

Language skills continue to be a strength. Mario creates his make-believe play activities with a wealth of language detail, and plays a role in these scenarios like an actor. He enjoys being read to, but has shown no interest in independent reading. His preferred quiet time activity is watching TV, particularly movies. He and his father spend many hours together watching videos, and the father is pleased that Mario watches either cartoon types of movies or more realistic movies. As with his play themes, he mostly enjoys movies with good guys and bad guys.

The family is intact. Mrs. Diaz described her relationship with her husband as loving, but not demonstrative. Both parents work full-time outside of the home. The mother is the primary wage earner, but also the primary caregiver for Mario. The father spends time with Mario in the evenings and on weekends.

Assessment

Mario was first observed in his home, in order to evaluate him in his best environment. He was not excited about playing with a stranger, and played only reluctantly and only with his mother during this assessment session. He did show the observer his stash of weapons, and the different capes he wore when playing. He did not want to play outside on the swings and when invited to go to the park he declined. His preference was to watch TV and let his mother and the examiner talk. The mother seemed quite comfortable with this situation and did not encourage Mario to interact. During the discussion between the examiner and mother, Mario interrupted only once, requesting juice. Informal observation was not fruitful given his reluctance to interact, move or play.

Mario and his parents live close to his aunt and cousins. He is fond of his cousins, and plays well with them. It was decided that further observation would take place in their house and yard, using them to motivate Mario to engage in activities.

Play at his cousins began outside on the swing set. Mario sat on the glider while his two cousins swung, climbed, and played to some extent. The mother remained close by, but did not interfere as the children engaged. The cousins invited Mario to climb and swing, but it was not until he decided they should be Batman, Robin, and Catwoman that Mario became more involved. After donning the appropriate outfits, the three engaged in a "catch the bad guys" activity that had them running, doing some climbing up the slide, and playing in the clubhouse at the top. While the cousins slid back down the slide Mario carefully walked down the ladder. Overall movements and skills seem to be within expected ranges, but it was difficult to be certain. All children were very animated in their pretend roles. The game came to a natural conclusion as all three children became bored. Mario wandered away from the swing set, indicating an interest in watching TV. Mrs. Diaz responded by suggesting all three children move inside to play. At the second request for TV, Mario was told no, that he and his cousins should find something else to play inside. Mrs. Diaz accompanied the children inside and worked at finding an activity that all would want to play.

Mario and one of his cousins decided to play with GI Joe dolls. Mario owns a cadre of these toys and their various accessories. It was clear he was very familiar with them. He was able to move the dolls, get them into position, put them in and out of vehicles and structures, and act out the activities. He had some difficulty dressing and undressing them for action, but this was to be expected at his age. He appeared very imaginative in his play with the dolls, but during discussion Mrs. Diaz indicated that his play scenarios are often very similar.

Throughout the discussion at the Diaz' home, and play at the cousin's house, Mrs. Diaz responded to Mario in a manner both encouraging and respectful. While she allowed him a great deal of TV during our initial conversation, it may have been what allowed Mario time to accommodate to the presence of the examiner. When at the cousins' house Mrs. Diaz tended to be involved to get things started, and then she pulled back to allow them to unfold. When Mario began to lose interest, Mrs. Diaz again intervened. She appeared very adept at guiding Mario through transitions, and making his world run smoothly.

Because his milestones appeared generally on time, and he did not seem to have developmental delays, no formalized early motor or language assessment had been carried out. However, given his mother's concerns about his limited display of gross motor skills at present, and his impending move to kindergarten, the Peabody Developmental

Motor Scales was administered. In addition, Mario's mother was given The Sensory Profile to complete, based on her concerns about Mario's difficulty engaging in activities and social events, and her suggestion of some sensory sensitivities.

Peabody Developmental Motor Scales (PDMS)

Fine and gross motor components of the PDMS were administered. Mario was generally cooperative with the assessment process, although at times he needed some encouragement from his mother to try or to continue with the process. At times his attention seemed to wander, and items were repeated. Overall the assessment was felt to be reliable, reflecting his actual skill level.

Mario's PDMS scores indicated that he performed just above the 50th percentile in gross motor skills, and right at the 50th percentile in fine motor skills. On the gross motor subtests his lowest area was Locomotion, primarily due to difficulties on balance and jumping items. His standard score was 8 (M of 10, SD of 3). In the fine motor area, Mario also scored below average but well within normal limits. For example, on the Grasping Subtest his standard score was 9. Of considerable interest was his unusual grasp pattern. Mario held the writing tools with fingertips of his right index, middle, ring finger and thumb. His grasp appeared very awkward, although his performance was adequate. This odd grasp pattern accounts for his relatively lower score in this area. No overall motor delays were notable.

Sensory Profile

Mario's responses on the Sensory Profile (SP) were compared with those for children age 4 (see below). At this age there are more differences in typical sensory processing than at older ages and a separate scoring profile is included in the manual.

First examining his scores by SP section scores, Mario demonstrates "definite differences" (poorest scoring category of scale) in Auditory, Tactile, and Oral Sensory Processing, and "possible difference" (2nd poorest scoring category of scale) in Vestibular Processing. He showed a "definite difference" in Emotional/Social Responses and Modulation of Sensory Input Affecting Emotional Responses, along with "possible difference" in Sensory Processing Related to Tone and Endurance, and Modulation of Movement Affecting Activity Level and Movement.

On the SP factor scores Mario showed a "definite difference" in Emotionally Reactive, Oral Sensory Sensitivity, and Sensory Sensitivity. Factors on which he demonstrated "possible difference" included Low Endurance/Tone and Fine Motor/Perceptual. There was no indication of Inattention/Distractibility or Poor Registration.

Impressions

Mario shows sensory over-responsivity to auditory and tactile sensation. This is demonstrated by his scores on the Sensory Profile and supported by behaviors he shows in play. He was observed to have a tendency to be more sensitive than would be expected to movement activities as well, confirmed by the probable difference score in this domain. Overall these sensory sensitivities lead to his reluctance to engage in play with a variety of materials, and a variety of friends. He is reported to be a difficult child to get to know, and a difficult child to enjoy playing with by adults outside of his mother and father. He tends to be very quiet, appears fearful, anxious, and cautious, and tends to use avoidance as a coping strategy. He interacts little in family events.

Mario also tends more often toward sedentary play activities, or activities in which he is in control. While the PDMS results do not support motor delays, he is qualitatively less skilled than other children his age in terms of balance and movement, and tool use. With tools (e.g., pens, pencils, scissors) his grip is light and awkward, although at present, skills with drawing and writing are within expected age limits. Mario appears to compensate for somewhat limited motor skills through creativity. His IQ was not tested.

Further, Mario's oral sensory sensitivities lead to his limited food choices, and tactile sensitivity leads to clothing intolerances. While these behaviors can be tolerated at home, and to some extent in day care, they present increasing challenges when Mario begins school. One might expect that when he gets to school the combination of a loud cafeteria environment and his limited food tolerance would make lunch a very difficult experience for him. Clothing limitations may become more of a social issue as Mario gets older.

Mario's sensory sensitivity appears linked to diminished social interactions, and a limited repertoire of emotional expression. His history suggests difficulty at the earliest emotional developmental level, that of shared attention and regulation. Engagement and relating with his parents was and is characterized by attenuated affect. Mario's ability to read and respond to the cues of others likewise appears limited, although his mother's ability to read and respond to Mario's emotional cues was very strong. Observationally it is difficult to determine Mario's ability to engage in integrated problem-solving in affective interactions as so few opportunities for such observation were present. The one behavioral pattern used most consistently in affective problem-solving was that of withdrawal or escape. He does not demonstrate insight into motivations for his actions, nor does he often use words to describe how he is feeling. His mother reports that she is working with him on putting words to his feelings, on the recommendation of his day-care teacher. Both of these adults sense that this helps Mario to get more involved with his peers. Globally, Mario's social and affective skills appear immature. The combination of sensory sensitivity with immaturity in social and affective expression characterizes Mario as a child with sensory over-responsivity, withdrawal subtype.

Mario's mother provides a great deal of support for him. She is artful at smoothing out transitions and creating environments in which Mario can best function. During this observation she did not encourage him to challenge himself with anything that might make him uncomfortable. The father was not available during this assessment, so these dynamics could not be assessed.

Conclusion

Mario presents with a primary Regulatory-Sensory Processing Disorder of Over-Responsive, Fearful, Anxious Pattern (201.). His diminished emotional expression and tendency toward constricted affect are consistent with this finding. His mother is adept at meeting his sensory needs, and allows him the freedom he needs to withdraw, while at the same time encourages him to become engaged in another activity. It is recommended that he be referred to an occupational therapist with experience in sensory-based approaches to treatment or another professional with knowledge of and skills in working with children with sensory modulation challenges and their families.

Contributed by: Shelly J. Lane, Ph.D., OTR, FAOTA

Emily: Case Illustration of a Mixed Regulatory-Sensory Processing Disorder

Emily, a 4 year, 3 month-old girl, was referred for an evaluation at the urging of her preschool due to concerns about her ability to follow the flow of school activities. Although Emily appeared to be a bright little girl who was highly verbal and imaginative in her own play, she had difficulty joining other children. She often appeared lost and in her own world. She tended to isolate herself on the playground and in the classroom. Transitions were difficult because she seemed to get confused or lost. It was hard to orient her to what was happening; she needed help with each step of the transition.

Background

Emily is the older child in an intact two-parent family. Her younger brother was born about ten months before the referral and has no reported problems. Emily's father is a psychology professor and her mother is a mental health professional. Emily was born full term following an uncomplicated pregnancy. She was slow to catch on to breast-feeding, but eventually was successful. Her early motor milestones occurred within an average age range and she was walking by 12 months. She has a history of frequent ear infections between 6 months and 2 years of age but she did not require surgical intervention. She is toilet trained for urine, but continues to have difficulty with bowel movements.

Her parents describe her as clumsy with frequent falls. She is not yet able to ride a tricycle. They report that she "W-sits" (the opposite of sitting cross-legged, so that her legs are folded back on their sides and look like w's, very hard on the hips) and she sometimes looks stiff when she is standing. They stated that her arms and hands seem weak. She prefers imaginative play with dolls and figures and avoids manipulative play and fine motor activities. She does not yet have a hand preference. Emily's parents are concerned about how difficult it is for her to connect to other children. They describe her as "spacey" and inattentive. She has trouble keeping track of her belongings and finding things in visually cluttered environments such as the preschool room. They were curious to find out why her ability to attend and connect varies from day to day and within different situations.

Evaluation

Emily was evaluated in the clinic with her mother present using the Pediatric Examination of Educational Readiness (PEER), (Levine, 1985) and clinical observations of her sensory and motor functioning. The PEER assesses a child's performance on 29 tasks in six different areas of development: orientation, gross motor, visual-fine motor, sequential, linguistic, and pre-academic learning. The child is also rated on selective attention and activity, processing efficiency, and adaptation. Emily's parents filled out the Sensory Profile (Dunn, 1999) and the examiner completed a school observation.

During the standardized assessment, Emily was cooperative but difficult to engage and poorly oriented. She was neither able to receive nonverbal social cues nor read body language. She became confused by directions presented at a conversational speed, but could respond if she was reoriented and time was unlimited. However, her ability on language items was at or above age level. Emily has a rich vocabulary, which is most evident when she is engaged in solitary imaginative play. In conversation, she has difficulty with language processing due to slow processing speed. Her expressive language is poorly organized and she has difficulty maintaining conversational reciprocity. Social pragmatics such as social referencing and use of non-verbal gestures are poorly developed. At times Emily seemed internally distracted, which increased with anxiety. Her attention could be sustained if the examiner used very high affect, slow speech, and physical support. This was striking for a child who performed at or above age level on pre-academic areas such as letters and numbers, naming days, and counting.

Emily's mother appeared anxious while observing the evaluation and frequently attempted to help focus her daughter by moving very close, holding her at the shoulders, and calling her name until she got eye contact. She spoke rapidly and with very high affect that was successful in breaking into Emily's self-absorption, but this interactive style at times appeared to be too much for Emily. The amount of language and the rapid delivery as well as the high intensity of the input seemed to get Emily's attention for a brief response, but shut down her ability to stay connected for continuous interactive flow.

Standardized Results on the PEER

Emily had difficulty with three of the five items on the Orientation subtest, which evaluates body awareness and localization of specific sensory input. She appropriately identified body parts. Finger movements were difficult with or without visual monitoring. She was poor at recognizing shapes drawn on the back of her hand (graphesthesia), but she did better matching blocks that were felt with her vision occluded (stereognosis). Her ocular smooth pursuits were impaired and she was unable to follow a moving object with her eyes unless her head moved.

Emily had great difficulty with gross motor tasks, particularly those that required balance and postural control, falling below normal limits on all six gross motor items. Her resting muscle tone was somewhat low, but her postural control during movement was remarkably poor due to lack of stability through the trunk as well as poor head control. She was unable to walk on her heels or her toes. While attempting these activities she demonstrated a transient increase in upper body tone with posturing that had a dystonic quality. She was unable to stand on one foot or to catch a ball. She lacked rotation through the trunk and was unable to sustain flexion or extension. She was also unable to maintain a stable, erect motor stance with arms extended and eyes closed, suggesting difficulty with vestibular/proprioceptive processing. Rapid pronation and supination were impossible for her to complete, suggesting cerebellar involvement. A marked asymmetry was noted, with the left side having greater impairment.

Emily also demonstrated weaknesses in visual and fine motor capacities. Emily demonstrated a weak, inconsistent grasp pattern with a pencil even within a task, ranging from a static tripod to a fisted grasp. The difference between her cognitive ability, which is at or above age level, and her delayed fine motor skills was notable. Emily copied vertical and horizontal lines, but could not imitate a circle or shapes using small sticks. Her difficulty manipulating the sticks indicated poor tactile and proprioceptive discrimination. When she dropped a stick she was unaware that the stick had fallen. She did better copying block constructions but had difficulty sustaining visual attention. She missed task details and lost track of the task, using the blocks to build her own buildings. Though her visual shape matching was age appropriate, the examiner had to structure her and use verbal redirection for her to focus on the task.

On the Sensory Profile, "Probable Differences" (sensory under-reactivity) were reported in Auditory Processing, Vestibular Processing and Multi-sensory Processing. Emily was age appropriate on the sensory modulation sections, but had scores of "Probable Difference" on Emotional/Social Response and fell in the range of "Definite Difference" on the section reflecting Behavioral Outcomes of Sensory Processing. The factor indicating "Probable Difference" was Inattention/Distractibility; "Definite Difference" factors were Emotionally Reactive and Fine Motor/Perceptual.

During testing, Emily responded well to structure and to well-defined demands for simple verbal responses, but she became anxious when asked to perform specific gross and fine motor tasks. She was able to have a conversation as long as she generated it. If the examiner tried to expand an idea or if a new idea was introduced, she became confused and exhibited silly or avoidant behavior.

In open-ended play, Emily responded best to sensory motor play more typical of a younger child, such as chase games. Her ability to sustain attention and interaction was best under conditions of high affect and no requirement for discrete skill output. In simple playful games she sustained reciprocal interaction for 15- 20 interactive turns. If the activity involved much language, moved quickly, or had much movement, she became disorganized. She had difficulty sustaining a play activity interrupted by motor planning or balance problems. Her activity level escalated when she moved though space. Her parents described her as "always on the move," but she was observed in this assessment to be withdrawn and slow to respond.

School Observation

In the school observation, it was clear how the impairments seen in the evaluation affected her school functioning. Emily's class had gathered in small groups where they freely moved among classroom activity centers. During this observation many of the children were playing actively around the climbing structure. The noise level was high but not overwhelming. Emily sat at a far corner of the room with her back to the rest of the group playing alone with a set of large dinosaurs. At one point a boy approached and attempted to join her play. When Emily did not respond to him he lost interest. Emily then stood up and looked in his direction as he moved across the room. She watched several groups from a distance and then moved over to the group of children playing house. She stood at the periphery, watched, and made one or two quiet comments but she was not successful in joining the group.

During a circle music activity, Emily needed adult direction to join the class, and external postural support provided by a teacher's assistant to be able to attend to the task. When the class stood for a movement song, Emily approximated the movements but was slow and out of sync with the group. When she lost her balance, she became disoriented and was unable to join back into the song. She was not able to use the help that the assistant tried to give her. Emily required adult direction to join the class line for a toilet break. She left with the children but did not return. A teacher finally found Emily looking at a bulletin board where she had become overly absorbed in the pictures.

Emily rejoined the rest of the class in a smaller room. She went to her favorite activity center and pulled out a box of materials that she examined with her back to the rest of the class. Another child tried to join her and was successful. She followed Emily's directions and the two had a nice interaction. When the other child made a suggestion, Emily became confused and tried to revert back to her previous play. Her play partner became frustrated and left. The teacher encouraged Emily to pick another area of the room. She avoided the art project and moved from one area to another, unable to settle and explore the activities. The teacher expressed her frustration at trying to get Emily to explore the various activities in the room, the difficulty they had with transitions, and the difficulty with getting her to interact with other children. The teachers feel that she is a bright, delightful girl who has trouble attending to interactions and learning. They expressed confusion and concern about her seeming day-to-day variability.

Social Emotional Functioning

Emily's social emotional functioning has been greatly impacted by her sensory processing and motor deficits. Her attention and regulation for a wide range of sensory experiences is constricted due to variable sensory reactivity and poor sensory processing that make it difficult for her to draw meaning from sensory events around her. Emily tends to be under-reactive to many sensations, but can be over-reactive to others. Her postural instability and difficulty with ocular control make it difficult for her to stabilize herself while standing to view the world around her and to follow the movements and actions of her peers. Her slow processing speed for visual and auditory input causes her to miss details needed to interpret the nuances in the flow of social interactions. Emily tends to over-focus on static objects in near space and to become absorbed in her own internal thoughts rather than to orient to the activity around her.

Emily initiates engagement and enjoys moments of rich engagement with her parents, but because Emily uses self-absorption as a coping mechanism, she can also be difficult to engage. She responds well to rich affect when is it delivered slowly and timed to her processing speed. It is important for those interacting with Emily to monitor the volume of their speech and to use facial expression and vocal intonation rather than loudness to bring affect to their interactions. Her engagement can be quite good when she is stable and the demand for postural control is low, but when she is upright and moving, it is difficult for her to sustain engagement. Emily is able to engage in two-way intentional affective communication when the timing and intensity of the interaction is a good fit for her processing abilities. She enjoys simple back and forth interactions and is best when the language and movement demands are low. The flow of her interaction and her ability to stay engaged for longer chains is easily disrupted by the demands of movement and balance, by motor planning challenges, by language processing challenges, and by gaps in her sensory processing. Unless she has a well-attuned partner, Emily quickly becomes confused and reverts to self-absorption. She has difficulty repairing breaks that occur in interactive flow and needs help to recover from interruptions. She can engage in brief islands of shared social problem solving, but the idea must be one that comes from her. She has difficulty incorporating others' ideas and shifting her own action and thoughts around others' ideas. This impacts her ability to play with peers. She does well when a friend follows her lead, but when a friend injects her own ideas into the play, Emily often becomes lost and disengages. Emily's slow processing speed and difficulty with social pragmatics also interrupt the flow of interaction with others because it can appear that she is not responding or is not still engaged. This can cause her play partner to disengage. However, if she is given time to respond, she often can continue the interaction. The inconsistency in Emily's responses makes it difficult for family and friends to know what to expect and how to respond to help her stay in the moment.

Emily has a relative strength in her capacity for solitary representational play. She can engage in long periods of representational play that at times have the beginnings of symbol content, e.g., acting out sequences of daily life and simple emotional themes such as care giving, dependency and simple conflicts or problems. She has difficulty letting others into her play and in logically bridging her ideas. Her own affect is not yet well differentiated and this is apparent in the constriction to the emotional content of her play.

Summary

Emily demonstrates a Regulatory-Sensory Processing Disorder characterized by (1) Self-Absorbed and Creative Patterns (203.2) and (2) Inattentive, Disorganized Patterns with contributing postural control problems and dyspraxia (205.4).

She is under-responsive to vestibular, tactile and proprioceptive information. At times she is alert to visual information and other times under-responsive to visual details in her environment. Visually, she functions better in near space than across space or while moving. This may be due to poor postural ocular functioning related to her postural disorder. Emily has auditory processing deficits for speech sounds and has slow processing speed. She is over-reactive to loud, unexpected sounds and has auditory discrimination difficulties.

The variability of her attention, awareness, and self-absorption suggests a modulation disorder rather than a discrimination disorder. Emily has marked deficits in motor functioning that are most apparent in her postural control, stability, balance, and control and gradation of gross and fine movements during functional activities. The motor planning deficits that accompany her postural issues are based on poor tactile and proprioceptive processing. Emily's postural instability has a significant impact on attention and orientation in busy environments and contributes to her self-absorption and anxiety.

A referral for a comprehensive DIR-based intervention program is recommended that focuses both on her regulatory-sensory processing challenges (i.e., occupational therapy) and her emotional, social, and educational challenges (e.g., a mental health professional to help construct a home program, consult to the school, and work with Emily and her family).

Contributed by: Beth Osten, MS. OTR/L

Axis I: Neurodevelopmental Disorders of Relating and Communicating[1]

300. Neurodevelopmental Disorders of Relating and Communicating

301. Type I: Early Symbolic, with Constrictions
302. Type II: Purposeful Problem Solving, with Constrictions
303. Type III: Intermittently Engaged and Purposeful
304. Type IV: Aimless and Unpurposeful

Other Neurodevelopmental Disorders (Including Genetic and Metabolic Syndromes)
Children Who Are Difficult to Classify

Neurodevelopmental disorders of relating and communicating (NDRC) involve problems in multiple aspects of a child's development, including social relationships, language, cognitive functioning, and sensory and motor processing. This category includes earlier conceptualizations of multisystem developmental disorders (MSDD), as characterized in *Infancy and Early Childhood* (Greenspan, 1992) and *Diagnostic Classification: 0-3* (DC 0-3) (Diagnostic Classification Task Force, 1994). Additionally, it includes the DSM-IV-R category of pervasive developmental disorders (PDD), also referred to as autism spectrum disorders (ASD). The main distinction between NDRC and the earlier conceptualizations is that the NDRC framework enables a clinician to more accurately subtype disorders of relating and communicating in terms of the overall level of social, intellectual, and emotional functioning and the associated regulatory and sensory-motor processing profile. This helps differentiate the profiles that children commonly considered on the autism spectrum present and helps define the variations seen among the children with the same diagnosis. This differentiation is important for both intervention planning and research purposes.

Since the description of MSDD in DC 0-3 and PDD in DSM-IV-R, the framework has been broadened to allow consideration of the full range of disorders of relating, communicating, and thinking. Thus, the large degree of individual variation in infants and young children who ultimately evidence common features of difficulties in forming relationships, communicating at preverbal and verbal levels, and engaging in creative and abstract reflective thinking can be captured. These children typically evidence a type of static encephalopathy (i.e., non-progressive central nervous system dysfunction) that interferes with the expected progression of these core capacities. Children within this broad category, however, evidence wide variation in the degree to which they relate to others and master early communicative and thinking skills, as well as in their most basic

[1] Since the description of multisystem developmental disorders in DC:0-3, a work group of the Interdisciplinary Council on Developmental and Learning Disorders (ICDL) has developed the current classification of NDRC. The work group members include Serena Wieder, Ph.D., Lois Black, Ph.D., Griffin Doyle, Ph.D., Barbara Dunbar, Ph.D., Barbara Kalmanson, Ph.D., Lori-Jean Peloquin, Ph.D., Ricki Robinson, M.D., M.P.H., Ruby Salazar, LCSW, Rick Solomon, M.D., Rosemary White, OTR, Molly Romer Witten, Ph.D., and Stanley I. Greenspan, M.D.

ways of processing sensation (e.g., some are sensory over-responsive and others are sensory under-responsive; some have relatively strong visual memory while others have relatively weak visual memory). Therefore, we believe it is important to have the broadest possible conceptual framework within which to capture the full range of individual variation.

As we look at this full range (i.e., at all possible subtypes), we discover that there are numerous biological and overall developmental pathways associated with these types of challenges. For example, difficulty in connecting affect to perception and motor action, and subsequent difficulty in relating, communicating, and thinking, may be the result of several neurodevelopmental pathways, each with its own genetic or constitutional-maturational variations. Therefore, we suggest a broad category of neurodevelopmental disorders of relating and communicating to facilitate advances in research, evaluation strategies, and clinical intervention programs.

Neurodevelopmental disorders of relating and communicating may be viewed as part of the broad neurological category of a non-progressive disorder of the central nervous system. The technical term in ICD-10 (the International Diagnostic System) is "static" (non-progressive) "encephalopathy" (disorder of the central nervous system). It is also important to understand how regulatory-sensory processing disorders differ from NDRC.

Although regulatory-sensory processing disorders involve deficits in processing capacities, unlike NDRC, they do not derail a child's overall relating and communicating. Disorders of relating and communicating combine regulatory-sensory processing problems with significant developmental delays and dysfunctions. The child's biologically-based processing difficulties contribute to, but are not decisive in determining, relationship and communication difficulties. A complete evaluation of the regulatory-sensory processing capacities is necessary to understand their contribution to NDRC.

In contrast, an important pattern to recognize involves developmental impairments resulting from severe environmental stress and trauma. For example, in failure-to-thrive syndrome, an infant's motor, cognitive, language, affective, and physical growth may slow down or cease altogether. Persistent abuse or neglect can produce a similar global disruption in development and functioning. A tentative diagnosis of neurodevelopmental disorder could be given, but in these cases it would be important to see what changes occur once a comprehensive intervention program is put in place. In some cases, intervention can reverse the developmental impairments and the child may get back on track with only residual problems or may recover completely. In severe cases, only partial recovery may be evidenced.

The Developmental, Individual-Difference, Relationship-Based (DIR) approach helps us understand the relationship between adaptive capacities and pathologic symptoms in each infant or child. For example, an infant's impairments in auditory-verbal, visuospatial, or perceptual-motor processing can make ordinary relating and communicating extremely difficult. Even reasonably stable, supportive, and empathic parents may lack the intuitive skills to find some special way to capture their child's attention, engage him, and interact with him. The resulting lack of appropriate human interaction likely prevents vital social learning during key periods of development. Between 12 and 24 months of age, for example, most children develop several critical skills at an especially rapid rate—reciprocal affective and motor gesturing, comprehending the "rules" that govern complex social interactions, pattern recognition, a sense of self, and early forms of thinking. A deficit in these skills can easily look like a primary deficit rather than a consequence of underlying biologically-based processing impairments.

The DIR model is especially helpful in understanding how genetic and/or other biological patterns interact with environment patterns in the formation of a disorder. An example of this is an infant with low muscle tone and sensory under-reactivity who becomes more and more self-absorbed because his caregiver is depressed and unavailable.

Interestingly, many families of children diagnosed with autism or related disorders report—and have videotapes to back it up—that in the first year of life, their child was engaged and beginning to participate in reciprocal interactions. Only in the second year did he begin disengaging, suggesting that for some reason he became overwhelmed and withdrew. We hypothesize that a combination of two events may derail the child's forward momentum between 16 and 24 months.

The first is the child's own emerging capacities for higher-level presymbolic, symbolic, and cognitive functioning. Because these new capacities are emerging on a vulnerable foundation (such as a weak capacity for intentional two-way affective communication), they contribute to the child's becoming overloaded with new information about the world. Around this time, for example, the toddler is developing a sense of his physical relationship to surrounding space, and this leads to a greater awareness of his potential vulnerability. Such cognitive advances may, paradoxically, overwhelm a child with severe vulnerabilities in earlier developmental capacities, causing him to regress in his behavioral organization, self-regulation, interpersonal patterns, motor control, and language abilities.

New capacities alone seem to be enough to derail some children. In many cases, however, a second event might occur. Careful history-taking reveals that during the same period of development, the child experienced one or more stresses, such as a serious illness or the loss of a caregiver. For children who already have biologically-based vulnerabilities and a tenuous hold on their interpersonal relationships and developmental competencies, the combination or cumulative effect of emerging capacities and physcial and environmental stresses may be overwhelming.

As the child becomes increasingly challenging, the parents may find him so confusing, frustrating, and anxiety-provoking that they disengage from him, ceasing their previous attempts at shared attention, engagement, and preverbal and verbal communication. Having disengaged, many parents report growing feelings of alienation, anger, fear, and loss. They may unintentionally behave in increasingly ambivalent ways toward their child. The child, as he loses whatever level of engagement and purposeful relating he had previously enjoyed with his caregivers, seems to spin more and more idiosyncratically out of control. Prerepresentational children may exhibit increasing motor and behavioral randomness, whereas children who have achieved some degree of representational capacity may begin using words and ideas in more fragmented and personalized ways or they may lose the capacity for speech and representation altogether. In either case, the lack of an intentional, organizing human relationship may further contribute to the child's biologically-based primary vulnerabilities.

We have recently formulated a new hypothesis to understand the core biological and subsequent experiential relationships in the developmental pathway leading to autism spectrum disorders. In this hypothesis, which we call the affect-diathesis hypothesis (Greenspan & Wieder, 1999; Greenspan & Shanker, 2004; Interdisciplinary Council on Developmental and Learning Disorders Clinical Practice Guidelines Workgroup, 2000), we suggest that the core biological deficit expresses itself as a difficulty for the infant in connecting sensory and affective experiences with motor and affective experiences.

Typically, infants evidence a sensory-affect-motor connection as they begin to attend to the world. For example, turning to look toward mother's smiling face and pleasurable vocalizations requires perception (taking in pleasurable sensations), pleasurable affect (the sound of her voice, the sight of her face), and motor action (turning toward the pleasurable face and voice). This sensory-affect-motor connection becomes especially important as the infant engages more and more in reciprocal social and emotional interchanges in the second half of the first year of life. In these interchanges, affect clearly guides purposeful motor actions, such as exchanging vocalizations, trading funny little grins, reaching for the piece of banana in mommy's mouth, and so forth.

By the early part of the second year, the child's ability to connect sensation, affect, and motor action becomes even more vital as the toddler engages in shared social problem solving—for example, taking a caregiver by the hand, gesturing to the toy area, pointing to a particular toy which is out of reach, and making numerous back-and-forth gestures to get the parent to pick him up to reach the desired toy. In such interactions, as in earlier developmental stages, the child's purposeful or intentional behavior is clearly fueled by his affect (e.g., the desire for that toy). Yet now the child's affect is involved in many back-and-forth interactions in a row, and in this way affect guides the relationship between perception (e.g., seeing the toy) and a complex, multistep social and motor action to get the toy. The vast majority of children with autism spectrum disorders, even when these disorders are diagnosed at later ages, are reported by their parents to have had difficulty in mastering this early capacity for shared social problem solving (i.e., a continuous flow of back-and-forth affective signals) (Greenspan & Wieder, 1997).

Therefore, we hypothesize that a biologically-based difficulty with forming an early sensory-affect-motor connection and subsequent difficulties with connecting affect to complex motor patterns to facilitate motor planning and sequencing and shared social problem solving is an important contribution to the pattern of challenges and symptoms we observe in autism spectrum disorders.

Children vary, however, in the degree to which this fundamental capacity is disrupted and also differ in basic motor, sensory modulation, visuospatial, auditory processing, and language capacities. However, without the capacity to connect affect or intent to these fundamental capacities, especially the initial motor capacities, these related capacities are not developed in an appropriate manner. For example, children with relatively strong auditory processing and verbal capacities may repeat whole books because of their strong auditory memory, but at the same time may be unable to use language meaningfully. Similarly, children with relatively strong motor capacities may line up their toys, but are often unable to engage in motor-based interactive problem solving. Children with relative weaknesses in these related developmental capacities may evidence little or no verbal behavior at all and only simple repetitive or aimless motor behavior.

We have found that children with relative strengths in their related developmental capacities tend to make progress more rapidly once we are able to engage them in a comprehensive intervention program that works with their core difficulty in connecting affect to sensations and motor actions. We have also observed that the relative deficit in connecting affect to sensations and motor actions is often improved with an intervention program that focuses on affective learning relationships that take into account the child's unique developmental profile. Children appear to have the flexibility to develop side-roads even when the main highway evidences relative impairment (Greenspan & Wieder, 1997; 1998; 1999).

As this discussion suggests, NDRC can be more fully understood from the perspective of a developmental biopsychosocial model. Applying the DIR model to NDRC has enabled the development of a classification system that attempts to capture individual subtypes based on a more complete understanding of the developmental pathways that lead to significant challenges in relating, communicating, and thinking. These pathways, characterized by individual processing differences, include:

- **Auditory Processing and Language:** the way in which we receive information and comprehend and express it.
- **Motor Planning and Sequencing:** how we act on our ideas or on what we hear and see.
- **Visuospatial Processing:** the ability to make sense of and understand what we are seeing.
- **Sensory Modulation:** the ability to modulate or regulate sensation as it is coming in.

We propose four types of NDRC which cluster the major profiles we have observed in children with significant challenges in relating, communicating, and thinking. Each type highlights the varied features of the subgroup, but it is important to remember that these types and their associated features are on a continuum. As children make progress, we see movement within each type as well as from one type to another as the child receives intervention and moves forward. Each type is described below, along with a brief clinical illustration. These illustrations highlight the main features and quality of the relationships and functioning and are not complete. The DIR approach to comprehensive assessments and intervention plans appear in Appendices I and II.

TYPES OF NEURODEVELOPMENTAL DISORDERS OF RELATING AND COMMUNICATING (NDRC)

301. Type I: Early Symbolic, with Constrictions

Children with Type I disorders exhibit constrictions in their capacities for shared attention, engagement, initiation of two-way affective communication, and shared social problem solving. They have difficulty maintaining a continuous flow of affective interactions before intervention and can only open and close about four to ten circles of communication in a row. A circle of communication is a back and forth interaction where the infant or child responds to the caregiver's gestures or overtures, and visa versa. Often, the child also evidences perseveration and some degree of self-absorption. At initial evaluation, one sees islands of memory-based symbol use, such as labeling pictures or repeating memorized scripts, but the child does not display a range of affect expected for his age and has difficulty integrating symbol use with other core developmental capacities and engaging in all processes simultaneously.

With an intervention program that addresses individual processing differences and promotes shared attention and reciprocal affective communication, children with Type I difficulties tend to make rapid progress. Often, one sees such a child move from constricted patterns of interaction, perseveration, self-stimulation, and self-absorption toward warm, pleasurable engagement and a continuous flow of affective interactions. The child begins initiating such interactions by spontaneous use of language and maintaining the flow of interactions at the levels of two-way problem-solving communication, creating ideas, and building bridges between ideas. Even when language is delayed, the child is able to sequence complex gestures (signs) and use toys to convey symbolic ideas until language is strengthened. Thus, the child moves toward abstract and reflective levels of symbolic thinking. His more robust capacities enable him to develop healthy peer relationships and participate in typical activities.

Eventually, with appropriate intervention, children with Type I difficulties can usually participate fully in a regular academic program. Often an aide may be required for a period of time to help with regulatory-sensory processing and related attentional challenges. In addition, because academic skills and abstract thinking depend on processing abilities, educational interventions to address specific learning difficulties may be required.

CLINICAL ILLUSTRATION OF TYPE I

David, age 2½ years, was self-absorbed, perseverative, and given to self-stimulation. He did not make eye contact with his parents or exhibit much pleasure in relating to them, nor did he play with other children. During his evaluation, David spent most of his time reciting numbers or the alphabet in a rote sequence, spinning and jumping around randomly, and lining up toys and cars while making self-stimulatory sounds. When he was extremely motivated, he could blurt out what he wanted. He occasionally showed affection by hugging his parents and tolerated their hugs though he never looked at them. He could imitate actions, sounds, and words, and recognized pictures and shapes.

David presented both challenges and strengths in his regulatory and sensory processing profile. He was a highly active child who was interested in learning about the world even though he could only do so in a fragmented and fleeting way as he flitted around the room flapping his arms searching for something familiar. His intense movement also served to increase his muscle tone and energy. When something captured his attention, he explored the object briefly, sometimes blurted out its label, but had no communicative intent. He could recite memorized letters and numbers which never changed, but could not process (comprehend) when others spoke to him. By his third year he became more and more self-absorbed and would resort to exciting himself with his recitations, but was unable to engage in any two-way communication or even respond to his name. David also demonstrated some visuospatial strength in that he could randomly discriminate objects in his environment and later locate them again. He sought out mirrors to reflect what he was doing and used them for visual feedback as he could not process incoming auditory feedback from others. He also manipulated toys, indicating he understood what they represented and could use them in simple sequences (e.g., to eat the pretend food or push the car), indicating he had the rudiments of connecting purposeful intent to motor planning. This was also seen in his ability to spontaneously imitate new actions with toys and ritualized movements to songs. It was also evident David had strong affect and showed great pleasure when happy—even in his self-absorbing pursuits—and intense anger or avoidance when thwarted. His ability to initiate and connect affect to intent was his strongest asset. While auditory and visual processing capacities were significantly challenged, he still showed relative strengths and weaknesses.

With a comprehensive intervention program, David quickly became more engaged, entered into a continuous flow of affective interactions, began initiating long pretend-oriented sequences, and gradually began using language purposefully and creatively. His early perseverative interest in cars transformed into their use for elaborate symbolic dramas and remained a special interest for several years during which he became the resident "expert" on brands and models. This gave way as he expanded his emotional range and emotional interests as well as motor planning abilities. He used Floortime sessions to spontaneously explore and rehearse new emotional themes and he became an abstract thinker. He could also reflect on his feelings and was highly empathic with others. (See Appendix II on Comprehensive Intervention Approaches). In the pattern of progress described above, his developing capacities enabled him to begin relating more to both parents and peers. At present, as a teenager, David attends a regular school, where he excels in English as well as math. He continues to have some difficulty with fine motor sequencing (e.g., with penmanship). While he did not become an athlete, he enjoys shooting baskets or playing tennis with friends and writes the sports feature in his school paper. He is still active and quite enterprising, now looking for opportunities to do "business." While he tends to become somewhat argumentative in competitive situations, he enjoys close friendships, has a great sense of humor, and shows insights into other people's feelings.

302. Type II: Purposeful Problem Solving, with Constrictions

Children with Type II disorder, when seen initially (often between ages 2 and 4 years), have significant constrictions in the third and fourth core developmental capacities: purposeful, two-way presymbolic communication and social problem-solving communication. They engage in only intermittent interactions at these levels, completing at most two to five circles of communication in a row. Other than repeating a few memorized scripts from favorite shows, they exhibit few islands of true symbolic activity. Many of these children show some capacity for engagement, but their engagement has a global, need-oriented emotional quality on their terms. They often evidence a profile of moderate processing dysfunctions in multiple areas.

Children in this group face greater challenges than those in Type I and make slower, but consistent, progress. Overcoming each hurdle requires a great deal of time and work. Over time, they can learn to engage with real warmth and pleasure. They gradually but steadily improve their capacities for purposeful interaction and shared social problem solving, learning to initiate and sustain a continuous flow of affective interactions. The slow development of this continuous flow prevents a more robust development of symbolic capacities; these also improve, but tend to rely on imitation of books and videos as a basis for language and imaginative play. As the children gradually progress through each new capacity, they begin creating ideas and may even reach towards building bridges between ideas in circumscribed areas of interest. However, they do not display an age-appropriate depth and range of affect, and their abstract thinking is very limited and focused on real-life needs.

Although many children in this group make continuous progress, most cannot participate in all the activities of a regular classroom with a large number of children. They can, however, benefit from appropriately staffed inclusion or integrated programs or from special needs classrooms in which language development is emphasized and the other children are interactive and verbal.

CLINICAL ILLUSTRATION OF TYPE II

Three-year-old Joey was extremely avoidant, always moving away from his caregivers and making only fleeting eye contact with them. He displayed considerable perseverative and self-stimulatory behavior, such as rapidly turning the pages of preferred books or pushing his toy train around and around the track. He also chose books and figures from his favorite shows, such as Barney or Winnie the Pooh, and had them board his trains. No one dared to touch his figures since he would tantrum instantly when he thought the figures would be taken away. He could purposefully reach for his juice, put out his arms to get dressed, or give and take an object from his parents, but he could neither negotiate complex preverbal interactions nor imitate sounds or words though he vocalized some. The only pleasure he showed with his parents was during roughhousing or tickle games and when his mother sang to him as he fell asleep.

Joey relied on visual information to deal with his environment and had a remarkable memory for things and places. He was under-responsive to words spoken to him, but over-responsive to sudden high pitched or vibrating sounds which continuously distracted or alarmed him and kept him vigilant. He relied on ritualized patterns in daily life and protested changes he could not understand. While he seemed to somehow find his favorite books or figures, he did not search for things in any planned way, leading to frustration and tantrums. He also found obstacle courses hard to do and rather than follow the other children in the gym, he would collapse on the floor and watch them. These patterns reflected the multiple sensory and motor processing challenges (auditory, visuospatial and motor planning), compounded by over- and under-responsiveness and low tone. Life became more and more challenging for him and his family as he grew and pulled away from relationships and their increasing expectations.

Joey's intervention program addressed each of the processing areas in individual therapies and a home program (see Appendix II). The emphasis was on expanding pleasurable interactions and establishing a continuous flow of interactions through affect cuing and problem solving. As he became more engaged and began to expand his play, it became evident that Joey had islands of receptive symbolic understanding suggested by his early interest in Barney riding his train. He began to use figures from various books and shows, first scripting and then recreating real life experiences such as birthday parties. Visual strategies and oral motor treatment helped reduce his frustration.

Now, at age 6½ , after nearly four years of intensive intervention, Joey can relate with real pleasure and joy and uses complex gestures and words to negotiate with his parents. He can describe what he wants in sentences ("Give me juice now, I'm thirsty!"); respond to simple questions ("What do you want to do?" "Go to Disneyworld on my trains!"). He can have conversations involving four or five exchanges of short phrases giving his opinion or making a plan for the day. He enjoys listening to and reading story books and is beginning to read sight words. He also engages in early imaginative play, throwing grand birthday parties, dressing up and making his action figures fly around the room with great joy and delight. Joey insists on being the superhero but does not always have a motive even when he has a destination (to get the "bad guy").

Although he cannot yet consistently answer abstract "why" questions, Joey can do basic real life reasoning about safety. He is able to play with peers and run with the crowd in the context of action or structured games and with some adult involvement. He is now in an inclusion kindergarten program and participates in pre-academic activities, with relative strengths in visual thinking and math. He also enjoys play dates with his classmates. Joey continues to make progress at a slow but consistent pace. Interestingly, Joey's perseverative, self-stimulatory patterns have largely abated and appear only occasionally.

303. Type III: Intermittently Engaged and Purposeful

Children in this group are very self-absorbed. Their engagement with others is extremely intermittent, having an "in and out" quality. They display very limited purposeful two-way communication, usually in pursuit of concrete needs or basic sensorimotor experiences (e.g., jumping, tickling). They may be able to imitate or even initiate some rote problem-solving actions, but they usually evidence little or no capacity for shared social problem solving or for a continuous flow of affective exchange.

With affect-based intervention, children with Type III difficulties can become more robustly engaged in pleasurable activities, but their capacity for a continuous flow of affective interactions improves very slowly. They can learn to convey simple feelings such as happy, sad and mad, but the "in and out" quality of their relatedness constricts the range and depth of affect they can negotiate. Over time, they can learn islands of presymbolic purposeful and problem-solving behavior. These islands may, at times, also involve the use of words, pictures, signs, or two- to three-step actions or gestures to communicate basic needs. Receptive understanding of often-used phrases in routines or when coupled with visual cues or gestures can become a relative strength.

Some children in this group use toys as if they are real, e.g., they try to eat pretend foods or feed a life-size baby doll, or put their feet into a pretend swimming pool as if they could go swimming. They do not usually reach the level of truly representing themselves using toys or dolls. Multiple severe processing dysfunctions, including severe auditory processing and visuospatial processing difficulties and moderate-to-severe motor planning problems, impede the continuous flow of purposeful communication and problem-solving interactions.

Some children in this group have severe oral-motor dyspraxia and do not speak more than a few words, if they speak at all; they may, however, learn to use a few signs or to communicate using pictures or a favorite toy.

Children in this group require very individualized educational approaches and may eventually learn to read words through motor pathways and to understand visuospatial concepts. It is important that they be included in hybrid programs to encourage social activities, ritualized learning, and the development of friendships.

CLINICAL ILLUSTRATION OF TYPE III

Sarah, age 3 years, ran into the playroom looking for Winnie the Pooh, climbed up on the stool in front of the shelves, but could not move the little figures in the basket around to search for her beloved character. The next moment, the basket was pulled off the shelf and all the figures fell out. Without bothering to look on the floor, Sarah began searching in the next basket. Her mom ran over before the second basket was dropped and offered to help. Sarah echoed, "Help!" and grabbed her mother's hands and put them in the basket. Her mother had to point to the Pooh figure before Sarah actually saw it. She grabbed it and ran off to lie on the couch. Mom then brought Tigger over to say hello; Sarah grabbed Tigger and ran to the other side of the room. She held her figures tightly and turned away when her mother came over again. Mom then took the Eeyore figure and started to sing "Ring around the Rosie..." while moving Eeyore up and down. This time, Sarah looked and filled in "down" to "all fall down." She then moved rapidly away and went over to the mirror. This pattern of flight and avoidance after getting what she wanted, followed by not knowing what to do next, was typical of Sarah.

With a comprehensive intervention program, Sarah slowly learned the labels for things she wanted. She learned how to protest rather than scream. She recognized and could say familiar phrases like "come and eat," "go out," and "bath time." She became quite engaged when involved in sensorimotor play and loved to be swung and tickled. She even began to play with toys, first dipping her toes into the water of the play pool and then letting Winnie jump in. She began to imitate more words and actions. She tried to initiate problem-solving interactions to get her figures, but only when she was very motivated or very mad and usually only after energetic sensorimotor play had pulled her in. Her expressive language expanded to include more and more phrases indicating what she wanted, but her weak receptive processing made it difficult for her to answer any questions, and she relied on visual and affect cues to understand what was said to her. This transferred to puppet play and even simple role-playing in which she took the part of a cook or doctor. Problem solving progressed very slowly because of Sarah's very poor motor planning, but she became more easily engaged and more responsive to semi-structured and structured approaches to learning. Between ages 4 and 5, she learned to count and to identify colors, and she loved to paint and cut with scissors. At age 6½, Sarah demonstrates some pre-academic abilities, including reading some sight words. She attends a special education class which integrates activities with typical peers. She enjoys being with other children and joins the crowd in running around, hiding, and chasing, but she does not yet play interactively. She has, however, learned various social rituals of greeting, sharing, protesting, and so on. Sarah can also spontaneously communicate with a big smile, "Feel happy!" or with a frown, "Feel mad!"

304. Type IV: Aimless and Unpurposeful

Children in this group are passive and self-absorbed or active and stimulus seeking; some exhibit both patterns. They have severe difficulties with shared attention and engagement unless they are involved in sensorimotor play. They tend to make very slow progress. Developing expressive language is very challenging.

With intervention, children with Type IV difficulties can become warmly engaged and intermittently interactive through use of gestures and action games. Through their ability to relate and interact, they can learn to problem solve. The goal is to challenge them to open and close many circles of communication in a row so that they can progress as much as possible in their problem-solving ability.

Some children learn to complete organized sequences of the sort needed to play semi-structured games or carry out self-help tasks, such as dressing and brushing teeth. Many such children can share with others the pleasure they experience when they use their bodies purposefully to skate, swim, ride bikes, play ball, etc. These meaningful activities can be used to encourage shared attention, engagement, and purposeful problem solving.

Children in this group have the most severe challenges in all processing areas. Many have special challenges in motor planning, including oral-motor dyspraxia. As a consequence, their progress is very uneven. They have the most difficulty with complex problem-solving interactions, expressive language, and motor planning. They may have periods of progression and regression. Regressions can occur for unknown reasons. Sometimes, regressions appear to occur because the environment is not sufficiently tailored to the child's processing profile.

Educational approaches should be very meaningful to the child in order to pull these children in. Both visual and motor pathways must be found to help the children focus and learn.

CLINICAL ILLUSTRATION OF TYPE IV

Harold progressed only very slowly to imitating sounds and words, even with an intensive program to facilitate imitation. He could say one or two words spontaneously when he felt mad or insistent on getting something, but otherwise he had to be prompted and pushed to speak. Every utterance was extremely difficult for him, and he would sometimes stare at a caregiver's mouth to try and form the same movements. His severe dyspraxia also interfered with his engaging in pretend play, although from his various facial expressions and the gleam in his eye when he engaged in playful interactions with his parents, it appeared he was playing little "tricks." He sometimes held onto toy objects like a soft sword or magic wand and used them in ritualized ways, but he could not use toys to sequence new ideas. He could become engaged and even initiated sensorimotor interactions involving the expression of pleasure and affection. Although games with his brother had to be orchestrated, he did enjoy running around the schoolyard and the pool with other children. In the second year of intervention, at age 5 years, he was able to interact and communicate with three or four back-and-forth exchanges about what he wanted (e.g., pulling his dad over to the refrigerator and finding the hot dogs). He could even retrieve a few words at such moments: "Hot dog." "What else?" "French fries." Harold became more consistently engaged over time, developed islands of presymbolic ability, and tuned in to more of what was going on around him. He no longer wandered aimlessly and could be observed picking up trucks to push, putting together simple puzzles, or engaging in other cause-and-effect play. He let others join him but invariably turned the interaction into sensorimotor play, which brought him great pleasure.

REGULATORY-SENSORY PROCESSING PROFILE FOR EACH NDRC SUBTYPE

As indicated, each subtype, in addition to being characterized by its functional emotional developmental capacity (Axis II), should also be characterized in terms of its regulatory-sensory processing profile (Axis III), as well as along the other axes (Axes IV -VIII). Axis III, which refers to this profile (and is further elaborated in the Axis I section on Regulatory-Sensory Processing Disorders [200s]), highlights the different regulatory-sensory processing domains that should be considered. A full clinical understanding of the child requires this profile, in addition to the subtype designation described above.

For research purposes, the regulatory-sensory processing profile can be simplified. For example, most children with NDRC (including autism spectrum disorders) evidence challenges in language and visuospatial thinking, but differ enormously in their auditory memory and visuospatial memory capacities, as well as their motor planning and sensory modulation capacities. Therefore, these features that capture important clinical and, most likely, etiological pathway differences, must be highlighted. The summary form at the end of this section summarizes both the subtypes and the regulatory-sensory processing profile in terms of these dimensions.

Other Neurodevelopmental Disorders (Including Genetic and Metabolic Syndromes)

The four subtypes described above (Axis I: 301 - 304) can be used to describe children with any type of non-progressive developmental disorder, including many of the well-known genetic syndromes. These syndromes involve problems with communicating and language, thinking (i.e., cognitive challenges), sensory and motor processing, and sometimes relating. Children born with these syndromes, including Down's, Rett, Angelman, Prader-Willi, Turner, Fragile X, and others, may have relative strengths in relating, but often have compromises to different degrees in various developmental capacities. As with the other NDRC disorders, it is important to evaluate auditory processing and language capacities; motor planning and sequencing, including oral motor; visuospatial processing; and sensory modulation. Only such a comprehensive evaluation permits the construction of an optimal intervention program. When a child evidences a well-identified genetic or metabolic syndrome, the syndrome should be identified as well as the subtype of NDRC that best describes the child's functioning. In this way, the child can be described both from the perspective of the etiology of his or her disorder and the developmental profile that characterizes it.

It should be emphasized, however, that as with all infant and early childhood disorders, attempts at categorization should not substitute for constructing a developmental profile of the child that includes the perspective reflected in each of the axes of the recommended multi-axial framework. This emphasis is especially important for many of the syndromes described in this category because, as indicated above, some children with a number of developmental challenges are very warm and engaged and have a real strength in their capacity for intimacy and, at the same time, evidence marked difficulties in motor functioning, language, and/or areas of cognitive functioning.

In addition, while many of the developmental disorders referred to above are best described in terms of the category of NDRC (in addition to their etiologically based diagnoses), some children may be best described in terms of their regulatory-sensory processing patterns and more closely approximate the criteria for this category. For example, a child may be very warmly related and comfortable with intimacy, using emotions or affect to signal, and may easily participate in back-and-forth reciprocal social interactions. However, he may also show marked motor and cognitive challenges, as well as language delays (using whatever language is at his disposal creatively and meaningfully). This child may best be described in terms of his etiologic syndrome and the regulatory-sensory processing categories that capture his unique individual differences.

Therefore, it is helpful to consider all non-progressive developmental disorders within the multi-axial framework presented in this manual. The goal is to describe each child's unique characteristics as a basis for constructing a comprehensive, developmentally-based intervention program.

Children Who Are Difficult to Classify

It is important to note that some children may give the initial impression of functioning only at the most fundamental levels seen in Types III or IV. However, with continued observation they appear to have patterns that are different and difficult to classify. Three such groups are suggested.

The first group is defined by children with severe oral motor and overall dyspraxia, who are severely impaired in expression with very limited outflow to express thoughts or feelings. They stand out in their strong interest in symbolic ideas gleaned from books and videos. Since they cannot talk, gesture, or use toys to communicate, it is not clear what they understand, but the gleam in their eye and the pleasure (or other affect) in the content are evident. They appear more related to their parents and persist in getting help. They have better receptive language and their choice of objects suggests islands of symbolic understanding. With augmentative support, these children may reveal stronger receptive abilities than was evident before and can progress into one of the higher levels of NDRC (Types I and II). When they are offered an augmentation system at school age (e.g., a voice output system, computer to type on), they actually begin to communicate quite rapidly and reach higher symbolic stages and academic learning. Some may begin to speak and others stay with typing. In a few cases even the most severely dyspraxic children with very limited repertoire of expression (Types III and IV) indicate their potential through some persistent symbolic interest, such as insisting on watching certain videos of highly charged emotional stories and, when communication improves, reporting their thoughts and feelings about the themes.

The second group is defined by children who crave extreme sensory stimulus and are continuously on the move, so that it is hard to assess what they are taking in and, when coupled with dyspraxia, it is often hard to know what they can produce.

The third group includes children who are extremely sensitive and over-responsive. They may get over-stimulated by the environment or overloaded by specific demands to conform or perform. They can dysregulate into self-injurious, highly disorganized, or "shut down" behavior.

All three subtypes of children may be difficult to classify and may be underestimated and classified as limited learners. It is important to develop a comprehensive program, for example with some children with augmentative communication, to determine the best pathways for them to learn and then observe their potential. Because these children may be difficult to classify initially, it's important to observe their progress with an optimal intervention program and be prepared to shift initial impressions and expectations according to progress over time.

The four subtypes described here provide a useful framework for organizing these initial impressions and for observing changes. What needs to be emphasized is the importance of exploring every avenue possible to enhance communication, because only in this exploration can the potential of the child be realized.

SUMMARY TABLES OF NEURODEVELOPMENTAL DISORDERS OF RELATING AND COMMUNICATING (NDRC)

Below is a very brief overview of the types of NDRC described earlier, along with motor and sensory processing patterns that are also helpful in profiling the child. This is provided as a summary to facilitate the use of this framework in a variety of clinical and research settings.

Table 1: Overview of Clinical Subtypes of NDRC and Related Motor and Sensory-Processing Profile

Type I - Intermittent capacities for attending and relating; reciprocal interaction; and, with support, shared social problem-solving and the beginning use of meaningful ideas (i.e., with help, the child can relate and interact and even use a few words, but not in a continuous and stable age-expected manner). Children with this pattern tend to show rapid progress in a comprehensive program that tailors meaningful emotional interactions to their unique motor and sensory processing profile.
Type II - Intermittent capacities for attention, relating, and a few back-and-forth reciprocal interactions, with only fleeting capacities for shared social problem-solving and repeating some words. Children with this pattern tend to make steady, methodical progress.
Type III - Only fleeting capacities for attention and engagement. With lots of support, occasionally a few back-and-forth reciprocal interactions. Often no capacity for repeating words or using ideas, although may be able to repeat a few words in a memory-based (rather than meaningful) manner. Children with this pattern often make slow but steady progress, especially in the basics of relating with warmth and learning to engage in longer sequences of reciprocal interaction. Over long periods of time, often gradually master some words and phrases.
Type IV - Similar to Type III above, but with a pattern of multiple regressions (loss of capacities). May also evidence a greater number of associated neurological challenges, such as seizures, marked hypotonia, etc. Children with this pattern often make very, very slow progress. The progress can be enhanced if the sources of the regressive tendencies can be identified.

Table 2. Overview of Motor and Sensory Processing Profile

Children with NDRC (which includes children with autism spectrum disorders) tend to evidence very different biologically-based patterns of sensory reactivity, processing, and motor planning. These differences may have diagnostic and prognostic value, and therefore it may be helpful to describe them. The child's tendencies can be briefly summarized in the framework outlined below. Note: Almost all the children with an NDRC diagnosis evidence language and visuospatial thinking challenges.

The patterns listed below are the ones that tend to differ among the children. Please check all boxes that apply and, if sufficient clinical information is available, also use the box to indicate the degree to which that characteristic applies on a 1 to 3 scale (with 1 indicating minimum and 3 indicating the maximum degree).

Sensory Modulation

☐ Tends to be over-responsive to sensations, such as sound or touch (e.g., covers ears or gets dysregulated with lots of light touch)

☐ Tends to crave sensory experience (e.g., actively seeks touch, sound, and different movement patterns)

☐ Tends to be under-responsive to sensations (e.g., requires highly energized vocal or tactile support to be alert and attend)

Motor Planning and Sequencing

☐ Relative strength in motor planning and sequencing (e.g., carries out many-step action patterns, such as negotiating obstacle courses or building complex block designs, etc.)

☐ Relative weakness in motor planning and sequencing (e.g., can barely carry out simple movements and may tend to simply bang blocks or do other one- to two-step action patterns)

Auditory Memory

☐ Relative strength in auditory memory (remembers or repeats long statements or materials from books, TV, records, etc.)

☐ Relative weakness in auditory memory (difficulty remembering even simple sounds or words)

Visual Memory

☐ Relative strength in visual memory (tends to remember what is seen, such as book covers, pictures, eventually words, etc.)

☐ Relative weakness in visual memory (difficulty remembering even simple pictures or objects)

Axis I: Language Disorders[1]

400. Language Disorders with compromises in

- 401. Self-Regulation and Interest in the World
  - 401.1 In Comprehension
  - 401.2 In Production
  - 401.3 In Both Comprehension and Production
- 402. Forming Relationships: Affective Vocal Synchrony
  - 402.1 In Comprehension
  - 402.2 In Production
  - 402.3 In Both Comprehension and Production
- 403. Intentional Two-Way Communication
  - 403.1 In Comprehension
  - 403.2 In Production
  - 403.3 In Both Comprehension and Production
- 404. First Words: Sharing Meanings in Gestures and Words
  - 404.1 In Comprehension
  - 404.2 In Production
  - 404.3 In Both Comprehension and Production
- 405. Word Combinations: Sharing Experiences Symbolically
  - 405.1 In Comprehension
  - 405.2 In Production
  - 405.3 In Both Comprehension and Production
- 406. Early Discourse: Reciprocal Symbolic Interactions with Others
  - 406.1 In Comprehension
  - 406.2 In Production
  - 406.3 In Both Comprehension and Production

Note: A child may evidence compromises at a number of levels

Language functioning involves many parts of the mind and the central nervous system working together. Sounds need to be perceived–which includes registration, sequencing and pattern recognition–and interpreted; speaking involves complex oral-motor patterns, as well as gestures and body movements that mobilize other parts of the motor system. The language-speaker also needs to formulate and comprehend complex ideas, which involves not just verbal skills but other aspects of the mind, such as visuospatial thinking and memory. The flow of thoughts and ideas that inform speech and create "language" also depend on one's affects or emotions: i.e., the motives, desires, wishes, etc., that inform what we want to say or communicate.

[1] Work group members include Sherri Cawn, M.A., CCC-SLP; Sima Gerber, Ph.D., CCC; Cindy Harrison, M.S.c., SLP; Diane Lewis, M.A., CCC-SLP; Jane R. Madell, Ph.D., CCC A/SLP; Stuart G. Shanker, D.Phil.; Amy M. Wetherby, Ph.D., CCC-SLP; Stanley I. Greenspan, M.D.

Each of these elements in the complex phenomenon of language functioning has its own developmental pathway, and, together with all the others, is characterized by developmental processes that orchestrate all of them into a cohesive whole at every stage in early development.

Historically, the full scope of the different parts of the mind, central nervous system, and developmental pathways that contribute to language functioning have not always been fully appreciated. Most important are the preverbal stages involving the various forms of communication that occur in the first 12-18 months of life. These early stages in pre-linguistic development have now been described and involve rhythmic synchrony, affective engagement, pattern recognition, different levels of affective signaling, and many levels of affective and socially-mediated gestural communication, including complex interactive communicative gesturing in the second year of life. This provides the communicative and experiential basis for understanding the meaning of symbols and words as well as the capacity to construct them.

The theoretical framework and practical guide used to classify language disorders, therefore, needs to incorporate the different dimensions of development that contribute to language. To facilitate this goal, ICDL created a working group to formulate a developmentally-based approach to characterizing healthy and disordered language functioning. The developmental model formulated is grounded in the concepts described above and builds on the important conceptual and research efforts of many pioneers as well as current investigators and clinicians. The model also builds on the recent advances in the field of psycholinguistics. Current approaches to language are also influenced by important historical trends. As is well known, psycholinguistics was fundamentally transformed in 1959 when Chomsky published his devastating review of B.F. Skinner's *Verbal Behavior*.[2]

Through a series of intricate arguments and examples, Chomsky took apart the behaviorist claim that a child learning language is simply being conditioned to chain words together. He showed that merely responding in a consistent manner to an utterance is not the same thing as *understanding the meaning* of that utterance, and that a behaviorist approach could never explain the most important aspect of language: its *creativity*.

Speech language therapists have incorporated Chomsky's contributions to understanding the structure of language (rather than his genetic hypotheses). In addition, modern approaches build on the work of other pioneering contributions, including the work of Bloom on the meaning of language (Bloom, 1973; Bloom & Lahey, 1978), Brunner and Bates on the social function of language (Bruner, 1990); Bates 1976), as well as many others.

Going beyond notions that a child learns how to speak by stringing together a series of discrete behavioral units, or as the result of exposure to a linguistic stimulus, clinicians and researchers have shown that a child only develops the ability to construct language,

[2] Chomsky, N. (1959) A review of B. F. Skinner's verbal behavior. Language 35(1): 26-58.

including comprehension and production, on the basis of having mastered a number of stages of development (Tomasello, 2003). In addition, contemporary models of language acquisition embrace the notion that the development of language is embedded in and cannot be disassociated from developments in other domains such as social, affective, and cognitive development (Bloom & Tinker, 2001). A number of developmental stages have been described that incorporate these different domains of functioning and serve as the basis for language and thinking (Greenspan & Shanker, 2004). These include the capacities to attend to sounds and self regulate; engage in relationships characterized by shared affective vocal experience (e.g., synchronizing vocalizations); initiate and respond to communicative gestures and use them for shared social problem solving and to recognize and produce linguistic patterns; engage in sustained joint attentional frames; and understand a caregiver's communicative intentions.

Traditionally, the goals of a speech, language, and communication assessment include:

- Screening to identify children who have a high probability of developmental delay in speech, language, and communication abilities and need further assessment
- Diagnostic assessment to determine the existence of a communication delay or disability and to identify a child's strengths and challenges by using formal tests and informal assessment instruments
- Assessment for individual program planning to determine a child's mastery of skills as well as developmental and functional needs

In order to accomplish these goals, the clinical assessment of young children's speech, language, and communication development typically encompasses formal testing, structured and unstructured observations, and/or language and play sampling and analysis. In the most frequently used approach, standardized tests are administered to determine the percentile ranks and age-equivalents of the child. In most tests, the assessment of language is dichotomized into receptive and expressive language abilities, which are defined on the basis of a series of sub-tests. For example, in the Clinical Evaluation of Language Fundamentals (CELF), receptive language subtests include sentence structure, concepts/directions and basic concepts; expressive language subtests include word structure, expressive vocabulary, and recalling sentences. These skills are tapped during administration of tasks presented by the examiner to the child. Besides the receptive and expressive sections, the CELF includes a section referred to as the Descriptive Pragmatics Profile. Here, the clinician is asked to comment on the child's understanding and use of facial expressions, gestures, turn-taking, expressing affection, initiating conversations, maintaining attention when another person speaks, etc.

On the positive side, establishing a child's age equivalent of communicative and language functioning helps to determine whether a problem exists and the child's eligibility for services. However, this type of information in and of itself provides minimal direction for intervention planning or for supporting caregivers.

Alternative approaches to assessment, which are more directly tied to intervention planning, include procedures such as the Communication and Symbolic Behavior Scales

(CSBS) and language sampling and analysis. The CSBS is a norm-referenced, standardized tool which is used for evaluating the communication, social-affective, and symbolic abilities of children who are functioning between 8 months and 2 years of age. The speech-language pathologist takes a direct sampling of the child's communicative behaviors in structured and unstructured play situations in the child's natural environment. Various domains of development are assessed including communicative functions, gestural communicative means, vocal communicative means, verbal communicative means, reciprocity, social-affective signaling, and symbolic behavior.

Language sampling and analysis involves recording a language sample of the child during a natural play interaction with a familiar adult. This sample is transcribed and analyzed relative to the comprehension and production of the components of language including morphology, syntax, semantics, and pragmatics. The goal here is to determine what the child knows, in other words, to determine the developmental level of the child's language. Those clinicians who assess language in this way, also often assess the child's play development using a paradigm of symbolic play development. Developmental language and play intervention goals can be directly generated from these types of analysis.

The assessment of the child's phonological system, articulation, and oral motor abilities is a standard part of a speech and language evaluation.

The purpose that we are trying to accomplish by developing a more comprehensive developmental framework for assessing young children's speech, language, and communication is to broaden the perspective on what one looks at when one is assessing a child's language and communication development. We are interested in helping clinicians consider those aspects of language and communication development that more closely represent the process of language acquisition rather than the products of language acquisition. For example, we would like to see speech-language pathologists observe the child during interactions with his caregiver and based on this observation, make comments on the child's affective engagement, reciprocity, and shared meanings, rather than focusing primarily on his production of words and sentences and his articulation. The question that underlies the process of assessment is what is language and what developmental achievements contribute to the acquisition of the ability to express one's ideas and feelings with other people in meaningful, interactive exchanges. In this sense, the process of assessment being proposed here is completely in sync with what language is and how children use language in their daily interactions as they move up and through the developmental stages.

The three goals of language and communication assessment can be accomplished using the developmental language paradigm being proposed here depending on how well-versed the clinician is with the categories of development and the behaviors which typically define each category. Initially, we would encourage clinicians to use this framework for their own educational purposes, and as a macroanalysis of the child's functioning to determine areas requiring further assessment and/or diagnostic intervention.

The following pages presents a framework that describes six early levels of language functioning. These six levels are:

- **Self Regulation and Interest in the World** (or self regulation and interest in sounds) (0-3 months).
- **Forming Relationships and Affective Vocal Synchrony** (2-7 months).
- **Intentional Two-Way Communication** (8-12 months).
- **First Words: Sharing Meanings in Gestures and Words** (12-18 months).
- **Word Combinations – Sharing Experiences Symbolically** (18-24 months).
- **Early Discourse – Reciprocal Symbolic Interactions with Others** (24-36 months and beyond).

Each level is characterized in terms of seven modalities:

- **Shared Attention.** In the beginning, involves a child's ability to maintain a calm regulated state and, as the child develops, can use eye gaze, gestures and sound to coordinate attention, follow his caregiver's focus of attention, shift his gaze between people and objects, and coordinate attention for long period of time.
- **Affective Engagement.** In the beginning, refers to the infant's ability to regulate her internal state in order to maintain interaction, and as the child develops, to engage in back-and-forth affective exchanges that become increasingly complex, and can come to comprehend and express a variety of affective themes and states.
- **Reciprocity.** In the beginning, refers to the infant's ability to participate in basic interactions with caregiver when regulated, and, as the child develops, to participate in increasingly complex affective exchanges and use appropriate repair strategies when not understood.
- **Shared Intentions.** In the beginning, refers to the infant's ability to exhibit his readiness to engage and to provide clues - e.g., through facial expressions - about his internal state, and as the child develops, to respond to others intentions and express his own intentions in an increasingly complex manner.
- **Shared Forms and Meanings.** In the beginning, refers to the infant's ability to respond to her name and discriminate and express different affect states, and as the child develops, her increasingly subtle abilities to respond to and express a variety of affects, by the age of 2, to understand a number of words and to use 2-3 word combinations, and by the age of 3, to have mastered a number of linguistic constructions and initiate logical conversations to share ideas.
- **Sensory Processing and Audition.** In the beginning, refers to the infant's regulation of arousal states and responsiveness to sounds, and as the child develops, to engage in distal communication, attend to a number of different sounds, and by the age of 3, to comprehend, organize and communicate logically connected symbols as a multi-sensory affective experience.
- **Motor Planning, including Oral Motor Functioning.** In the beginning, refers to basic motor functions and the timing and rhythmicity of motor movements, and, as the child develops, become increasingly controlled and lead to complex pattern-recognition and production skills.

The framework presented in this section provides assistance for the clinician in constructing a detailed profile of the child's current level of functioning and the child's relative strengths and weaknesses in the different modalities that contribute to language functioning. It also provides a short-hand way of describing a child that goes significantly beyond current approaches to simply indicating the child's language age or whether or not there is an expressive or receptive disorder. The language picture or profile allows the clinician to choose an appropriate diagnosis that describes the child's specific needs and plan an appropriate intervention program.

A language disorder can be considered a primary diagnosis when a neurodevelopmental disorder of relating and communicating is ruled out. If a language problem accompanies a regulatory or interactive disorder, then it can serve as an additional diagnosis and justifies treatment of both or all disorders.

HOW TO SELECT THE APPROPRIATE DIAGNOSTIC SUMMARY STATEMENT AND CODE FOR LANGUAGE FUNCTIONING

The summary statements embodied in the diagnostic codes listed at the beginning of this section (401.1 - 406.3) characterize the different subtypes of language challenges. They indicate the developmental level or levels evidencing challenges and the clinician should refer to these codes in his or her summary narrative. They also provide an opportunity to note whether comprehension, production, or both are involved in the difficulties. The specific modalities that operate at each level are not listed in the diagnostic code, but should be described as part of the narrative and in the summary formulation. It is essential to identify challenges in terms of developmental levels and modalities because both are needed to plan a comprehensive, developmentally-based language intervention program.

To illustrate how the diagnostic codes may be employed, consider a child of 18 months. She evidences challenges in both comprehension and production only at the level of First Words: Sharing Meanings in Gestures and Words (not at earlier levels). This would be designated with the diagnostic code 404.3. If, however, she also evidenced challenges in both comprehension and production at the two prior levels (Intentional Two-Way Communication and Forming Relationships), then the appropriate codes would be 404.3, 403.3, and 402.3.

To enable the clinician to construct a diagnostic profile and formulation, and select an appropriate code, we have described each of these developmental levels of language functioning and the modalities operating at each level (see Table 1). This table is intended to enable the clinician to determine which levels have been mastered, which levels evidence challenges, as well as describe the specific modalities that require special attention. Two case illustrations follow at the end of this section to illustrate how the table is used.

For many clinicians, the developmental approach embodied in the following table is quite familiar and, perhaps, helpful in systematizing observations and other data. For some clinicians, this developmental approach may provide a relatively new way of understanding a child's language functioning. In either case, a critical attribute of this developmental approach is that it orients the observational and diagnostic processes toward identifying the developmental foundations for competent language functioning and for planning an intervention program that takes the critical building blocks of language into account.

Self-Regulation and Interest in the World (0-3 months)		
Modality	**Comprehension**	**Production**
Shared Attention	• Can maintain a calm, regulated state • Able to gaze at caregiver • Cries to indicate discomfort, hunger, displeasure • Reacts to sound and can turn head to caregiver's voice	
Affective Engagement	• Infant regulates internal state in order to maintain interaction • Infant able to vocalize vowels and use cooing to engage communicative partners • Participates in affective exchanges with caregiver (e.g., cooing, smiling, gazing)	
Reciprocity	• Reciprocity dependent on regulation • When regulated the infant can participate in basic interactions with caregiver (e.g., gazing, smiling, cooing)	
	• Responds to interaction of others (e.g., smiling, gazing)	• Initiates interaction with others (e.g. smiling, cooing, crying)
Shared Intentions	• Illustrates readiness to engage (e.g., smiling, gazing)	• Shares intentions by giving her communicative partner clues about her affect state (e.g., cooing, smiling, gazing, crying, etc.)
Sensory Processing and Audition	• Early regulation of arousal and physiological states to adapt to the environment • Recognizes caregiver's voice • Alerts to sound. Distracted by sound while nursing.	

[2] Material contributed by Sherri Cawn, M.A., CCC-SLP; Sima Gerber, Ph.D., CCC; Cindy Harrison, M.S.c., SLP; Diane Lewis, M.A., CCC-SLP; and Amy M. Wetherby, Ph.D., CCC-SLP

Self-Regulation and Interest in the World (0-3 months)		
Modality	**Comprehension**	**Production**
Motor Planning, Including Oral Motor Functioning	• Timing and rhythmicity of interactions and caregiver patterns play an important role in laying the foundation for regulation. • Food is primarily from the breast or bottle. Oral reflexes (e.g., rooting and suckling) are present and necessary for survival. • The jaw, tongue, and lips move as a unit. • Breathing is rapid and primarily abdominal.	

<table>
<tr><th colspan="3">Forming Relationships: Affective Vocal Synchrony (2-7 months)
(Note that some stages overlap in ages and some do not)</th></tr>
<tr><th>Modality</th><th>Comprehension</th><th>Production</th></tr>
<tr><td>Shared Attention</td><td colspan="2">• Is much more regulated and available for interaction
• Uses eye gaze with gestures, sounds, and words to coordinate attention
• Shifts gaze between people and objects</td></tr>
<tr><td>Affective Engagement</td><td colspan="2">• Regulates internal state
• Is able to tune in to the affect state of others using affect cues (e.g., smiles, frowns, angry voices etc.)
• Participates in affective exchanges with caregiver</td></tr>
<tr><td rowspan="2">Reciprocity</td><td colspan="2">• Participates in affective exchanges with caregiver (e.g., gazing, smiling, cooing, with simple consonants emerging at the end of this period)
• Vocalizations become part of two-way affective exchanges</td></tr>
<tr><td>• Responds to others' attempts to initiate interaction</td><td>• Initiates interaction with others using basic gestures (e.g., reaching, babbling, or cooing)</td></tr>
<tr><td>Shared Intentions</td><td>• Responds to others' intentions to regulate behavior and turns to caregiver for comfort
• Understands basic gestural repertoire of others and can begin to interpret his caregiver's affect state
• Begins to respond to others' intentions to draw attention to objects/toys</td><td>• Begins to express communicative intents (e.g., sadness, anger, happiness)
• Begins to develop a gestural repertoire (e.g., reaching, grabbing, scowling, smiling) to share intentions with others
• Uses basic gestures and facial expressions to express interest in people and favorite toys/objects</td></tr>
</table>

Forming Relationships: Affective Vocal Synchrony (2-7 months)
(Note that some stages overlap in ages and some do not)

Modality	Comprehension	Production
Shared Forms and Meanings	• Responds to name • Able to discriminate caregiver affect states (e.g., mad vs. happy)	• Shows emergence of joint attention • Vocalizes pleasure and displeasure • Varies volume and pitch of vocalizations
Sensory Processing and Audition	• Is able to localize sounds from further away • Is able to engage caregiver across space (e.g., get daddy's attention from across the room) • Attends to sounds around him. Comforted by mother's voice. May be comforted by music. May be distressed by loud sounds.	
Motor Planning, Including Oral Motor Functioning	• From 2 – 5 months, oral-motor functioning is very similar to what is seen in the latter portion of previous level • From 4 – 5 months, child starts to integrate the primitive reflexes as a result of developing more mature, true patterns of sucking and swallowing. • Around 5 – 6 months when child begins to sit and develop rotation along the body axis, the pattern of breathing slows down to one breath per second and the pattern shifts to abdominal/thoracic. • Begins to suck food from a spoon. • Begins babbling (combining consonants and vowels)	

<table>
<tr><th colspan="3">Intentional Two-Way Communication (8-12 months)</th></tr>
<tr><th>Modality</th><th>Comprehension</th><th>Production</th></tr>
<tr><td>Shared Attention</td><td colspan="2">• Follows caregiver's focus of attention
• Looks at people regularly
• Shifts gaze between people and objects</td></tr>
<tr><td>Affective Engagement</td><td colspan="2">• Engages with caregiver and responds to changes in caregiver's affect
• Shares and indicates positive and negative affective state
• Participates in back-and-forth affective exchanges with caregiver</td></tr>
<tr><td rowspan="2">Reciprocity</td><td colspan="2">• Participates in back-and-forth interactions with caregiver
• Uses repair strategies (e.g., can initiate additional gestures to be understood when not understood)</td></tr>
<tr><td>• Responds to interaction of others</td><td>• Solicits (i.e., initiates) interaction with others</td></tr>
<tr><td>Shared Intentions</td><td>• Responds to other's intentions to regulate behavior (e.g., responding to a "no-type" vocal tone or gesture or "give-it-to-me-type" vocal tone or gesture)
• Responds to others' intentions to draw attention to themselves (e.g., responding to Dad waving "bye-bye"; looks at Mom when she calls her name or uses an inviting vocal tone)
• Responds to others' intentions to draw attention to objects (e.g., looks at an interesting object that Mom holds up and shows; looks at what Mom points to in front of her)</td><td>• Expresses intentions with gestures and/or sounds to:
– Regulate behavior (e.g., reaches open hand to request bottle, pushes away, or shakes head to protest)
– Draw attention to self (e.g., reaches to Mom for comfort; tugs on Mom's pant leg to call her attention)
– Draw attention to objects of interest (e.g., holds up and shows interesting object; points to interesting event across room to direct attention to it)</td></tr>
</table>

Intentional Two-Way Communication (8-12 months)		
Modality	**Comprehension**	**Production**
Shared Forms and Meanings	• Responds to intonation, other forms of affective variation, facial expression and gestures • Toward latter part of this stage, responds to a few words or phrases in familiar contexts	• Uses intonation, consonant +vowel combinations, facial expressions, and gestures such as pointing, showing, and reaching • Imitates variety of identifiable actions and sounds spontaneously • Uses variety of objects conventionally • Uses variety of conventional gestures • By end of this period, child begins to produce early word approximations
Sensory Processing and Audition	• Localizes to caregiver's voice • Responds to name • Localizes to sound • Attends to loud and soft sounds • Attends and responds to speech and non-speech sounds • Shared attention to sound • Recognizes caregivers' voices • Recognizes intonation and tone of voice (e.g., happy, angry "No") • Attends to auditory stimuli for about 15 minutes • May be distressed by loud sounds	• Can look at and/or focus on caregiver's mouth and different vocal patterns • Responds to name and familiar words • Responds to some familiar commands (e.g., where's mommy, how big is the baby etc.) • Uses voice to get attention

<table>
<tr><th colspan="3">Intentional Two-Way Communication (8-12 months)</th></tr>
<tr><th>Modality</th><th>Comprehension</th><th>Production</th></tr>
<tr><td rowspan="2">Motor Planning, Including Oral Motor Functioning</td><td colspan="2">• Uses thumb and forefinger to pick up objects in a pincer-type grasp
• Tracks food using the eyes. Sits up in a high chair.
• Toward the end of this stage, holds the cup and spoon independently
• Begins to separate jaw movements from tongue and lip activity with the emergence of the more mature suck-swallow patterns
• Transfers food transferred from the side of the mouth to the center of the tongue and from the center of the tongue to the sides
• Eats finely chopped food and softer solid foods (e.g., crackers, cheese, etc.)
• Begins to suck from a straw
• Uses upper teeth to clean food from the lower lip
• Has more lip closure while swallowing liquids and solids
• Has well-controlled and graded bite with ability to control the force of biting through softer solid foods
• Toward the end of this stage, can use a straw to suck in liquids
• Shows sound production is progressing to longer, more complex strings of vowels and consonants, including jargon-like speech</td></tr>
<tr><td>• Focuses on caregivers’ motor and affective gestures</td><td>• Communicates with gestures, including sounds, across space
• Demonstrates motor behaviors to share intentions and emerging meanings</td></tr>
</table>

<table>
<tr><th colspan="3">First Words: Sharing Meanings in Gestures and Words (12-18 months)</th></tr>
<tr><th>Modality</th><th>Comprehension</th><th>Production</th></tr>
<tr><td>Shared Attention</td><td colspan="2">• Follows caregivers' focus of attention
• Uses eye gaze with gestures, sounds, and words to coordinate attention
• Shifts gaze between people and objects</td></tr>
<tr><td>Affective Engagement</td><td colspan="2">• Engages with caregiver and responds to changes in caregivers' affect
• Shares positive and negative affective state
• Participates in affective exchanges with caregiver EASILY</td></tr>
<tr><td rowspan="2">Reciprocity</td><td colspan="2">• Participates in circles of back-and-forth interactions over many turns with caregiver
• Uses repair strategies by adding gestures, sounds, words, or behavior when not understood</td></tr>
<tr><td>• Responds to familiar verbal and nonverbal bids for interaction</td><td>• Initiates interaction with others using gestures, sounds, and words</td></tr>
</table>

First Words: Sharing Meanings in Gestures and Words (12-18 months)		
Modality	**Comprehension**	**Production**
Shared Intentions	• Responds to others' intentions to regulate behavior (e.g., responds to "don't touch" said with a warning vocal tone or "get your bottle") • Responds to others' intentions to draw attention to themselves (e.g., responds to Mom saying "bye-bye" or "come give me a hug"; looks at other people who call their name) • Responds to others' intentions to draw attention to objects (e.g., looks at what Mommy has as she holds up an object; looks at what Mom points to behind him)	• Expresses intentions with gestures, sounds, and a small number words to: – Regulate behavior (e.g., says "baba" to request bottle; says "no" and shakes head to protest) – Draw attention to self e.g., (says "bye-bye" and waves or shows off to get someone to laugh) – Draw attention to objects of interest (e.g., uses a show or point gesture to get another person to look at an interesting object; shows a dog and says "doggie" for joy of sharing)
Shared Forms and Meanings	• Responds to intonation, facial expression, gestures, and other contextual cues • Responds to a variety familiar words and phrases in everyday contexts for a variety of meanings (e.g., object names, person names, body parts, action words) • Responds to name	• Uses varied intonation patterns and differentiated speech sounds to express meaning • Uses varied facial expressions and a variety of conventional gestures (e.g., pointing, showing and reaching) to express meaning • Spontaneously imitates a variety of familiar and new actions, sounds, and words • Uses 10 to 50 different words to express a variety of meanings (e.g., more, all gone, bye-bye, that, no, cookie, doggie, mommy, up, go) • Uses a variety of familiar objects conventionally when playing alone and with others

First Words: Sharing Meanings in Gestures and Words (12-18 months)		
Modality	**Comprehension**	**Production**
Sensory Processing and Audition	• Responds appropriately to loud and soft sounds • Attends and responds to familiar and unfamiliar speech and non-speech sounds • Recognizes and responds to caregiver's voice • Identifies some familiar objects using auditory cue alone (no visual or situational prompt) • Attends to unfamiliar sounds • Attends to soft sounds • May be distressed by unfamiliar sounds • Attends to auditory information consistently • Can be distracted from play when called	
Motor Planning, Including Oral Motor Functioning	• Has the motor capacity to share attention, affective engagement, and reciprocity (e.g., has adequate trunk support and coordination of movement to use facial expression, gestures, body orientation, sounds and words)	
		• Drinking skills become more refined. Can drink from a cup independently. Less spilling. • Movements of the jaw are more refined and are smoother and more coordinated during chewing. • Diagonal movements of the jaw during chewing. • A wider variety of foods and textures is introduced.

First Words: Sharing Meanings in Gestures and Words (12-18 months)		
Modality	**Comprehension**	**Production**
Motor Planning, Including Oral Motor Functioning		• The corners of the lips and cheeks assist in controlling food in the mouth. • The tip of the tongue can be lifted to the roof of the mouth independently. • Drooling is more controlled. • Feeds independently using fingers or a spoon. • Upper lip moves downward to contact the edge of the cup for drinking. • Swallowing occurs with lip closure and easy tongue-tip elevation • Speech is produced using all vowels and bilabial sounds /m/, /b/ and alveolar sounds /d/, /t/, /n/ and the /h/ sound. • Speech is generally intelligible by the end of this stage.

Word Combinations – Sharing Experiences Symbolically (18-24 Months)		
Modality	**Comprehension**	**Production**
Shared Attention	• Able to coordinate attention between the task and persons during activities, including many back-and-forth exchanges	
Affective Engagement	• The child sustains affective engagement over lengthy gestural and emerging verbal communicative interactions and a range of emotions. Emotions include positive and negative feelings, curiosity, flirtatiousness, seeking protection, etc.	
Reciprocity	• Is able to comprehend the cues of others in a continuous flow of back-and-forth interaction that is sustained (e.g., ability to continuously perceive communication cues including gestures and words of others as the basis for ongoing interaction).	• Takes the initiative and responds to communicative cues both gestural and verbal with the intent of influencing the behavior of the other person. This includes expressing his own novel wishes and desires.
Shared Intentions	• Responds to others' intentions to regulate behavior (e.g., responds to "don't touch" said with a warning vocal tone or "get your bottle") • Responds to others' intentions to draw attention to themselves (e.g., responds to Mom saying "bye-bye" or "come give me a hug"; looks at other people who call her name • Responds to others' intentions to draw attention to objects (e.g., looks at what Mommy has as she holds up an object; looks at what Mom points to behind him)	• Expresses intentions with many gestures, words, and word combinations to: – Regulate behavior (e.g., says "Gimme my bottle" to request bottle; says "No bedtime" or "Put me down" to protest) – Draw attention to self (e.g., says "bye-bye" and waves or showing off to get someone to laugh) – Draw attention to objects of interest (e.g., "Look my doggie" to get another person to look; asks "What's that?" while pointing to a picture in a book)
Shared Forms and Meanings	• Understands a growing number of words and phrases (100s) in everyday contexts across all semantic categories with helpful nonverbal cues • Understands and responds to routine forms of	• Coordinates varied intonation patterns, facial expressions, and conventional gestures with jargon and intelligible words to express meaning

Word Combinations – Sharing Experiences Symbolically (18-24 Months)		
Modality	**Comprehension**	**Production**
	"who" "what" and "where questions • Comprehends a variety of instructions with two to three words, (e.g., "Get your shoes") • Understands word combinations with meaning, such as "agent + actions," "agent/action + location," "agent + attribute" • Understands "me/mine" • By age 2, understands words and phrases without significant contextual cues, i.e., only words, vocal, and facial expression	• Obvious increase in vocabulary growth to express a variety of meanings (e.g., agent, action, attribute, possession, location) • Uses 2-3 word combinations to express a range of meanings (e.g., "More cookie," "Baby all gone," "That doggie," "No night night," "Mommy go outside") • Asks questions with rising intonation ("What's that?" or "Doggie?") • Engages in simple pretend play with short sequences of actions about familiar routines
Sensory Processing and Audition	• Integrates sensory experience in order to comprehend and construct multi-sensory affective symbols. Modulates sensation (i.e., is not overwhelmed by sensory reactivity). • Responds to "Show me____________" for body parts • Identifies some familiar objects using auditory cue alone, with no visual or situational prompt • Attends to soft sounds • Attends to unfamiliar sounds • May be distressed by unfamiliar sounds • Can be distracted from playing when called	

Word Combinations – Sharing Experiences Symbolically (18-24 Months)		
Modality	**Comprehension**	**Production**
Motor Planning, Including Oral Motor Functioning	• Is able to focus on and comprehend relationships among a number of actions or sequences (i.e., perceive patterns). For example, can search for objects hidden in different areas of the room and understand novel situations. Language builds on understanding of the world in terms of patterns rather than discrete skill sets.	• Is able to carry out the pattern. Can execute early two-part pretend sequences, such as putting something in a location and taking it somewhere • Has skilled eating patterns, with eating occurring independently • Uses the tongue to clean the lips. • Uses the tongue and cheeks to transfer food across the midline of the mouth. • Continues refinement of feeding

Early Discourse – Reciprocal Symbolic Interactions with Others (24-36 Months and Beyond)		
Modality	**Comprehension**	**Production**
Shared Attention	• The child is able to coordinate attention with another person for long periods of time, while working on activities, enjoying play, exchanging ideas.	
Affective Engagement	• Can comprehend a variety of affective states symbolically during interactions and play with words as well as with gestures	• Can express a wide variety of affective themes and states (e.g., dependency, curiosity, power, anger, cooperation, etc.) during interactions and play
Reciprocity	• Responds to gestures and words of another during talking, social interactions and play around a range of emotional themes with logical bridges between the child and caregiver's communication in conversations and play. That is, reciprocity is now making logical symbolic sense. Reciprocity extends beyond small islands and into longer logical chains.	• Initiates long chains of reciprocal interactions using words and gestures
Shared Intentions	• Responds to a range of intentions expressed by others • Responds to requests for information about the "here and now" and the "not here and now" • Responds to requests for confirmation or clarification to repair • Responds to peers' social bids to plan and negotiate	• Expresses a range of intentions with an increasing variety of gestures, word combinations, and sentences • Requests information about the "here and now" the "not here and now," and later about what someone else has said • Requests confirmation or clarification to repair • Provides or reports information about past and future events • Makes plans and negotiates with peers

Early Discourse – Reciprocal Symbolic Interactions with Others (24-36 Months and Beyond)		
Modality	**Comprehension**	**Production**
Shared Forms and Meanings	• Understands a growing number of words (from several hundred to several 1000 words) and phrases that are not in the "here and now" • Understands a greater range of who, what, and where question forms • Understands and responds to simple, causal "why?" questions, e.g., "Why is your face all dirty?" • Comprehends more complex direction such as "Get the bottle and put it in the refrigerator," "Before you get your shoes, put on your socks" • Understands three-term relations such as agent-action-object (e.g., "The dog is eating the bone" by age 3 • Understands less predictable directions such as "The dog is riding in the car" • Understands locatives (e.g., in, on, under, behind, next to, in front of) • Comprehends grammatical morphemes including: present progressive (ing); plural (s); possessive ('s); irregular past (came, went) • Understands more complex syntactic relations, such as temporal causal, and additive • By late in this stage, understands a variety of sentence constructions such as declarative, interrogative, imperative and complex sentences • Understands the make-believe of the other person when pretending in play about less familiar routines (birthday party, doctor's office)	• Coordinates varied intonation patterns, facial expressions and conventional gestures with word combinations and sentences • Uses word combinations and subject-verb-object structures to express a variety of meanings (e.g., "That's a bike," "I go car," "I want book," "Baby up there," "Mommy eat a cookie") • Produces coordinated meanings (e.g., "I wanna go outside," "That's the baby's bike," "Mommy's eating a big cookie") • Later, produces successive clauses, conjunctions, (e.g., and, so, because) to form complex sentences and eventually sentence complements (e.g., "I don't know what color," "Look what I found," "I want Mommy to get up," "Mommy's eating cookie and I want one," "I wanna go outside cause it's hot" • Asks questions such as: "What's that?" "Who's that?" "Where man go?" and later "What's he doing?" "Why?" "Why is he crying?" • Morphemes such as plural "s" (boats), "ing" (running), possessive " 's" (mommy's shoe); irregular past, (ate, came) and third person "s" (baby eats), articles (a, the), regular past "-ed" (jumped); "is" (This is red) • Engages in more complex play with longer sequences of actions around less familiar events. Begins to take on familiar characters such as mommy, baby and dog.

<table>
<tr><th colspan="3">Early Discourse – Reciprocal Symbolic Interactions with Others (24-36 Months and Beyond)</th></tr>
<tr><th>Modality</th><th>Comprehension</th><th>Production</th></tr>
<tr><td>Emerging Discourse</td><td colspan="2">• Shows increasing ability to initiate topics in conversation
• Uses more contingent utterances that relate and begin to add to prior utterances
• Shows increasing ability to maintain topics by adding new information
• Begins to adapt to the listener with intonation, polite words (e.g., please, thank you) and “baby talk” to younger children</td></tr>
<tr><td>Sensory Processing and Audition</td><td>• Is able to comprehend, organize and communicate emerging symbols and logically connected symbols as a multi-sensory affective experience without becoming compromised or distracted by challenges in sensory reactivity. Experiences can be described by their many features (e.g., a dog by its bark, body shape, etc.)</td><td>• Identifies familiar pictures, objects, body parts using auditory cue alone, with no visual or situational prompt. Consistently attends to sound. Responds when called from a distance. Responds when called when there is competing noise. Can participate in conversation when there is competing noise.</td></tr>
<tr><td>Motor Planning, Including Oral Motor Functioning</td><td>• Shows ability to gradually comprehend logical connections in the sequences of symbolic play and to follow the sequences of ideas in the play as well as in a short conversation.</td><td>• Is able to execute motor sequences related to symbolic, language production. Can maintain his portion of the conversation. Can verbalize action sequences.
• Uses the tongue to clean cheek pockets, between gums and teeth
• Grades jaw opening according to the thickness of food presented
• Moves jaw up and down and in a circular rotary pattern
• Is able to eat wide variety of regular foods.</td></tr>
</table>

Case Illustration of a Child with Language Challenges

History and Concerns

Janie was referred to this clinician by her mother who was concerned that Janie "is not talking." Janie, now 26 months, attended the evaluation with her mother, Diane.

Diane reported that she had an unremarkable pregnancy with an uncomplicated vaginal delivery. She also reported that Janie had significant difficulties with breast feeding, and following a number of consultations with lactation consultants, Janie's parents decided to stop breastfeeding and to move to formula. Janie's mom reported that while they had more success bottle feeding, they "had to use many different nipples to find one that worked, and even then her daughter found eating really tiring."

Diane reported that Janie was a very placid baby who rarely fussed, was easygoing and was "content to entertain herself most of the time." Janie's parents began to have concerns when they noticed that Janie would "squeeze her eyes shut" for significant portions of the day. When they addressed these concerns with their pediatrician, they were referred to a pediatric ophthalmologist who determined that she had severe strabismus in her right eye. Surgery was the recommended course of treatment; however, it could not be scheduled until Janie was 7 months old. The surgery was successful and Janie's mother reported that she and her husband noticed Janie focusing on objects and on people with greater consistency.

When Janie was 6 months old, her parents became concerned that she was not meeting developmental milestones at the same rate as her infant cousins or her peers. When they addressed these concerns with her pediatrician, they were told that they "should not worry" and that they "should not compare Janie with other children."

At 8 months, Janie's parents approached the pediatrician again. The pediatrician remained unconcerned about Janie's development. Shortly after Janie's first birthday, her parent's sought the opinion of a developmental pediatrician who immediately referred her to the local children's hospital for a complete evaluation. This evaluation identified significant delays in the following areas: speech/language and communication, fine and gross motor skills, and cognition. Janie was placed on a waiting list for therapy. Her parents were not given any guidance specific to programming for Janie at home.

When Janie was 23 months old, her parents became increasingly frustrated and decided to seek private services for their daughter. They attended an evaluation with a practicing DIR speech language pathologist and a practicing DIR occupational therapist.

Sensory and Regulatory Profile

Sensory Reactivity

Janie presents with a mixed pattern of reactivity. Her predominant pattern is underreactive with difficulties in modulation. Janie was observed to shut down when overwhelmed during the evaluation and would lie down on the mat in the therapy room and close her eyes. It was observed that Janie had a tendency to become overwhelmed when her environment was "visually noisy." It is likely this is related to the visual difficulties she experienced as an infant. Janie's hypotonia and motor planning challenges appear to have made a significant impact on her regulatory profile.

Motor Planning

Low muscle tone, poor visual motor integration, and poor processing of vestibular information made it challenging for Janie to reach for toys, co-ordinate shifts in gaze, etc. Janie was observed to become disorganized when she was required to plan more than one step. For example, she picked up a toy, gazed at it and then dropped it. During this session, Janie's ability to motor plan was positively affected if her play partner guided her (e.g., her mom held out her hand with an expectant look and said, "Give it to Mommy!"), and if she was given significant time to mount a response.

Oral Motor

Janie explores toys and objects orally and according to her mother "is always shoving things in her mouth." Low muscle tone, motor planning challenges and poor trunk control all impact negatively on oral motor abilities. Janie's mom reports that she has a very limited diet, gags frequently, is texture sensitive, and often has "food falling out of her mouth." She demonstrates a preference for crunchy, salty foods and attempts to limit her diet to these types of foods.

Visuospatial and Visual Motor Processing

Janie's occupational therapist reports that she has significant challenges in this regard. Janie's mom reported that her daughter "spent the first 6 months of her life with her eyes shut because her strabismus made it so unpleasant to look at anything."

Auditory Processing

This appears to be an area of relative strength for Janie. She was observed to track items auditorally and would frequently look for the toy that was making noise. She was interested in toys and noisemakers in the evaluation room and was able to hand her mother a drum stick to have her bang on a drum. When Janie's mom stopped banging, Janie vocalized and looked expectantly at her mom as if to say, "More, Mommy." Janie's mother reports that Janie "loves to listen to music and loves it when I play our toy instruments."

Speech, Language, and Communication

During the evaluation for Janie, the clinician utilized the Diagnostic Framework to provide a summary of Janie's strengths and challenges in the areas of speech, language, and communication. The following observations were made.

Self-Regulation and Interest in the World

Shared Attention

Janie is able to maintain a calm, regulated state for periods of time. Janie's mother describes her as a "very good baby" who "really never fussed very much." Observation of Janie interacting with her mother revealed a toddler who has a tendency towards under-reactivity. She was observed to gaze at her mother; however, this was somewhat fleeting. Janie's mother reports that Janie did not really develop the "differentiated cry that I saw with my older child" and that it was often difficult for her to determine whether Janie needed food, changing, or comfort.

Affective Engagement

Janie was observed to engage in affective exchanges with her mother (e.g., looking at her, smiling, sound play, etc.). It is significant that Janie's ability to sustain affective engagement is constricted by her tendency to under-reactivity and challenges with visual motor integration and motor planning. Often, her mother would be unsuccessful in keeping her engaged in affective exchanges beyond one or two circles of communication.

Reciprocity

Janie's ability to be reciprocal appears very much dependent on her regulation. Janie's mother was observed to be skillful in interacting with Janie in a way that addressed Janie's tendency toward under-reactivity and self-absorption. Janie was a better "responder" to her mother's attempts to engage in affective exchanges (e.g., smiling back at mommy) than she was an "initiator." It is likely that this is due, in part, to her challenges with motor planning. Janie also did not readily initiate the affective exchange. This is due, in part, to her tendency towards under-reactivity, but also in part to significant motor planning issues.

Shared Intentions

Janie's affect cueing system was observed to be constricted. Her mother reports that "since she never really gets emphatic about anything, it can be kind of tough to know what she wants." Janie was observed to illustrate more robust clues as to her affective state when she was happy (e.g., smiling, laughing) than when she was unhappy.

Motor Planning

This was observed to be an area of challenge for Janie. She was observed to struggle with the timing and rhythm of interactions. Janie's mother was skillful at recognizing when Janie had "dropped out" on an interaction and would work to re-engage her. The occupational therapist working with Janie reported that even when Janie was calm, regulated (not under-reactive), and engaged, her significant motor planning challenges had an impact on her ability to respond to the affect cues of others and to give clues about her own affective state.

Forming Relationships/Affective Vocal Synchrony

Shared Attention

Janie's availability for interaction is constricted by her sensory profile (tendency to under-reactivity), and motor planning challenges (often by the time she mobilizes in order to engage in interaction, the moment has passed). These issues also have an impact on her ability to be reciprocal and to engage in affective exchanges with her communication partner. In turn, this affects Janie's ability to gain the experiential learning that flows from this reciprocity and engagement. As a result of her challenges at the lower developmental levels and in motor planning, Janie must work very hard to engage with her communication partner. It is through this engagement and through reciprocity that shared intentions, (e.g., responding to and beginning to express communicative intents) and shared forms and meanings (e.g., responding to name, joint attention) begin to develop. Compared to a typically developing child, Janie does not have the richness of experience in this regard.

Shared Intentions

Janie's mother describes her as "extremely easy-going and independent." She reports that Janie does not often seek her out for comfort or hugs but does seek her out when she is hungry. Janie's mother reports that Janie does not fuss when she is tired, but is more likely "to lie down on the floor to go to sleep." It is significant that Janie demonstrated some ability to respond to her mother's basic gestural repertoire (e.g., when her mom held out her arms and said "Hug, please," Janie responded by giving her mother a hug). Janie was not observed to respond to other gestures such as her mother shaking her head "no" and say "uh uh" when Janie was about to touch something that she should not be touching. Janie did not respond to her mother's attempts to draw her attention to toys and objects.

During the evaluation Janie was observed to express happiness on a few occasions such as when her mom played the toy drum. Janie was observed to smile, laugh, and clap, but would then quickly become overwhelmed and would move away from the play area. Again, Janie's sensory system interfered with her ability to "stay in the play" and to be reciprocal around a favorite activity.

Shared Forms and Meanings

Janie was observed to respond to her name; however, this was inconsistent. She did not demonstrate the ability to discriminate between the affect state of her mom (e.g., when mom changed her tone and inflection to say "No!" when Janie was about to pull an electrical cord out of the socket). Janie was observed to vocalize pleasure when her mom was playing with the drum, but was not observed to express displeasure. Janie's mom did report, however, that Janie has begun to fuss a little at night when it is time for bed and that "she would rather be up playing than sleeping." Janie was observed to utilize the same cvcv (/baba/) for all labels. Little variation in volume and pitch of vocalizations was observed during the evaluation. Janie's mom reports that she sometimes engages in babbling at home.

Sensory Processing and Audition

Janie was able to localize sounds from further away. For example, when the clinician turned on the video camera, Janie immediately looked up, identified the source of the whirring noise and moved across the room to look at the camera. Interestingly, Janie was also observed to respond to sounds, music, and noise with greater consistency than her response to voice. She did, however, work to get the clinician's attention when the video camera was turned off and she wanted it to be turned on again. This appears to be a relative strength for Janie.

Intentional Two-Way Communication

Shared Attention

Janie demonstrated significant challenges in her ability to follow the gaze of her caregiver, and to shift her gaze between people and objects. She was observed to glance at her mother during play, but that was fleeting.

Affective Engagement

Again, Janie was observed to interact with her play partner, however, this typically required support like engaging in sensory play to buffer her tendency to under-reactivity. With coaching, Janie's mom was able to amend her interactions with Janie (e.g., high affect, using voice to catch her attention, giving Janie time to respond, etc.) to address her individual differences. During these interactions Janie's affective interaction improved significantly.

Reciprocity

As noted previously, Janie is a better responder than an initiator. This improved when her play partners were mildly playfully obstructive regarding objects and games that Janie likes (e.g., singing "Zoom Zoom" and pausing so that Janie would request that the song continue).

Shared Intentions

As previously noted, this is an area of challenge for Janie. Again, if Janie's play partners approached her with high affect and focused on areas of interest for Janie, she was able to demonstrate the following intentions: to request a noisemaker by banging on the container that holds the instruments; to protest by pushing mom's hand away when mom attempted to wipe Janie's nose; to draw attention to an object by vocalizing and referencing this clinician when the video camera was turned off. Janie continued this until the camera was turned back on and then she smiled and moved away.

Shared Forms and Meanings

As previously noted, Janie was observed to utilize a cvcv vocalization to call attention to a favorite object (e.g., the video camera). No other indicators appropriate to shared forms and meaning were noted during the evaluation.

Comments

Janie, a 26-month-old girl, is demonstrating significant delays in speech, language, and communication. These challenges appear to be related to her sensory profile, motor planning challenges, and challenges in comprehension and production of language.

During the evaluation, Janie was observed to demonstrate skills at the first three levels of communication (i.e., self regulation and interest in the world, forming relationships - affective vocal synchrony and intentional two-way communication). It is important to note that there were constrictions at each of the above levels.

The Diagnostic Framework

While this diagnostic framework is not intended to be used as a standardized method of evaluation, it does assist the clinician in determining not only where the strengths and challenges lie, but also the degree of presence or absence of these challenges. It draws attention not just to the absence or presence of the skill, but the degree to which the skill is present and under which circumstances. This is a valuable indicator as it can inform and guide the treatment plan.

In Janie's case, the diagnostic framework allows the clinician to identify the aspects of the individual profile and the impact of each of these areas on the development of speech, language, and communication. It informs the work of the clinician by drawing attention to the challenges at the earlier levels of speech language and communication development and their impact on higher levels. For example, Janie's motor planning challenges make it difficult for her to respond in a rapid and continuous manner when her play partner attempts to engage her. This makes it very difficult for Janie to enter into continuous back and forth affective exchanges.

Intervention Program

The diagnostic framework also informs the treatment plan in that treatment goals can be established that follow a developmental sequence and that focus on addressing the individual differences within that developmental sequence.

To illustrate this point, the following treatment goals were established for Janie:

- To provide coaching and support to Janie's play partners to encourage them to use high affect to lure Janie in (e.g., since Janie loves noisemakers, try placing

favorite noisemakers on their heads or in their mouths to encourage her to look at them and to attempt to retrieve the toy. This can lead to back-and-forth games where Janie gets the noisemaker and they playfully get it back so that she can attempt to get it again
- To focus on keeping Janie engaged with her play partner for significant periods of time by approaching her in a way that addresses her individual differences - sensory play, noisemakers, positioning himself so that he is in front of her, giving her time to respond, decreasing the load on her visual system by not moving rapidly while communicating with her, etc.
- To provide coaching to Janie's play partner to be sure to give her significant periods of time to respond, but to stay connected to her during this time in an effort to prevent her from dropping out of the interaction
- To enhance communicative intent by utilizing favorite games, sensory play, and high affect toys/objects
- To strengthen Janie's non-verbal, gestural communication, both in production and comprehension

Summary

Janie, a 26-month-old girl is presenting with a significant speech, language, and communication delay. A typically developing child of this age would have mastered word combinations (Level 5) and would be demonstrating skills in the early levels of Level 6 -Early Discourse. At present, Janie is demonstrating skills at the first three developmental levels of communication.

It is important to note that Janie has a very supportive family that is committed to a developmental course of treatment. Based on observations of Janie and her mother, and the impact of the changes the mother was able to make with coaching, it is expected that Janie will continue to move up the developmental ladder.

The ICDL-DMIC diagnostic codes that would summarize Janie's language disorder indicate compromises in language functioning (both comprehension and production) at her expected age level and all prior levels, with partial mastery of some skills at the first three levels. Therefore, Janie evidences a Language Disorder with compromises in:

- Word Combinations: Sharing Experiences Symbolically (in both comprehension and production) - 405.3
- First Words: Sharing Meanings in Gestures and Words (in both comprehension and production) - 404.3
- Intentional Two-Way Communication (in both comprehension and production) - 403.3
- Forming Relationships: Affective Vocal Synchrony - 402.3
- Self-Regulation and Interest in the World - 401.3

Contributed by: Cindy Harrison, M.Sc., SLP, Reg. CASLPO

Case Illustration of a Language Disorder

Background Information

Rachel, a 16 month-old girl, was born full term via Caesarian Section and is the first child in an intact family. Rachel's mother was on bed rest for her entire pregnancy due to orthostatic/postural hypertension. No complications were reported during delivery. Rachel remained in hospital for six days due to a diagnosis of jaundice.

Rachel was diagnosed with reflux which lasted until she was 9-10 months old. She was put on Prevacid and Reglan to help with reflux symptoms and was slow to gain weight during this period. No extraordinary medical illnesses were reported.

Motor milestones were reported to be within normal limits, but mother reports that Rachel stopped babbling between 4-5 months old. A formal auditory assessment was done at that time and revealed normal range for hearing sensitivity bilaterally.

When she was 8½ months old Rachel was evaluated at this clinic for reflux and feeding difficulties. First impressions revealed an adorable baby who had an under responsive response to affective engagement. She was visually curious with a very slow reaction to auditory-verbal language. Her affect was neutral with a somewhat confused look on her face.

It was difficult for her parents to have continuous reciprocal exchanges with their daughter and no vocalizations were recorded at all during the initial visit. The family was seen and parents were told about and then coached on using DIR/Floortime and encouraged to use this approach at home.

After several months, a meeting with the family resulted in increasing Rachel's' therapy time to a weekly appointment where more time could be devoted to parent training and individual speech therapy sessions. Although repeated concerns were raised about her under-responsivity, Rachel's parents were not ready to have an OT evaluation done at that time.

At one year of age the *Rossetti-Infant Toddler Scale* was administered to Rachel with her mother as the respondent. Results indicated that at Rachel's receptive language skills fell between 6-8 months (with scatter above and below that) and her expressive language fell between 3-6 months (with scatter here as well).

Additionally, parts of the CSBS (Wetherby, Prizant, 1993) were informally incorporated into the assessment. Rachel demonstrated an underdeveloped ability to gaze shift or share positive affect. Her ability to follow a gaze point was judged to be emergent.

Rachel's frequency of communication acts was judged to be constricted with minimal social interaction and joint attention observed. Conventional gestures were judged to be in emergent development with pointing and giving the most consistent. Distal gesturing was not recorded during that session at all.

Rachel's lack of vowel + consonants or a differentiated inventory of consonants was significantly depressed. Furthermore, vocalizations were not paired with communicative acts. Rachel's comprehension skill was observed during book reading with her mother asking where something was located in the book and Rachel pointing to the correct picture. No generalization of picture identification was observed to familiar toys in the therapy room. Rachel was able to perform several action schemes (e.g., feed the baby, blow bubbles and roll a ball), but no other use of objects was observed.

Rachel's parents contacted the early intervention program several months ago. According to the results of their evaluation, Rachel qualified for occupational and speech therapy. It is interesting to note that the speech and language evaluation results concluded that Rachel's receptive language skills were within normal limits for her age.

Using the dynamic developmental speech and language assessment, Rachel's receptive and expressive communication skills were described using the developmental levels and modalities as follows.

I. Self Regulation and Interest in the World: Shared Attention

Shared Attention and Affective Engagement

Due to Rachel's under-reactivity, it is difficult to see what is and what is not dysregulation. Although she cries when she is in discomfort or unhappy, she is able to recover quickly. She is able to have a brief interaction with her parents and therapists.

Reciprocity/Shared Intentions

Rachel does not typically get dysregulated for extended periods of time. She responds to others in her environment with a smile and a gaze, but is unable to sustain the interaction.

Sensory Processing and Audition

Rachel presents as under-responsive to auditory-verbal stimuli, as well as non-verbal gestures and affective signals. However, she is over-responsive to movement across space and visual stimuli (e.g., people, objects, small pieces on the floor). She alerts to sound and to her mother's voice. Her vestibular process appears to be underdeveloped especially in the area of swinging, and climbing equipment.

Motor Planning and Oral Motor Functioning

Timing and rhythmicity have been challenging since Rachel began at this clinic. Rachel's mother has to work very hard to get Rachel to share attention which usually involves throwing her in the air.

II. Forming Relationships and Affective Vocal Synchrony

Shared Attention and Affective Engagement

Rachel is challenged in her ability to sustain visual gaze with gestures, sounds and words. She does not consistently tune in to the affect of others. She is able to return a smile but not continue with the affective engagement.

Reciprocity

Rachel can respond to simple reciprocal exchanges and can initiate with a smile. Recently she has begun to laugh with the therapist when she playfully obstructs their interaction. This has taken several months to establish.

Shared Intention

At the level of comprehension Rachel turns to her mother for comfort and appears to have emergent understanding of the intentions of another. There has been brief awareness to respond to another's intention around an object or a toy (e.g., books, Sesame Street characters).

At the expressive language level, Rachel is able to demonstrate the non-verbal gestures and affects of pointing and smiling to share her intentions with her parents and therapists. At this time, she does not demonstrate a wide range of affects (e.g., happiness, frustration, etc.).

Shared Meanings

At the level of comprehension Rachel consistently responds to her name. Her mother reports that she does not respond to reprimands ("no, no, don't touch!").

At the level of production, Rachel does not demonstrate joint attention. Her parents have been coached regarding the concept of joining her as opposed to teaching her, yet both parents tend to be more directive toward her in their interactive styles. Recently Rachel has begun to vocalize pleasure and displeasure.

Regulatory-Sensory Processing and Audition

Rachel's sensory processing continues to be a concern. Earlier in treatment she was not able to localize sounds in the environment. Over the past 6 weeks she has begun to engage her mom across space and is comforted by her mother's voice. She does not get distressed by loud sounds but responds less to verbal language when she's in a noisy environment (e.g., big gym at the clinic).

Motor Planning

Rachel has difficulty organizing and sequencing her affective responses. Although she is responsive to her caregiver and therapist, she cannot persist with an interaction. She does not move away from people and often cannot remain connected with them.

Rachel's minimal sound development, as well as her limited vocalizations, are of significant concern. While she is able to vocalize pleasure and displeasure she does so with limited variations of sounds. Recently she began vocalizing with some bilabial sound patterns ("up," "moo," "baa").

Very few early developing consonants have been recorded. Her mother reports a small increase in her sound play at home. Very little imitation has been observed in therapy or reported by her mother. Rachel prefers open syllable sequences (such as "baa," "up," "moo," and "neigh").

III. Intentional Two-Way Communication

Shared Attention

Rachel can follow a caregiver's focus of attention for a brief period of time. She is able to shift between people, but she is not able to shift between people and objects.

Affective Engagement

Rachel is able to share both positive and negative behavior for brief periods of time, but not in back-and-forth exchanges.

Reciprocity

At the level of comprehension, Rachel is able to respond to others but she is better when some distance is between herself and her mother. Mother is able to get some back and forth interactions when she rough houses with Rachel (e.g., throwing her up in the air or piggy back rides).

Rachel's mother has taught her some sign language. At this time, Rachel is able to sign "drink," "more," "eat," "open" and "all done." However, if Mom does not prompt her, Rachel does not use the signs. Her mother often says, "Rachel show me what you want."

At the level of production, Rachel uses some gestures (e.g., pointing, giving) spontaneously, but Mom cues her frequently using words and signs to try to understand her intentions. Rachel is unable to pair a sign with a social reference even when prompted to sign to do so.

At times Rachel is able to initiate an interaction with others but it usually to request something, such as reaching a toy, or reading a book. It is difficult to engage her in joint activity routines.

Shared Intentions

At the level of comprehension, Rachel is occasionally able to respond to her mother's intentions to regulate her behavior, draw attention to herself or to an object. However, there is a significant delay in her response.

At the level of expression, Rachel is able to use simple non-verbal gestures to signal to her mother when she wants to be picked up (she's now using the word "up"), and to bring her mother a toy or a book. When she brings a toy over to show her mother she usually drops it into her lap. When she wants a book read she hands it to her mother and then sit down in her mom's lap. This is not accompanied by a social reference or affective engagement.

Shared Meanings

At the level of comprehension, Rachel responds to high affect and big gestures. It takes longer for her to respond appropriately to more neutral or negative affect. She can become fussy if a toy is removed but recovers in less than 10 seconds. She has recently demonstrated consistent response to simple environmental questions ("come here," "get your shoes," "bring me the book," "let's dance").

At the level of expression, Rachel is demonstrating some underdeveloped skills. Her use of intonation and consonant vowel combinations are underdeveloped. She is able to demonstrate pointing, showing and reaching but these are recent developments (not emerging until after 12 months of age).

Rachel's ability to imitate is also underdeveloped, although she is able to imitate signs and use them when there is an external verbal prompt. She does not respond to high affective verbal responses like "oh-oh," "Oh-No," and "Oops."

She explores toys but does not play with them in the conventional sense. If her mother asks her to feed the baby or give Elmo a drink, she responds appropriately.

Regulatory-Sensory Processing and Audition

Rachel continues to have mixed reactivity to background noise. She is easily distracted by movement and visual objects. She is under-responsive to non-verbal, gestural and verbal language. She is able to attend to music for short periods of time, but does not imitate or turn to familiar children's songs. Very little distress is ever noted to loud background noise. She is more dysregulated by visual movement.

At the expressive language level, Rachel does not attend to her mother's mouth when she's talking. Mom and Rachel do play in the mirror with very little imitation.

Rachel responds to her name, familiar words and familiar commands. She does not use her voice to get attention except when she is upset. Rachel's mother reports that she does not call her when she awakens in the morning or from a nap.

Motor Planning and Oral-Motor Functioning

Rachel is not able to sequence and organize gestures, affect and vocalizations to sustain social engagement for long periods of time.

Rachel's early history of minimal babbling certainly raises the concern that she might be challenged in the area of expressive language. Whereas Rachel is able to respond to some affective gestures, she certainly is below expectations for her age at this time

At the level of expression there is significant concern about her lack of development of differentiated sound progression, as well as her ability to use motor behavior—both verbal and non verbal—to share intentions. In addition there has been minimal progress in her use of jargon as well as an increase in consonant use.

Rachel's feeding skills appear to be progressing within developmental age criteria.

Diagnostic Impressions

While based on her age, Rachel would be expected to be mastering the fourth stage in language development - First Words: Sharing Meanings in Gestures and Words - she has not yet reached this level. She is working on overcoming challenges in the first three levels of language development. In the narrative we've described Rachel's language patterns in terms of her strengths and challenges at each of these stages. It is also useful to consider her profile in the context of the diagnostic summary statements and codes for language functioning in the ICDL-DMIC. The appropriate codes for this child would be Language Disorder with compromises in:

- First Words: Sharing Meanings in Gestures and Words (comprehension and production) - 404.3
- Intentional Two-Way Communication (comprehension and production) - 403.3
- Forming Relationships: Affective Vocal Synchrony (comprehension and production) - 402.3

Recommendations

1. Continue to mobilize her intentions while maintaining reciprocity.
2. Expand communicative intentions to include possession, attribution, action and action-relations.
3. Continue to encourage playful interactions that support intentionality but are mindful of specific vulnerabilities, i.e., auditory processing and motor planning.

4. To expand ability to code relations between objects and emerging syntax.
5. To increase conceptual and lexical knowledge relative to environmental experiences.
6. To be aware of phonological processes and oral-motor vulnerabilities that
7. are decreasing intelligibility and begin to support them in a more formal process.
8. To continue to strengthen and build sound repertoire.

Within the context of speech and language therapy the following Floortime goals have been established:

1. Continue to maintain mutual engagement while in an affective state (excitement, disappointment, fear, worry, etc.).
2. Continue to support, and embrace a variety of affective states while in an interaction.
3. Continue to encourage sensory games where she is able to tolerate and enjoy the role of being "done to" and not always the "do-er."
4. Increase the number of communicative circles regarding a specific idea that takes into account both non-verbal gestures and verbal language.
5. Continue to support pre-symbolic behaviors in light of her motor planning issues.
6. Continue to encourage initiation, but at the same time support Rachel's ability to maintain an interaction while understanding simple causal relationships (e.g., getting hurt, making a birthday cake, car out of gas).
7. Continue to create problems to solve while supporting flexibility in play particularly in light of motor planning issues.

Contributed by: Sherri Cawn, MA, CCC-SLP

Axis I: Learning Challenges[1]

500. Learning Challenges

Emerging Learning Challenges with compromises in

501. Functional Emotional Developmental Capacities
502. Auditory Processing and Language
503. Visuospatial Capacities
504. Regulatory-Sensory Processing Patterns
505. A Combination of the Above Areas

Early Challenges in Reading and Language Arts with compromises in

506. Functional Emotional Developmental Capacities
507. Auditory Processing and Language
508. Visuospatial Capacities
509. Regulatory-Sensory Processing Patterns
510. A Combination of the Above Areas

Early Challenges in Math with compromises in

511. Functional Emotional Developmental Capacities
512. Auditory Processing and Language
513. Visuospatial Capacities
514. Regulatory-Sensory Processing Patterns
515. A Combination of the Above Areas

Early Challenges in Reading Comprehension with compromises in

516. Functional Emotional Developmental Capacities
517. Auditory Processing and Language
518. Visuospatial Capacities
519. Regulatory-Sensory Processing Patterns
520. A Combination of the Above Areas

Early Challenges in Written Communication with compromises in

521. Functional Emotional Developmental Capacities
522. Auditory Processing and Language
523. Visuospatial Capacities
524. Regulatory-Sensory Processing Patterns
525. A Combination of the Above Areas

Early Challenges in Organizing Capacities (Executive Functioning) with compromises in

526 Functional Emotional Developmental Capacities
527. Auditory Processing and Language
528. Visuospatial Capacities
529. Regulatory-Sensory Processing Patterns
530. A Combination of the Above Areas

Note: A child may evidence early challenges in a number of areas (e.g., reading, math, and organizing capacities)

---

[1] The ICDL Work Group on Learning Challenges includes: Pat Lindamood, M.S., CCC-SLP, Robert L. Hendren, D.O., Joan Mele-McCarthy, D.A., Kytja Voeller, M.D., Harry Wachs, O.D., Serena Wieder, Ph.D., and Stanley I. Greenspan M.D.

The section on Learning Challenges describes the developmental capacities required for mastery of reading, math, written expression, and organizing (executive functioning). As seen in the outlines that follow, there are certain critical accomplishments that must be met on the developmental pathway leading to these capacities. It is possible to identify strengths and weaknesses in these nodal points on these pathways during the first 3 to 5 years of life. In the near future, as we are able to integrate what is known about genetics and brain development with real-world clinical issues, it is likely that we will be able to identify risk factors even earlier in development. However, even at this stage of knowledge, we are now in a position where we don't have to wait for a child to demonstrate a learning problem. Rather, we can identify challenges as they are emerging because we are able to observe how a child is progressing on the particular developmental pathway leading to reading, math, writing, or organizing abilities.

Therefore, we are introducing a new approach—the identification of learning challenges in the early years of life, based on both clinical observations and emerging research on the developmental pathways involved in early learning and eventual mastery of reading, math, writing, and organizing. These early learning challenges involve emotional and social capacities, auditory processing and language (including memory and retrieval), visuospatial processing, perceptual motor, and motor planning (including visual memory, sequencing, and what is often referred to as nonverbal learning) capacities, and sensory modulation.

Learning early in life, as well as later, including the mastery of specific academic abilities, involves all of these capacities working together. For example, math involves the capacity to comprehend the concept of "quantity," which depends on understanding spatial relationships (e.g., the difference between a long line of blocks and a short line of blocks), and auditory processing and language (e.g., applying number symbols to these different quantities of blocks, for example, two versus four). More advanced math, such as understanding a graph, depends on more complex understanding of spatial relationships. The manipulation of numerical symbols and verbal problem solving depends on more complex language and visuospatial capacities working together (e.g., matching verbal symbols with visualized print or written symbols). It also involves investing both with meaning and performing a variety of problem-solving sequences (e.g., sequencing or executive functioning). The capacities just cited, in turn, depend on early emotional and social experiences that lead to engagement with the world; early purposeful, emotionally-directed actions with the world; reciprocal interactions with the world (e.g., cause-and-effect preverbal thinking); and longer problem-solving social interactions that lead to complex pattern recognition, sequencing capacities, and investing the world of people and physical objects with meaning.

As with math, reading skills involve the abilities to observe patterns (visuospatial processing); distinguish sounds, letters and words (auditory processing, language, and communication capacities); track words across the page (visual-motor capacities); and isolate sounds, words, and word patterns from their background on a printed page (without being overloaded by sensory input—sensory modulation). Therefore, a comprehensive approach to the most common learning challenges requires a developmental framework that looks at the different areas of functioning. For each area, it is vital to have a road map or developmental pathway that reflects age expectations, beginning in the early months of life.

Typically, we have identified major developmental emotional and social challenges in infancy and early childhood, but not looked sufficiently for subtle features of what may later contribute to learning problems in reading, math, writing, or organizing abilities. Now that there is greater understanding of the different components of the mind and brain that contribute to learning capacities, it is possible, as indicated above, to identify the early steps in the learning process. When these early steps are not fully mastered, we can identify learning challenges before they become full learning disorders. We can identify these learning challenges in each of the components (i.e., each developmental pathway) that contribute to such complex capacities as reading and math. As we embark on this new line of inquiry, we create a unique opportunity for preventively oriented interventions early in life involving the strengthening of the basic building blocks of learning. There is mounting research suggesting that interventions for learning problems that appear later in childhood involving the foundations that contribute to that learning capacity (rather than simply drilling on the overall capacity itself) are especially helpful.

The approach we are presenting is based on clinical observations and research demonstrating that each complex learning capacity, such as reading, involves many different mental processes, and that identifying and working with these processes offers the most promise for helping children with learning challenges.

To illustrate the points made above, consider dyslexia, which is probably the best-studied learning disability. There is now an enormous body of research that strongly supports the notion of early identification. That dyslexia runs in families has been known since the late 19th century (Hinshelwood, 1907; Morgan, 1896; Stephenson, 1907) and the high degree of heritability has been amply confirmed in numerous modern genetic studies (DeFries, Olson, Pennington, and Smith, 1991; DeFries and Light, 1996; Willcutt et al., 2002; Stevenson, Graham, Fredman, and McLoughlin, 1987). There are likely several different genes that result in reading disability and there is a spectrum of severity. Not everybody who has the genetic trait is severely disabled. However, about 70% of children who come from families with dyslexia experience difficulty in learning to read (Lyytinen et al., 2001; Lyytinen et al., 2004; Snowling, Gallagher, & Frith, 2003). In addition to the anatomical and functional abnormalities reported in neuro-imaging studies, a characteristic feature of dyslexia is the impairment in processing of speech sounds which is observed across the life span (Ruff, Marie, Celsis, Cardebat, & Demonet, 2003). At birth, as well as at different points in the first year of life, infants from dyslexic families have been shown on electrophysiological testing to process speech sounds differently than infants from families of typical readers (Molfese, 2000; Richardson, Leppanen, Leiwo, & Lyytinen, 2003). Over the first 2½ years of life, except for the differences in speech sound processing, these at-risk infants perform like infants from families of typical readers on developmental test batteries. At 24 months of age, the at-risk group was noted to have shorter maximum length of utterances than the control group, but it was only at around 30 months that differences in language processing begin to be apparent. Interestingly, children who were slow to acquire speech at 24 months continued to be slow in acquisition of language at 42 months, but only if they came from dyslexic families. By 42 months of age, some of the characteristic deficits of phonological processing begin to emerge in the children from dyslexic families. A subset of these at-risk infants also showed delays in the realm of gross motor development, which are associated with greater language impairment, manifested by reduced vocabularies and shorter utterance length (Viholainen, Ahonen, Cantell, Lyytinen, & Lyytinen, 2002; Lyytinen et al., 2001). By age 5 years weak letter-sound knowledge, naming, and phonemic awareness are clearly apparent in children who evolve into patterns of dyslexia by school age (Scarborough, 1984; 1991; Maurer, Bucher, Brem, & Brandeis, 2003; Catts, 1991; Menyuk et al., 1991; DeFries et al., 1991; Pennington & Lefly, 2001).

In addition, a reasonable question is how individuals with various learning problems or other developmental disorders differ from one another. Based on the information flowing out of neuroscience research, it is apparent that different developmental disabilities and learning disorders have distinctive neuro-anatomical and functional neuro-imaging characteristics. Although there is tremendous variability in normal brain development from one child to another (Gogtay, et al., 2004), there are numerous examples demonstrating the association of characteristic structural and functional neuro-imaging features which are reflected in the cognitive profiles of these children. For example, how do children on the autism spectrum differ from dyslexics? Behaviorally it is quite obvious. However, one can also see this in functional processing characteristics of the brains. Although the visual pathway for processing letters and faces travel along the same pathway during the initial phase of processing (both involve the visual system), individuals on the autism spectrum, who have specific difficulty in the processing of faces but not letters, have been shown to have inactivation of the fusiform face area. In contrast, dyslexics, who are generally good at face-processing but poor at letter-processing show deficits in letter-processing but not face-processing when compared to controls (Tarkiainen, Helenius & Salmelin, 2003).

However, to avoid over-simplifying the situation, there are a number of factors that interact with genetic risk and early neurobiological patterns. These include: (1) environmental factors, (2) the child's intellectual abilities and language, and (3) genetic risk for other neuropsychiatric disorders. Environmental factors include the parents' educational level and the early exposure of the child to language and symbolic play. In the first 6 to 12 months of life, language acquisition is embedded in social interaction and requires the presence of both visual facial movements and auditory information to be effectively learned (Kuhl, 2004). In the second year of life, exposure to symbolic play and language is a contributor to language development. In one study, children of mothers who were normal readers showed enhanced comprehension skills when they were in the 14 to 18 month age range. This was associated with the mother's use of symbolic play and language when interacting with the child. Mothers, who were themselves dyslexic, did not use as much symbolic language and gesture during play and comprehension skills in their children were not as well developed. Finally, in the toddler and the child in early elementary school, phonemic awareness is clearly and strongly dependent on alphabetical exposure. Illiterate Portuguese women (who had stayed home to raise their younger siblings and never had the opportunity to attend school) were compared to their younger sibling who had learned to read and write. When examined as adults, they were able to repeat real words but had considerable difficulty repeating non-words. Neuro-imaging revealed less activation in brain areas involved in phonological processing, compared to their siblings who had attended school (Castro-Caldas, Petersson, Reis, Stone-Elander, & Ingvar, 1998).

Therefore, the quality and character of early interaction patterns has an important influence on eventual reading capacities. Lack of exposure to spoken and written language results in restricted neuronal development in brain areas underlying phonological processes. In a child at risk for dyslexia, a lack of appropriate experience would further disrupt the development of the neuronal circuitry that underlies phonological processing. Alternatively, preventively oriented interactions may have significant positive effects. Our proposed framework provides a basis for developing and studying preventive approaches.

The Learning Challenges diagnoses are based on a framework that recognizes the different parts of the mind and brain that contribute to reading, math, writing, and organizing capacities. As described above, there is now an impressive literature that supports longstanding clinical observations and shows that these academic abilities require a child to utilize many different parts of the mind and brain together.

In the outline, we extend the descriptions of these pathways into childhood to show the continuity between the early points on the pathways and their later manifestations. Because children in infancy and early childhood are not yet expected to actually engage in reading, math, or writing exercises, this framework is intended to be used as a way to observe the earliest signs of learning challenges. Most importantly, it enables parents, educators, and clinicians to begin working with a child to strengthen these critical building blocks, even before a learning problem or learning disorder is ever formally diagnosed.

In this section, we describe the developmental pathways for all the major learning capacities and challenges together. As the earlier example for math and reading illustrated, each complex learning capacity involves emotional and social patterns; auditory processing and language capacities; visuospatial, motor planning, and perceptual motor capacities; and the ability to modulate sensations. Clearly, however, some of these basic foundations are a bit more essential for certain learning capacities than others. For example, auditory processing and language is especially important for reading. Visuospatial processing is especially important for math. Sequencing capacities are essential for organizational or executive functioning skills. Yet, while each area of learning may emphasize certain foundations, all these developmental pathways contribute to each of the core learning capacities, and compromises in any one of them may contribute to a challenge. Therefore, all these areas need to be addressed.

MULTI-DIMENSIONAL APPROACH TO EARLY LEARNING PATTERNS

As indicated, we are looking at early learning from multiple perspectives in order to incorporate the different dimensions of mental functioning that influence what eventually become the capacities to read, write, understand math, organize, and problem solve. We, therefore, look at the infant and young child's learning capacities from the perspective of the necessary foundations required in the following areas of functioning:

1. Functional Emotional Developmental Capacities
2. Auditory Processing and Language
3. Visuospatial Capacities
4. Regulatory-Sensory Processing Patterns

We describe each of these areas of functioning beginning with an overview of its importance to early learning and, later, academic skills, followed by a more systematic framework to facilitate and identify competencies and vulnerabilities on the pathways involved in mastering early learning and later academic capacities.

Since the goal is to identify learning challenges and emerging academic challenges in the early years before the child is fully involved in academic work, the multi-dimensional framework presented in this section may be helpful in two ways. First, it may be used to understand and profile a child who is beginning to show challenges in the skills involved in the early stages of reading, math, writing, or organizing. For example, a 4 year-old child who has a hard time knowing that two cookies is more than one cookie, and using simple numbers, like one, two, and three to indicate preferences may be demonstrating early math difficulties, even before school requires him to add and subtract. Similarly, a 3½ year-old child who is still "fisting" the pencil or crayon and finding it hard to copy even simple shapes like a line may be demonstrating an early sign of difficulty with the fine motor skills necessary for writing. A 3 year-old who constantly mispronounces words, confusing the "b" sound and the "d" sound, for example, and by age 4 doesn't yet have a capacity to match one or two sounds to one or two letters may be providing an early sign of language and reading challenges.

In such instances, the framework presented in this section can be used to figure out which of the dimensions are contributing. This can be indicated in the multi-dimensional diagnostic approach. The area of challenge is indicated (e.g., reading, math) and the contributing dimension or dimensions are listed. The clinician should go further to determine the specific steps that need additional work in each of the contributing dimensions and plan an appropriate intervention program. The multi-dimensional diagnostic framework, however, provides a guide to identify the areas of functioning that need to be looked at more closely.

The second way this framework can be used is to identify emerging learning challenges significantly before there is even a hint of a difficulty with reading, math, writing, or organizing. By monitoring the child's progression in each of the dimensions outlined, the clinician can observe if there are steps not being fully mastered. To use the framework in this way, the clinician would indicate emerging learning challenges, and then indicate the dimensions that were contributing (e.g., emerging learning challenges with contributions from visuospatial capacities and regulatory-sensory processing capacities).

Next, we will describe each of the dimensions that should be considered in understanding a child's learning profile. For example, are the main contributing dimensions function emotional developmental capacities, visuospatial capacities, language, or all three?

Functional Emotional Developmental Capacities

The functional emotional and developmental capacities are described below and involve the infant or young child's abilities to be regulated and attend to the outside world, engage in relationships that provide the basis for investing in the world outside oneself, and mastering such crucial abilities as communication and causal thinking. Mastering these functional emotional developmental capacities is the basis for pattern recognition and symbolic thinking, as well as the vehicle through which the child connects what he sees, what he hears, and what he does together (i.e., integrates the different parts of the mind and brain). All the basic academic abilities, including reading, math, writing, and organizing, require mastery of these critical abilities to attend to the outside world, engage in interactive relationships, participate in complex social interactions that lead to pattern recognition, construct such meaningful symbols, and connect the different realms of experience together. In addition to the outline below, also see Axis II, which describes the functional emotional developmental capacities.

Table 1: Functional Emotional Developmental Capacities

Functional Emotional Developmental Level	Examples of Importance for Early Learning and Academic Skills
Level 1 Shared Attention and Regulation (Begins at 0-3 months)	Necessary for attention to sights and sounds and, later, to words, letters, numbers, etc.
Level 2 Engagement and Relating (Begins at 2-6 months)	Necessary for engaging with the world (not being self-absorbed), learning about "reality," and mastering all cognitive skills.
Level 3 Two-Way Purposeful Emotional Interactions (Begins at 4-9 months)	Necessary for "cause-and-effect" preverbal and verbal thinking and high levels of logical thinking.
Level 4 Shared Social Problem Solving (Begins at 9-18 months)	Necessary for: • Pattern recognition, including discriminating quantity (more vs. less or bigger vs. smaller) as well as the recognition of number (quantity) • Recognition of deviation from a pattern and constructing new patterns, such as finding an object that's hidden and bringing it into one's visual range. • Multi-step problem solving

Table 1: Functional Emotional Developmental Capacities *(continued)*

Functional Emotional Developmental Level	Examples of Importance for Early Learning and Academic Skills
Level 5 Creating Ideas (Begins at 18-30 months)	Necessary for forming and using symbols in language, reading, math, planning, and problem solving
Level 6 Building Bridges Between Ideas: Logical Thinking (Begins at 30-48 months)	Necessary for all learning, including: • Symbolizing quantity concepts • Matching symbols to letter patterns • Comprehending written and oral communication
Level 7 Multi-Cause, Comparative, Thinking (Begins at 4-6 years [48-72 months])	Levels 7-9 are necessary for all learning, including: • The manipulation of numerical symbols in terms of relativistic gray-area thinking (e.g., multiplication, division) and thinking off an internal standard (e.g., algebra and, later on, calculus). • Comprehending sentences, paragraphs, and essays.
Level 8 Emotionally differentiated gray-area thinking (Begins at 6-10 years)	Being able to construct patterns of ideas at progressively higher levels of creativity and logic.
Level 9 Intermittent reflective thinking, a stable sense of self, and an internal standard (Begins at 9-12 years and beyond)	Self evaluative thinking evidenced in analyzing one's own or another person's oral or written communication, considering different options, creating "experiments" to prove or disprove a hypothesis, and using judgment.

Auditory Processing and Language

Auditory processing and language capacities are also essential for early learning and later academic skills. For example, reading requires the capacity to distinguish sound patterns (phonemes), combine sound patterns into words, and match sound patterns to letters and, eventually, words. Mounting research supports the importance of the infant and young child's ability to discriminate and recognize sound patterns, and later the identity, number, and order of individual sounds within words, as the basis for reading and spelling (Calfee, Lindamood, & Lindamood, 1973; Shankweiler & Liberman, 1989; Heilman, Voeller, & Alexander, 1996; Lindamood & Lindamood, 2005). Obviously, language skills are also essential for listening, comprehending, and discussing all school subjects, as well as for participating in social interactions and mastering higher levels of abstract verbal reasoning. In addition to the outline below, which highlights elements of auditory processing and language functioning that are especially important for reading and other academic skills, please also see the section on language functioning described in the section on Axis I: Language Disorders.

Table 2: Auditory Processing and Language

Age and Level	Examples of Auditory Processing and Language Skills
0-3 months Shared Attention and Regulation	Attends to the world of speech sounds and their production, e.g., • Attention to caregiver's mouth and tongue actions • Attention to caregiver trill sounds and tongue clucking sounds • Attention to additional sounds
2-6 months Engagement and Relating	Synchronous sound productions with increasing capacity to: • Discriminate and make sounds (e.g., tonal variation, vowel sounds with synchronous consonant sounds and mouth movements • Synchronize sound and mouth movements with caregivers' vocal rhythms
4-9 months Two-Way Purposeful Emotional Interactions	Reciprocal exchange of expanding sound productions, e.g., • consonants • vowels • syllables, such as "dada" "gaga" "baba,," etc. • beginning emergence of words up, out, etc.
9-18 months Shared Social Problem Solving	Increasing reciprocal use of vocal patterns, including words , e.g., • expansion of verbs • expansion of nouns • use of two-word phrases • compliance with two-word commands. Beginning comprehension of spoken language. *For all, but specifically for math:* Coordinates touching and quantifying to judge specific quantity
18-30 months Creating Ideas	Combining words into ideas Begins to form visual images for word meanings. Increasing comprehension of spoken language and, eventually, complex ideas.
30-48 months Building Bridges Between Ideas: Logical Thinking	Exchanging ideas (e.g., why, how, when, etc.) Perceives the parts/whole concepts of sound patterns in words (e.g., syllables) both receptively and expressively.

Table 2: Auditory Processing and Language *(continued)*

Age and Level	Examples of Auditory Processing and Language Skills
4-6 years [48-72 months] Multi-Cause, Comparative, Thinking	Begins to connect sounds (duration, pitch, and elements) and expressively. Begins to connect sounds, words and shapes, including letters, e.g., • Creates a multisensory motor experience of the basic shapes (e.g., walks, pantomimes, or draws straight line, curves, slants as named). • Identifies, then copies and names shapes and designs • Writes some letters • Follows 4-step communication Names and identifies sounds and letters of alphabet in and out of sequence (for all, but specifically for reading and language arts) <u>Between 4 - 5 years:</u> Begins to integrate awareness of auditory, visual, and motor components of speech sounds and place and manner of articulation. <u>5 years (60 months) on:</u> Becomes aware of nature of errors enabling monitoring and self-correction *(for all, but specifically for reading and language arts)* *For all, but specifically for reading comprehension:* Comprehension of written language as reading ability develops
6-10 years Emotionally Differentiated Gray-Area Thinking	Integrates awareness of auditory, visual, and motor components of speech sounds and place and manner of articulation: • Lips vs. tongue actions • Unvoicing vs. voicing • Plosive vs. continuant air streams • Self-corrects own articulation of these features in words • Begins to associate speech sounds and letters that represent them • Begins to perceive identity, number, and order of sequences of sounds within spoken words <u>Begins at 6 years</u> *For all, but specifically for reading comprehension:* Development of critical academic thinking skills, e.g., main idea, conclusion, inference, prediction, evaluation, etc., for higher order thinking

Visuospatial Capacities

Visuospatial capacities are often attended to in considering early learning and academic skills, but not in the sufficient depth or scope required for a full understanding of their importance. For example, understanding math even at its most elementary level of addition and subtraction requires comprehending one-to-one correspondence. This means that the child doesn't simply count, but can match the number he says to the number of objects he sees in front of him, and can manipulate these objects and see how a change in their pattern would relate to a change in the number he applies to them. Once a child has mastered one-to-one correspondence, he is able to understand, for example, that four blocks lying flat on the table in the form of a snake is more than three blocks stacked on top of each other like a tower. The child who doesn't yet have one-to-one correspondence may think the tower has more blocks simply because it looks bigger to him. Similarly, the child with one-to-one correspondence understands that eight beads arranged in a circle are more than seven beads arranged in a straight line, even though the seven beads take up more physical space on the table. Developing visuospatial capacities, however, involves a developmental pathway with many components and steps. It involves, for example, an infant and young child developing:

- Body Awareness and Sense
- Awareness of the Body in Space
- Understanding of Physical Objects in relationship to oneself and other objects and other people
- Conservation of Space (i.e., its different dimensions)
- Visual-Logical Reasoning
- Representational Thought (e.g., drawing, visualizing, and thinking)

Each of these different components of visuospatial processing has its own developmental steps, which can be observed and, more importantly, can be strengthened if needed. The following table outlines these components of visuospatial processing and the steps that should be mastered at the end of each year for the first five years of life. Axis V describes these visuospatial capacities in more detail. The clinician should use the more detailed description of these components of visuospatial processing and the steps involved in their mastery described in the section on Axis V for constructing the child's learning profile.

Table 3: Visuospatial Capacities

Visuospatial Capacities
1. Body Awareness and Sense Year 1: Purposeful, coordinated movement, guided by vision and sound. Year 2: Purposeful movement for interactive play (rolling a ball back and forth) Year 3: Awareness of body boundaries of self and others Year 4: Awareness of body affecting others in space and time Year 5: Awareness of body for coordinated actions

Table 3: Visuospatial Capacities *(continued)*

Visuospatial Capacities
2. Location of the Body in Space Year 1: Beginning movement in space Year 2: Observes things move in space in relationship to self Year 3: Purposeful movement in relation to other moving objects Year 4: Planning and organization of movement prior to the action Year 5: Becoming a team player
3. Relation of Objects to Self and Other Objects and People Year 1: Reciprocal interactions with people and things Year 2: Self-control in relation to other people and things Year 3: Development of symbols Year 4: Rules and expectations Year 5: Boundaries and membership
4. Conservation of Space Year 1: Space is uni-dimensional Year 2: Space is three-dimensional and movement in space is alterable Year 3: Relationship of object in three dimensional space Year 4: Relationship of object to object in space Year 5: Combining time and space
5. Visual Logical Reasoning Year 1: Knowledge through sensorimotor action Year 2. Moving from action knowledge to planning the actions Year 3: Understanding the cause and effect of the action Year 4: Stability of early visuospatial thinking Year 5: Logical thinking to solve problems
6. Representational Thought (Drawing, Thinking, Visualizing) Year 1: Direct representation Year 2: Words, pictures, gestures and toys Year 3: Early imaginative play Year 4: More purposeful representations Year 5: Matching space to representational thought

Regulatory-Sensory Processing Patterns

Regulatory-sensory processing patterns also contribute to the child's early learning and later academic skills. For example, some children evidence sensory modulation challenges where they are over-responsive to sensations, such as certain sights, sounds, and touch. Children who are extremely visually over-responsive sometimes find the contrast between dark print on a white page too dramatic and find it difficult to focus in on individual letters, syllables, words, or phrases. As one child with this difficulty put it, "All I see is a blur of different shapes." When exposed to less dramatic contrast between the letter and the page (e.g., softer colors), this child was able to read very well. Over-responsivity to sounds can contribute to making it difficult for some children to discriminate sound patterns and, therefore, connect sounds to letters and, eventually, words. Children who are under-responsive to sensation such as sound, sight, and touch may tend toward self-absorption (e.g., the teacher's voice doesn't attract their attention) and find it hard to listen or follow directions. In the extreme, self-absorption can compromise attention to the outside world and, therefore, comprehension of reality and logic (e.g., the child escapes into fantasy). Children with motor planning problems (dyspraxia) may find it difficult to carry out the sequence of motor actions required for writing, lining up columns in math, or following directions.

There is a range of regulatory-sensory processing patterns that contributes to learning and later academic skills. Most of these regulatory-sensory processing patterns are observable in infancy, as well as early childhood and childhood. Sometimes they change in a favorable direction and, at other times, they may change in an unfavorable direction, intensifying the child's challenges. Most importantly, these regulatory-sensory processing capacities can be worked with and strengthened towards the healthier end of the continuum with proper interventions.

Three basic regulatory-sensory processing patterns need to be observed, including those involving sensory modulation, sensory discrimination, and sensory-based motor performance (including postural control problems and dyspraxia). These broad patterns and the specific regulatory-sensory processing disorders that involve them, as well as a guide for observing them, can be found in the section on regulatory-sensory processing disorders under Axis I: Regulatory-Sensory Processing Disorders. That section should be used as a reference for observing this component of the child's early learning and later academic capacities. It should be emphasized that each of the differences in regulatory-sensory processing described in the section referred to above occurs on a continuum, from the relatively adaptive expression of individual differences to clinically disordered patterns.

Case Illustration of a Child with Learning Challenges

This case illustration represents a unique opportunity to observe the growth and development of a child who received periodic instruction in sensory-cognitive functions underlying speech and spoken/written language development. The intervention was provided from early childhood to early adulthood at the Lindamood-Bell Learning Processes Center in California. It illustrates the multidimensional approach taken to assess and work with the child's severe challenges and bring her to the point of success in her young adult life.

Jill, a Caucasian female born in 1984, was first seen for speech pathology services when she was 22 months of age. With a history of several developmental challenges evident during the first year of life, extensive records have been kept on diagnostic testings, and the results of preventive and remedial efforts. These culminate in the most recent testing and instructional efforts when Jill was 20 years of age and a community college student. Her developmental profile is described in detail, a summary speaks to the diagnostic and intervention implications, and a projection is made regarding Jill's future developmental profile.

At birth, Jill was a quiet baby with such dark pigmentation in comparison to her parents that two pediatricians questioned her mother extensively regarding alcohol use, etc. during her pregnancy. (There had been no substance abuse of any kind.) After determining the dark coloring was due to an overabundance of red blood cells, Jill was transfused to relieve the situation. She did not have a normal cry, due to weak ligaments that had not matured around her larynx. Her tear ducts had not opened, and eye drops were needed until surgery cleared the tear ducts at 1 year of age. Because Jill's staring behavior interfered with her parents' efforts to engage her attention, questions were raised about her hearing acuity. A check on her hearing indicated no problem. Her tongue had to be clipped to aid her in nursing. Until she was 6 months of age she had extreme gastrointestinal pain, would nurse only on her right side, and had severe lengthy inconsolable crying episodes during which few people could hold and comfort her. This seriously interfered with her engagement and relating. Her growth and weight gain were slow, but genetic testing revealed no abnormalities.

Between 6 and 9 months, her parents attempted to engage her with very exaggerated facial expressions, peek-a-boo, and eye contact. This resulted in some appropriate smiles and random physical movement of arms and legs, but no vocal engagement or mirroring of a range of facial emotions. Between 6 and 12 months she sat up, crawled, and walked. By 18 months she had only a few single words and her caregivers could not talk with her. Her parents began telling her what to do in short phrases, and she was difficult to discipline. Too much language input caused Jill to scream "No, no, no!" indicating a severe over-responsiveness to spoken auditory input. She definitely preferred physical interaction. She still cried inconsolably for long periods, sleep walked, and had night terrors. There was evidence of pattern recognition and deviation from pattern and quantity, (e.g., she wanted to do whatever her big brother did, have the same thing he had at meals, knew if she needed more to match his quantity, etc.).

At 22 months Jill was still not combining words to create ideas, and was seen by speech-language pathologist Pat Lindamood who specialized in the development of phoneme awareness and sequencing, a foundational skill underlying the development of speech and language. Jill engaged readily with Pat, but only when Pat limited the amount of language she used with Jill and set up tasks in very small, gradual steps also involving motor activity. Engagement and relating were difficult for Jill when that relating included language input. Jill and her mother were patterned in various activities which drew attention to Jill seeing and feeling the motor features of speech sounds while the adult labeled them (e.g., lip poppers, lip coolers, etc.). Ways were devised to represent speech sounds' sameness/difference, number and order when they were spoken in sequences (e.g., representing speech sounds with colored blocks, with gestures, etc.). Syllables were also counted and physically represented in various ways as they formed words. Weekly sessions with daily follow-up at home over a period of three months resulted in the family reporting definite improvement in the amount and clarity of speech and language production, as well as a reduction in frustrations and tantrums during communication.

At 2½ and into 3 years of age, expressive language was beginning to be minimally functional in combining two words to express physical needs and wants. However, Jill wanted chiefly outdoor play and had little language interaction, combining words into ideas, and connecting and exchanging ideas involving who, what, and why questions, even though she and her mother attended a parent-participation preschool where other children were role models for that language interaction. Significantly, Jill strongly resisted being read to. This usually comforting and intimate interaction between parent and child was aversive to her because of her extreme sensitivity to the constancy of language input. It overloaded her and paralleled her earlier negative reactions to conversational language.

From 4 years of age, when Jill entered an early intervention public school program, through high school, she received traditional speech therapy services. From fourth grade on she also qualified for special education resource room services. In addition to the routine district-wide testing each year, and the required periodic special education testing, speech pathology services also provided assessments. Jill passed all routine hearing screenings. Extensive documentation of Jill's development from kindergarten through high school can be summarized as follows.

Repeating kindergarten enabled Jill to gain in ability to work independently, complete tasks, follow oral instructions, and orally give her phone number and address. Socially, she had few friends and played largely alone. It was difficult for her to understand and follow standard social behavior. Her language included no references to past or future, and she did not use multi-cause comparative thinking in situations where it was needed.

She recognized eight colors, identified four basic shapes, orally identified upper and lower case letters out of order, could orally count to 20, identify those numerals out of order, and sequence them from 0 to 12. The standard large and small muscle skills foundational for the demands of first grade were an area of strength. However, to work preventively, the parents arranged diagnostic testing in mid-first grade at Lindamood-Bell Learning Processes.

Although reading skills had been reported as satisfactory, severe deficits were revealed in reading comprehension, and receptive and expressive oral language processing. Her expressive vocabulary was at the bottom of the normal range, but her receptive vocabulary was two years above her age. She was scheduled for a month of sensory-cognitive intervention, one to two hours daily, to begin development of visual imagery for language comprehension, and to further develop her phoneme awareness as a support for the continued development of decoding skills.

At age 7 years, 11 months, ending first grade, she was reported to be at grade level in reading accuracy, mathematics, and language skills. She only needed improvement in working independently, following directions, using time wisely, and completing assignments. These four skills had improved into the satisfactory range on ending second grade, and her self-confidence was reported as strengthened. However, she could not comprehend "If..., then..." gray area thinking.

On ending third, fourth, and fifth grades, reports began to change. Problems were cited consistently in reading comprehension, math reasoning, oral language, and knowledge of history and geography. At age 11 years, 5 months, during fifth grade, Jill's parents were concerned about her academic difficulties. She had just told her mother, "Mom, I think I just figured out what 'early' means!" This was possibly the beginning of reflective thinking for Jill. Her parents requested the school to do a battery of testing to assist educational planning for the middle school years. The special education team used standardized tests in areas of neurological screening, intelligence, written language, visual and auditory memory, visual-motor perception, and social behavior. Jill was found to be functioning academically at grade level, but with much assistance and directed teaching from the classroom teacher. Difficulties were evident in organizing visuospatial material. Her pattern of looking at the internal parts rather than the wholeness of a design indicated visual sequencing, spatial and visual planning problems. She showed a preference for concrete, rote learning, and did not generally do reflective thinking for dealing with concepts or abstract reasoning. Interestingly, Jill showed an eventual ability for, and interest in, math. Although her math reasoning skills were weak, she showed a relative strength in math computation. Jill continued to show challenges in math areas where language input was required (e.g., word problems), but in pure computational areas she was quite good. The Special Education team recommended exploring the possibility of Jill receiving resource specialist intervention in middle school, and that she be closely monitored to assure that her academic program met her individual needs. The behavioral analysis indicated she related more easily socially to adults than she did to her peers.

At the end of fifth grade, to work preventively toward sixth grade demands in middle school, Jill's parents had her tested again at Lindamood-Bell. She was found to need further development of phoneme awareness into the multi-syllable level, and further development of concept imagery to enable reflective thinking and comprehension of more abstract concepts from an internal standard. This further intervention was provided in the summer before she entered sixth grade, and on her second semester sixth grade report card she received all A and B grades, except for a C+ in History and in Science.

At age 13 years 8 months, the same Special Education team that assessed Jill in fifth grade reassessed her abilities in March of the seventh grade with the same tests. However, because of Jill's documented language-based learning disability, the team selected a non-verbal measure of intellectual functioning (Test of Non-verbal Intelligence-TONI) in place of the Wechsler. On this measure, Jill's intellectual functioning was within the average range and some of her correct answers were in the 18-20 year-old range. The team regarded this measure to be a more realistic reflection of her capabilities, as she had always performed better academically than intellectual assessments would indicate. Academically she was near grade level in all areas. When she was asked which of her subjects was her favorite, she indicated math. At home, Jill was being provided with many enriching educational experiences. Behaviorally, Jill was reported to be shy, and seldom initiating social contact at school. Overall, the team reported, "Jill has shown tremendous growth since the last testing. She still has difficulty with some areas of language processing and continues to qualify for special education in speech and language."

As Jill progressed through middle school and high school, periodic school district, special education team, and speech pathology assessments continued. Her performance varied during that period. In tenth grade, on the Woodcock-Johnson-III Tests of Achievement, her Story Recall was at the 5th percentile, but Written Expression was at the 84th percentile. On The WORD Test, her expressive vocabulary was at the 8th percentile, but on the Peabody Picture Vocabulary Test her receptive vocabulary was at the 34th percentile. Academically, her skills were in the average range, and the assessment team considered Jill's achievement scores and academic performance to be a more valid indication of her level of functional cognitive processing. She was in the college prep curriculum with some accommodations, such as extra time on course testing and prompts and paraphrasing. She could also request Resource Room help on course assignments. Her grade point average of 3.57 at graduation thus reflects her diligent efforts and the use of accommodations.

During twelfth grade, Jill's parents again requested an assessment at Lindamood-Bell. They wanted to determine whether further intervention should be scheduled before Jill attended community college. In March of her senior year in high school, Jill completed the Learning Ability Evaluation. A previous pattern of written language stronger than oral language, and receptive vocabulary stronger than expressive vocabulary, had been found throughout Jill's elementary and secondary school speech-language and Special Education assessments. This pattern was again indicated. Jill had increased her receptive vocabulary from the 34th to the 42nd percentile, but her expressive vocabulary was still in the 5th to the 8th percentile range. She still needed extended time to convert oral or written input to verbal output. Her reading (64th percentile), spelling (66th percentile), word attack (94th percentile), and context reading accuracy (84th percentile) continued to be contrasting areas of strength. This decoding/encoding strength was supported by underlying processing skills of phoneme awareness intact at the complex single syllable level, and symbol imagery accuracy on 41 of 50 items. Reading comprehension (16th percentile) continued to be a contrasting area in need of development. The oral directions measure (25th percentile) was at the bottom of the average range and in contrast to Jill's receptive vocabulary at the 42nd percentile.

SUMMARY

This profile clearly indicated Jill was a person with spirit who was willing to persevere and who had the potential for further development. Another positive in her situation was that throughout the school records there were comments about the degree of emotional and engaging and relating support she had from her family. The recommendation with this profile of strengths and weakness was an intensive period of intervention with the Visualizing and Verbalizing Program (four hours per day for six weeks). Because of the severity of Jill's language deficits, it was not expected that this amount of intervention would be sufficient, but retesting, clinical notes, and her own subjective experience would inform the further plan to be made at the end of the first intervention period. The goal was to increase Jill's receptive and expressive language skills by developing her ability to form visual images for the concepts expressed by language. It would be highly desirable to do this before she enrolled in a community college program. Jill did not make that choice. In the year following her graduation from high school she took two community college courses. She experienced so much difficulty that she decided to follow the recommendation, and she completed 124 hours of concept imagery training at 20 years of age.

The findings on retesting were as follows. Jill's receptive vocabulary improved from the 42nd to the 53rd percentile. Her expressive vocabulary improved from the 5th to the 16th percentile. This was an increase of two standard scores, and the first significant increase in expressive vocabulary in all the years of testing. It is not enough, but it indicated a beginning that would continue to build. There was also an improvement in oral directions from the 25th to the 37th percentile. Her phoneme awareness increased to the 77th percentile, which involved multi-syllable processing in addition to single syllable processing. In reading comprehension, she was unstable. There were gains on one reading test from the sixth grade level through the twelfth grade level. On another reading test, her accuracy increased from the 84th to the 91st percentile,and her fluency increased from the 50th to the 61st percentile, but her comprehension went from the 16th to the 9th percentile. This score can be expected to pick back up and increase further as she gains additional experience with concept imagery.

A projection that Jill's receptive and expressive language processing will continue to improve is based on years of experience with the role of concept imagery in language comprehension. At this time Jill's ability to form connections was very weak and she encountered vocabulary and knowledge gaps in information which interfered with her processing. Her family reported a dramatic increase in her social awareness, participation in conversations, and her ability to ask clarifying questions. She has begun making consistent eye contact during conversations. Her grandmother commented that she had a delightful phone conversation with Jill and that her usual responses of "yes," "no," and "maybe" had been replaced by complete sentences, jokes, laughter, and questions. A second period of intervention with concept imagery was planned, because Jill could now access this sensory-cognitive function to support continuing growth in her spoken and written language.

Diagnostic Summary Impression

Jill was first seen at the Lindamood-Bell Learning Processes Center when she was just 22 months old. At that time, we felt that she evidenced combinations of challenges that could now be characterized in the Interdisciplinary Council on Developmental and Learning Disorders (ICDL) Diagnostic Manual for Infancy and Early Childhood (DMIC) system as:

- Emerging Learning Challenges (500) with compromises in:
  - Functional Emotional Developmental Levels (501)
  - Auditory Processing and Language (502)
  - Regulatory-Sensory Processing Patterns (504)

She evidenced marked challenges in auditory processing (she couldn't separate the phonemes in continuous speech into their word patterns) (502) and, therefore experienced sensory overload (504) from continuous language. As a result of these difficulties, Jill evidenced compromises in her ability to attend, engage, and relate (it was hard to engage and maintain her attention). She wasn't able to engage in purposeful interactions involving language and social problem solving. Because we were unable to communicate well with her, we weren't able to assess whether or not she was creating ideas (501), which would have been her age-expected functional emotional developmental level at that time.

Jill was assessed again at Lindamood-Bell when she was in the first grade. At that time, she could have been appropriately characterized as having Early Challenges in All Learning Areas with compromises in:

- Functional Emotional Developmental Levels (526.)
- Auditory Processing and Language (527)
- Regulatory-Sensory Processing Patterns (529)

When Jill was assessed in the third, fourth, and fifth grades, in school testing, it was discovered that she also evidenced challenges in the visuospatial area, and we could have added the new diagnosis of Early Challenges in All Learning Areas with compromises in Visuospatial Capacities (528.)

Throughout the course of her preschool, elementary, and secondary school program and her treatment, descriptions of Jill's capacities in the categories of Learning Challenges (500s) varied, depending on the changing levels of task demands. Some areas would be stronger at some times and diminished at others and in various situations. She functioned academically at grade level as she got older, but required much assistance in organizing her efforts and approaches to her work, even though she was able to spell and use punctuation so appropriately that she performed above-average on tests of written language expression. The sequencing of the tasks and ideas was the difficult part for her (529. Regulatory-Sensory Processing Patterns). In seventh grade, she was still behaviorally shy, seldom initiating interactions with peers. In the tenth grade, however, she was finally able to engage and have friendships with a few children in the band and chorus, of which she was a part, because of their common bond in music as a based for communication.

Additional diagnostic testing in 12th grade indicated Jill's need for higher levels of expressive vocabulary and higher order thinking skills in order to be successful in community college. After further work (126 hours) of concept imagery application through spoken and written language processing, Jill has come full circle in her learning challenges. She has had a dramatic change in her comfort and ability to initiate, engage, and relate to other individuals in shared social problem solving, and is spontaneously and joyfully engaging in interactions in all five learning areas identified in the ICDL-DMIC system. Jill is planning to work on further concept imagery development for mastery of higher order thinking skills in auditory processing and language.

Contributed by: Pat Lindamood, MS, CCC-SLP

A Case Illustration of a Child with Visuospatial Processing and Motor Challenges

When Robbie was first seen, at age 4 years, 11 months, he was a very attractive, well-built child with severe developmental gaps—enough so that it made it very difficult for him to perform educational activities at school.

He had some language, as evidenced by his ability to follow simple directions (e.g., being asked to sit in a chair) and to respond to his parents' offering him a snack, as well as being able to choose between different possible snacks. However, he appeared reluctant to speak and often only verbalized simple phrases, such as "I don't want to." At home, however, his parents reported that he was a bit more verbal, though it was difficult to have a long back-and-forth conversation with him.

When we placed him at a developmental age using the Wachs' Analysis of Cognitive Structure (a standardized test of intellect that focuses on visual-motor and visuospatial capacities), he varied in the testing from below 3 to almost 4 years, with an overall score of first percentile. In other words, 99% of children his age functioned better than he did.

In terms of his graphics (e.g., the ability to draw circles, a square, a cross, and follow the instruction "Copy this design" requested both visually and verbally), he was far below age-expectation and what would be required for writing and all academic work. Some of the tasks used to test this ability were: "Can you make a line between these two parallel lines without going over them?" (he couldn't), "Connect these two dots," and "Draw a person." He clearly wasn't ready for school. If attempts were made to put him there, it would be enormously stressful in light of his challenges.

Robbie had the general movement skills and control of a 2½ year old. Specifically, he could not draw a circle, square, triangle, cross, or rectangle in response to an auditory request ("Draw a circle for me, please,") or a visual presentation (e.g., pointing to a circle and indicating that he should draw the same). He fisted (the Palmer Grasp) his writing implement (a pencil) and had very little control of it. He was certainly not ready for writing of any sort. When asked to draw a person, Robbie produced only scattered scribbles, some of which he identified as an eye, an ear, or a nose. However, none was in its proper order and they were scattered around the page.

Robbie's visual thinking was rated at 3 years 11 months, far below requisite for mathematics and reading. Using blocks and pegs, he wasn't able to complete patterns at age-expected levels (e.g., match a three-block design or replicate a diagonal, vertical, or horizontal line with pegs.) These capacities are necessary for understanding shapes and their relationships to one another and, therefore, they provide a foundation for reading and math.

Because of his challenges with perceiving visual relationships, as indicated above, his world of "sight" was at a much younger age than his almost-five-year-old body. Such a difference often causes a child to feel confused and frustrated.

We discovered because of his receptive/expressive language skills, he couldn't follow a two-step command (e.g., "Take the red block and put it under the green block"). Also, he had compromised ocular control. For example, if a person moved a pencil across his face with the instruction to "Follow the pencil with your eyes," his eyes would stay still or move in another direction or he'd move his head to follow the moving pencil. He certainly was not ready for any stressful near vision activity (e.g., anything done within 20 inches from his eyes). This doesn't mean he couldn't do it, but rather that it would be very stressful for him and he was already under a great deal of stress. His visual logic was impaired. For example, he couldn't lay out a sequence of blocks in a yellow/green/yellow/green pattern. He couldn't do one-to-one correspondence and had no concept of number.

Robbie's visual-auditory skills were also significantly below age expectations. For example, he was unable to match sounds to shapes or to discriminate or sequence sounds. He might have been able to learn to recognize letters or words with a great deal of drilling, but he wouldn't be able to learn to use phonics or read in any sort of meaningful way.

Robbie presented with certain primitive reflex actions that are usually inhibited in the first year of life as an infant learns to be more purposeful. These early reflex actions showed an immaturity in Robbie's body functions. To help him move out of those primitive reflex states, we gave him experiences that would allow him to use his automatic reflexes purposefully, for example, pretending to walk like different animals. Until he could get rid of those natural born reflexes, he couldn't work in a purposeful, coordinated manner.

Robbie was unable to turn his feet in or out and could not hop while moving forward, backward, left, or right. These movement dysfunctions render any motor task quite difficult.

Robbie also seemed to be emotionally immature. For example, when presented with a challenging task, he generally used avoidance tactics (e.g., getting up to walk around the room, becoming silly, or simply trying to play with some of the materials). Sometimes he would become self-absorbed and seem to daydream.

Robbie's parents were successful attorneys and he had received considerable and multi-disciplined therapies for several years prior to his first visit with us. There is no organic or physical impairment. Robbie was a healthy but very unhappy little boy who had severe social difficulties and was not able to fully enjoy playing with other children or cooperate and follow expectations in a mainstream preschool class.

Robbie attended our center to focus on his visual-motor and visuospatial challenges, as well as his visual-auditory difficulties for almost three years, with periodic leaves of absence throughout. During that time, we focused on strengthening each of the areas that evidenced below-age expected functioning. The intervention program was organized around helping Robbie by building from the "bottom up." This worked on the foundations for purposeful sensory-motor actions, perceptual motor problem-solving, visuospatial logic, and integrated multi-sensory problem and symbolic capacities. He evidenced gradual progress. Most importantly, he strengthened the fundamental building blocks for learning, rather than simply trying to compensate or use memory-based drilling approaches to substitute for them.

On Robbie's last progress evaluation in October 2004, there was considerable improvement in affect as well as developmental functioning. He is now able to match block designs almost at age expectancy. He is using a proper tripod grasp for drawing or writing.

He has resolved the early reflex patterns and is able to turn his feet in and out at will. His ocular tracking, convergence, and binocularity are excellent. Robbie is now in mainstream classes with very few accommodations. He's very appropriately verbal, constantly smiles, and is extremely cooperative. His draw-a-person function is no longer a series of scribbles but is almost age appropriate.

Robbie's visual logical reasoning is much improved. For example, he can match complex block designs, understand one-to-one correspondence and other higher level conservation tasks, hold a logical, and often creative, conversation and is now a happy, cooperative, successful child.

This case illustrates the importance of looking at visuospatial processing, along with auditory processing and language, emotional and social development, and regulatory-sensory processing to identify early learning challenges and develop an appropriate intervention plan.

Diagnostic Impression

To characterize Robbie in terms of our ICDL-DMIC system, we would say that he evidenced an Emerging Learning Challenge with compromises in Visuospatial Capacities (523.)

Contributed by: Harry Wachs, O.D. and Melinda Carlson

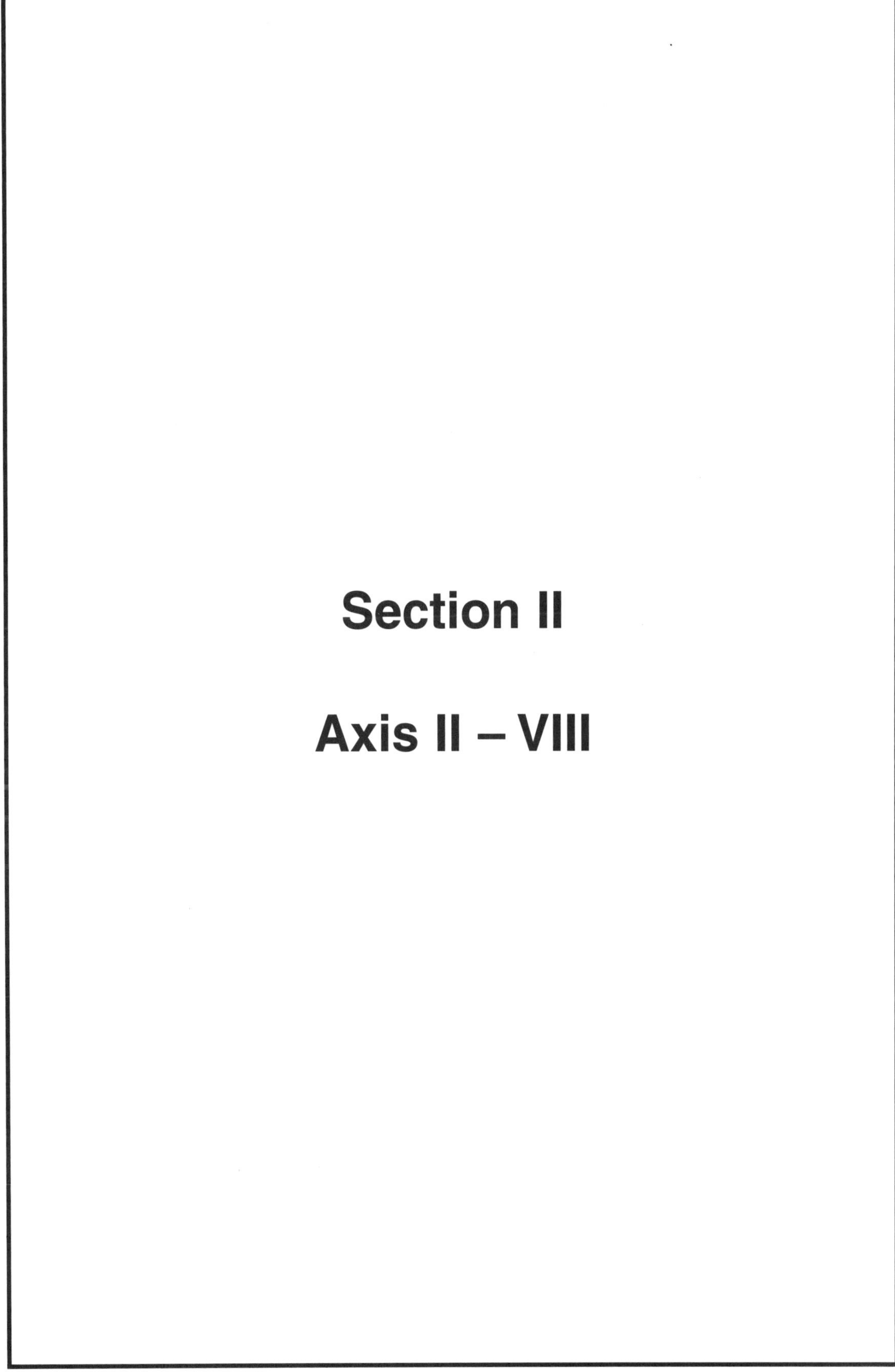

Section II

Axis II – VIII

Descriptions of Axis II to VIII

The following sections describe Axes II through VIII. As indicated earlier, a complete profile of each child and family necessitates characterizing the child's and family's functioning from the perspective of each of the axes outlined below. Some of the axes are only described briefly (e.g., Axis VIII: Other Medical and Neurological Diagnoses), and other axes are described in more detail (Axis II: The Functional Emotional Developmental Capacities and Axis V: Visuospatial Capacities).

In addition, two of the axes refer to the descriptions already presented in Axis I under primary diagnoses (i.e., Axis III: Regulatory-Sensory Processing Capacities and Axis IV: Language Capacities). For regulatory-sensory processing capacities and language capacities, the descriptions of the primary diagnoses are also well suited to serve as the descriptions for the axes. However, when using either one of these as an "axis description," the clinician has an additional option of making an overall clinical demarcation (rating) to reflect the degree to which this capacity is compromised. However, this is not a substitute for the clinical narrative and formulation.

The following sections describe each axis in the order in which it should be considered.

Axis II: Functional Emotional Developmental Capacities

The diagnosis of infants and young children cannot be undertaken without a developmental perspective of emotional functioning and a developmentally-based approach to the classification and diagnosis of emotional problems. In a developmental model, the infant's constitutional-maturational patterns, and the infant's environment, including caregivers, family, community, and culture, contribute to the child-caregiver interaction patterns in a dynamic interactive process. These interaction patterns are the vital structure that builds aspects of emotional functioning. Emotional functioning includes capacities for self-regulation; different levels of relating to others; emotional cueing and signaling evident of preverbal affective reciprocity and communication; co-regulated social problem solving; symbolizing or representing wishes and emotions; elaborating emotional themes in pretend play; reasoning about feelings; reflecting on one's own feelings and empathizing with the feelings of others; and reality testing. The infant/child-caregiver interaction experiences determine the child's capacity for relative mastery (or non-mastery) of these six core functional emotional developmental capacities or levels as they are developed and build upon each other in the course of early life.

The functional emotional developmental levels also serve as an organizing construct for integrating the other aspects of development, including motor, sensory, language, and cognitive functioning. For example, when we describe the child's capacity for two-way interactive emotional communication at around 8 months (reciprocal affect-cueing), we take into account the cognitive component (cause and effect interaction), the motor component (reaching), the language component (exchanging vocalizations that convey affect), and the sensory component (using sight, touch, and perception of sound as part of a co-regulated reciprocal emotional interaction). Thus, the functional emotional developmental level provides a way of characterizing emotional functioning and, at the same time, a way of looking at how all the components of development (cognition, language, and motor skills) work together in a functional manner (as a mental team) organized by the designated emotional goals at each level. One can look not only for what the infant or toddler is evidencing (e.g., specific emotions or symptoms), but also for what he is not evidencing. For example, the 8-month-old who is calm, alert, and enjoyable, but who has no capacity for discrimination or reciprocal social interchanges, may be of more concern than an irritable, negativistic, food-refusing, night-awakening 8-month-old with age-appropriate capacities for differentiation and reciprocal social interchanges.

Each developmental level involves different tasks or goals. The relative effect of the constitutional-maturational, environmental, or interactive variables, therefore, depends on and can only be understood in the context of the developmental level they relate to. For example, as a child negotiates the formation of a relationship (engaging), his mother's tendency to prefer "talking" over "holding" may make it harder to become deeply engaged in emotional terms. If he has muscle tone and is under-responsive to touch and sound, his mother's intellectual style may be doubly difficult, as neither she nor the child is able to take the initiative in engaging the other. He may be able to negotiate this early phase of development with the support of others, e.g., father "wooing" him. Then at age 3, when the developmental phase and task are different, he may have an easier time, even though his mother hasn't changed. She may be highly creative and enjoy pretend play as well as give-and-take logical discussions. The task is no longer forming a relationship, but of learning to represent (or symbolize) experience and his mother's verbal style is now quite helpful to him. It is important to note that all levels embrace a widening range of emotions as child develops.

The goal of Axis II is to look at the child-caregiver interactions at different stages of development, consider what influences their interaction, and determine whether emotional functioning leads to adaptive or maladaptive organizations at each developmental level. There are six early organizational levels of experience. Each is described below with expected emotional functioning and examples of challenges.

Table 1: Functional Emotional Developmental Capacities

Level	Expected Emotional Function	Developmental Level
1	Shared Attention and Regulation	Readily observable between birth and 3 months
2	Engagement and Relating	Readily observable between 2 and 6 months
3	Two-Way Purposeful Emotional Interactions	Readily observable between 4 and 9 months
4	Shared Social Problem Solving	Readily observable between 9 and 18 months
5	Creating Symbols and Ideas	Readily observable between 18 and 30 months
6	Building Logical Bridges Between Ideas: Logical Thinking	Readily observable between 30 and 48 months

LEVEL 1: SHARED ATTENTION AND REGULATION

(Readily Observable between Birth and 3 Months)

The first level of development involves self-regulation and shared attention, that is, the capacity to attend to multisensory affective experience and, at the same time, organize a calm, regulated state (e.g., looking at, listening to, and following movement of a caregiver). In the early stages of development, the caregiver normally provides sensory input through play and caretaking experiences such as dressing and bathing and soothes the young infant when distressed to facilitate state organization. It is an interactive process of mutual co-regulation whereby the infant uses the parent's physical and emotional state to organize himself. The early regulation of arousal and physiological states is critical for successful adaptation to the environment and for learning self-calming, attention, and emotional responsivity. The optimal level varies considerably and depends upon the infant's threshold for arousal, tolerance for stimulation, and ability to self-control arousal. The caregiver needs to tailor interactions to sensory modulation differences (e.g., under- or over-responsivity to touch or sound), as well as motor planning capacities (e.g., turning to look at the caregiver). See Axis III: Regulatory-Sensory Processing Capacities for more information. The baby who calms down is learning the means for obtaining dependency and comfort. The baby who is interested in the world can, with a certain posture or glance, let his primary caregiver know he is interested in visual, auditory, and tactile sensations. Infants who have difficulty calming are uncomfortable and may not be able to organize the affective domains of joy, pleasure, and exploration as well as goal-directed movement or social behaviors. Even when the infant is quite competent from a regulatory standpoint, a depressed or self-absorbed caregiver might fail to draw a baby into a regulating relationship. A caregiver who is impatient with dysregulation, or who reacts with abuse or withdrawal, may encourage ineffective patterns of behavior.

Summary

- Capacity to show calm interest in the world by looking and listening when talked to or provided with appropriate visual, auditory, movement and tactile experiences
- An interactive process of mutual co-regulation whereby the infant uses the parent's physical and emotional state to organize himself and learns self-calming, attention and emotional responsivity
- The ability of the dyad to attend to one another and remain calm and focused for a reasonable period of time increases with the age of the infant, e.g., 5+ seconds by 3-4 months, 30+ seconds by 8-10 months, 2+ minutes by 2 years of age, and 15 minutes by 4 years

LEVEL 2: ENGAGEMENT AND RELATING

(Readily Observable between 2 and 6 Months)

Once the infant has achieved some capacity for regulation and interest in the world, between 2 and 4 months of age, she becomes more engaged in social and emotional interactions. There is greater ability to respond to the external environment and to form a special relationship with primary caregivers. Engagement is supported by early maturational abilities for selectively focusing on the human face and voice and for processing and organizing information from senses. A type of synchrony of relating is evident in both the way the infant and parent use their senses, motor systems, and affect to resonate with one another to orchestrate highly pleasurable affect in their relationship. Clinically, some infants are not able to employ their senses to form an affective relationship with the human world, such as when sounds, touch, and even scents are avoided either with chronic gaze aversion, recoiling, flat affect, or random or nonsynchronous patterns of brightening and alerting.

Functional relationships organize a widening range of emerging affect as development unfolds from positive affect such a joy and pleasure, to assertiveness, curiosity, protest, anger, etc. Major limitations are evidenced by flat or shallow affect or under stress.

Summary

- Ability for mutual emotional engagement, seen in looking, joyful smiling and laughing, synchronous arm and leg movements, and other gestures which convey a sense of pleasure and affective engagement
- As the relationship evolves, the infant evidences a growing sense of security and comfort, and interest and curiosity in the caregiver
- As development proceeds, the fuller range of emerging emotions becomes part of this capacity, e.g., protest and anger at caregiver are tolerated along with positive affects of pleasure and joy
- Over time this capacity embraces the full hierarchy of emotions including frustration, disappointment, sadness, fear, jealousy, competition, fairness, etc.

LEVEL 3: TWO-WAY PURPOSEFUL EMOTIONAL INTERACTIONS

(Readily Observable between 4 and 9 Months)

The next stage involves purposeful communication consisting of intentional, pre-verbal communications or gestures (i.e., opening and closing a number of circles of communication in a row). These gestures convey affective communication seen in facial expressions, arm and leg movements, pointing, vocalizations, and postures or movement patterns. This stage indicates processes occurring at the somatic (sensorimotor) and emerging psychological levels once the infant is able to discriminate primary caregivers and differentiate his own actions from their consequences. One can see cause-and-effect signaling with the full range of expected emotions. For example, the 8 month-old infant shows pleasure with smiles and love of touching when cuddling, shows curiosity and assertiveness reaching for a rattle, shows anger and protest as he throws his food on the floor in an intentional manner and looks at his caregiver as if to say, "What are you going to do now?" and may protest and even bite as an expression of anger. With the lack of reciprocal responses from their caregiver, the infant may evidence affective dampening and despondency or sadness even after he has shown earlier joyfulness and an adaptive attachment.

The child demonstrates mastery of this stage by using purposeful gestures, such as facial expressions, motor gestures (e.g., showing you something), or vocalizations in a reciprocal back and forth manner. It is important to note whether the infant/toddler initiates such gestures (i.e., opens the circle of communication) and if she in turn responds to the parents' counter-gesturing with a further gesture of her own (i.e., closes the circle of communication). Aimless behavior, misreading of the other person's cues, fragmented islands of purposeful interaction, self-absorbed behavior, indicate challenges at this level. In addition, the ability to be purposeful around some affects, but not others (e.g., around love, but not assertiveness), also indicates limitations.

Summary

- Ability to interact in a purposeful, intentional and reciprocal manner, both initiating and responding to the other's signals

- The capacity for cause-and-effect interacting involves both sensorimotor patterns (e.g., arm and leg movements, vocalizations, body postures) and different emotional inclinations (e.g., reaching out to be picked up, curiosity and exploring, pleasure in putting a finger in mommy's mouth, expressing anger and protest, etc.). This may be thought of as opening and closing circles of communication. The infant initiates, for example, looking at an object (opens the circle of communication), and the parent responds with picking up the object and putting it right in front of the infant with a big smile and says, "Here it is!" When the infant either vocalizes or reaches or changes her facial expression in response to the parent, she is closing the circle of communication by building on the parent's response. This capacity is usually established by 10 months.
- Number and complexity of interactions increases as the child grows and more circles are expected in a continuous flow of interactions, from closing 3-4 circles by 8-10 months, to 10-30 circles by 12-16 months, to 30-to a "continuous flow" of circles by 20-24 months.
- This capacity should increase as the child grows from 2-3 years to 3-4 years, etc.

LEVEL 4: SHARED SOCIAL PROBLEM SOLVING

(Readily Observable between 9 and 18 Months)

This capacity is evidenced by engaging in a continuous flow of circles of communication. These are now complex organized problem-solving, affective interactions (e.g., the 14 month-old who can take his mother's hand, walk her to the refrigerator, bang on the door, and, when the door is opened, point to the desired food). The toddler now sequences many cause-and-effect units related to wishes and intentions into a chain or organized pattern and takes a more active role in developing and maintaining the reciprocal relationship with his parent's interactions. He can now use and respond to social cues to achieve a sense of competence and autonomy (i.e., sense of self). The piecing together of many smaller cause-and-effect units of experience involves a widening range of experience, such as pleasure, assertiveness, curiosity, and dependency, into an organized pattern. For instance, a toddler may start out cuddling with parents, shift to a pleasurable, giggly interchange with them, imitate a little hand game, and then get off their laps and invite them to engage in an assertive chase game in which he runs to a room that is off-limits and turns to look at the parent. When the parent says, "No, you can't go in there," protest and negativism may emerge. The toddler uses emotional signals to figure out whether behaviors related to exploration, aggression, and limits are acceptable. The toddler runs back to the playroom, picks up the play phone to call Mommy (indicating functional understanding of objects used in a semi-realistic way but not yet imaginary play. guided by mental representations or ideas), and then sits on his parent's lap, pleasurably exploring pictures in his favorite book. Had someone unfamiliar come into the room he might be wary or fearful, discriminating his affiliations, but able to regain security in proximity to his parent who responsively signals he is okay. Had he been across the room feeding the doll babies, distal emotional signals from his parent (e.g., smiling and talking in a friendly voice) would allay his concerns. Here the child has gone full circle, suggesting that he has connected the many affective-thematic areas in multiple circles of communication.

The different gestures reveal the range and type of affects from assertive, competitive, and mildly aggressive behavior to explosive and uncontrolled rage, or promiscuous emotional hunger to mild affection, and a sincere sense of warmth and compassion. Basic emotional messages of safety and security vs. danger; acceptance vs. rejection; approval vs. disapproval; can all be communicated through facial expressions, body posture, movement patterns, and vocal tones and rhythm. Words enhance these more basic communications, but gestures convey emotional messages even before the conversation gets started and may discount the words. Gestural communication also relays what aspects of our own emotions are being accepted, ignored, or rejected. The raised eyebrows and head nods we perceive quickly tell us whether the person hearing our message is reacting with excitement, anger, curiosity, or detachment. The nonverbal, gestural communication system is therefore a part of every dialogue contributing to our sense of who we are and what we perceive. In the second year of life, toddlers can make their intentions known and are learning to comprehend the intentions of others through opening and closing many circles of communication in a row (30 or 40).

The importance of the presymbolic gestural level of communication cannot be overestimated. The clinician who only focuses on a person's words may miss an underlying, critical lack of organized gestural communication. Our gestures, in part, help us define our feelings (e.g., muscle tension and anger) and also are a form of expression of feelings. Even when children move onto symbolic levels, the lack of gestural variation removes the early warning system. Children don't learn to modulate their behavior because there is no graded gestural feedback or internal signaling system, only all-or-nothing punishments, much like the all-or-nothing quality of their own behavior. A child may not establish this distal communication capacity because a parent is overanxious, overprotective, or overly symbiotic. Or the child may not have optimal use of the distal modes because of a unique maturational pattern or processing problem. He may not decode the emotional intent or tone of Mother's statement, "That's a good boy." Or, he may have difficulty reading facial gestures or interpersonal distance. Or, he may have to be held to feel secure. Most worrisome is the toddler who pulls away entirely from emotional relationships or becomes constricted, e.g., the child who never asserts himself, is always negative, has difficulties with affiliative behavior, does not form the intermediary warning and delay capacities that complex internal affects are used for, tends to see people only as fulfilling their hunger for physical touch or candy, cake, or other concrete satisfactions. Problems at this stage of behavioral organization are chronic temper tantrums, inability to initiate even some self-control, lack of motor or emotional coordination, chronic negativism, sleep disturbance, hyperirritability, withdrawal, delayed language development, and relationships characterized by chronic aggressive behavior.

Summary

- Reciprocal affective interactions increase in complexity, purpose, and number of steps as the infant is able to sequence together many cause and effect units related to wishes and intentions into an organized behavioral pattern through gestures., e.g., the 14 month-old who can take his mother's hand, walk her to the refrigerator, bang on the door, and when the door is opened, point to the desired drink.

- Takes a more active role in initiating and maintaining the interactions through affect-based gestures which involve a range of experience such as pleasure, assertiveness, curiosity, etc.
- Utilizes and responds to emotional signals and social cues, which encourage a sense of competence and recognition of approval, safety, humiliation, e.g., the toddler invites a chase game, picks up the signal not to go downstairs, protests but runs the other way, until "caught" and cuddles and kisses
- Closer to 18 months, the toddler is able to use objects according to their functional properties (e.g., talk on the phone or comb hair) in semi-realistic way (not yet imaginary play)

LEVEL 5: CREATING SYMBOLS AND IDEAS

(Readily Observable between 18 and 30 Months)

The next level involves the creation, elaboration, and sharing of meanings seen in the toddler's ability to represent experience in pretend play, the verbal labeling of feelings ("I feel happy"), and the functional use of language. Now affect or emotions invest symbols and give them meaning. Meaningful symbols are quite different from memorized ones or labeled objects or pictures. The child can express and interpret feelings rather than simply act them out ("me mad") and can also express a variety of needs and ideas.

Pretend play is, perhaps, an even more reliable indicator than language of the child's ability to represent experience, especially when the child may have language delays. Infants progress from engaging in actions with themselves (e.g., feeding self) to using themselves as the agents to act upon others (e.g., toddler uses a doll to feed another doll). The elaboration of ideas or representations gradually becomes more complex as does the sense of self which now involves symbols, not just behaviors. Initially, the elements in the complex drama *may not be logically connected*, but expand to include a range of themes, including dependency, pleasure, assertiveness, curiosity, aggression, self-limit-setting, and eventually empathy and love. If for any reason the child is not getting practice through interactive pretend play and/or functional language use, deficits or constrictions may occur because the mother or father becomes anxious in using ideas in emotionally relevant contexts. For example, the child may be afraid of emotional fantasy, especially specific themes such as separation or rejection, aggression, or assertiveness. Parental anxiety often leads to intrusive, over-controlling, undermining, over-stimulating, withdrawn, or concrete behavioral patterns, i.e., "Let's not talk or play; I will feed you." As a result, he may not use ideas to reason but regresses to a concrete pre-representational behavioral action pattern of acting out. If his parents ignore elevating aggression to the representational plane, they are leaving aggression to the behavioral discharge mode. Other children may never learn to use the representational mode and show impulsive or withdrawn behavior or limit symbolic modes to dominance and aggression and show little elaboration in the pleasurable or intimate domain.

Summary

- Capacity to represent or symbolize experience, as evidenced in functional use of language, pretend play, and the verbal labeling of feelings for communicating emotional themes and ideas. For example, the child using words to ask for candy or juice, pretending to feed or put the doll to bed, repair crashed cars with hammer, etc. at 18 to 24 months. More elaboration and simple language to express feelings (e.g., "me mad," "love you,") appear by 30 months.

- At first gestures and language may be concrete and functional, related to daily experiences and routines and then elaborated through longer, more logical sequences (e.g., drama of doll playing in park, comes home for dinner and goes to bed).
- Over time ideas begin to go beyond the basic needs and simple themes to convey two or more emotional ideas at a time in terms of more complex intentions, wishes, or feelings, (e.g., themes of closeness or dependency, separation, curiosity assertiveness, anger, etc.)
- The ideas need not be related or logically connected to one another, (e.g., trucks are crashing and then load up blocks to build a house)

LEVEL 6: BUILDING LOGICAL BRIDGES BETWEEN IDEAS: LOGICAL THINKING

(Readily Observable between 30 and 48 Months)

The next level involves *creating logical bridges* between ideas and feelings, and differentiating those feelings, thoughts, and events that emanate from within and those that emanate from others through pretend play and reality based conversations. As logical bridges between ideas are established, reasoning and appreciation of reality grow, including distinguishing what's pretend from what's believed to be real, what's right and wrong, and learning to deal with conflicts and finding prosocial outcomes. As children become capable of emotional thinking, they begin to understand relationships between their own and others' experiences and feelings (e.g., "I am mad because you took my toy"). As they develop, they balance fantasy and reality taking time and space into account

Pretend play often begins with feeding or hugging scenes suggesting nurturance and dependency. Over time, however, the dramas the child may initiate (with parental interactive support) expand to include scenes of separation (e.g., one doll going off on a trip and leaving the other behind), competition, assertiveness, aggression, injury, death, recovery (e.g., the doctor doll fixes the wounded soldier since good guys never die), and so forth. At the same time, the structure of the fantasy/drama becomes more and more logical and causally related. The "He-Man" doll is hurt by the "bad guys" and therefore "gets them" riding his super rocket ship which can go on land, sea and outer space. It is at this stage that the young child develops the capacity to share differentiated meanings. He can not only communicate his own ideas, but also build on the ideas and comments of the other person, whereby he explores a wider range of feelings. Parents who confuse their own feelings with the child's feelings, or cannot set limits, may compromise the formation of a reality orientation. Children at this stage also begin to negotiate the terms of their relationship with others in more reality-based conversations, e.g., "Can I do this?" or "Can I do that?" "What will you do if I kick the ball into the wall?" They begin to engage in debates, opinion-oriented conversations, and/or elaborate, planned pretend dramas.

Summary

- Capacity to elaborate, in both make-believe and dialogues, a number of ideas that go beyond the basic needs and simple themes typical of early representational communication above.
- Evidences the capacity to use symbolic communication to convey two or more emotional ideas at a time in terms of more complex intentions, wishes, or feelings which are *logically connected*, e.g., themes of closeness or dependency, separation, exploration, fear, assertiveness, anger, aggression, self pride or showing off.
- By 36 months, the child can close symbolic circles of communication in pretend play as well as in actual conversations.
- At the upper end (42-48 months), the play or direct communication involves three or more ideas that are logically connected. The child can distinguish between reality and fantasy, and take into account concepts of causality, time, and space. He usually can distinguish the real from the unreal, is able to switch back and forth between fantasy and reality with little difficulty, and can plan "how," "what," and "why" elaborations that give depth to the drama or reality-based dialogues.

SUMMARY OF AXIS II

Axis II identifies six basic functional emotional developmental capacities, which depend on critical affective interactions. These capacities initially emerge in a developmental progression at the ages indicated. In optimal development, as a child grows, he or she continues to develop each capacity to a higher level. Yet, each child may first evidence these processes at ages that are later than expected and/or to different degrees.

GUIDELINES FOR ASSESSING AXIS II

(Also see Appendix I)

The assessment of this axis should be based on observations of the infant or young child interacting with the caregiver for at least 20 minutes. Toward the end of the evaluation the diagnostician should do some "coaching" and/or evaluate the quality of his or her own interaction with the infant to observe the infant's capacities under the most supportive conditions possible at the time.

Infants and young children vary in the length of time they can sustain these processes, as well as the conditions needed for optimal engagement (e.g., to maintain the quality of the relating). For example, infants who are highly reactive or sensitive to various sensations and distractions may not be able to sustain mutual attention or reciprocity unless the parent changes to a quieter environment and woos them back into interaction. Infants who are under-responsive to input, or may over-focus on playing with toys rather than with their parents, may not become affectively engaged as evidenced by mutual gaze and pleasure, unless the parent provides sensorimotor support such as deep pressure, tickling, rough housing and/or high energy affective wooing to establish some mutuality.

Specifically, the clinician needs to observe and consider the following for each level. Also see Table 1 which follows.

1. Has child reached expected his age expected capacities with a full range of affect states in a stable manner?
2. Has the child reached age-expected capacities, but with constrictions? Constrictions are not in keeping with age-expected forms of the capacity, e.g., relates but immaturely, or not functioning across the full range of emotions, the full range of age-expected motor and regulatory-sensory processing capacities (e.g., uses vision, not sounds), or inconsistently (e.g., capacity is not yet stable).
3. Capacity is not yet present though expected for age.
4. Not applicable because the capacity is not yet expected for the child's age.

Table 2: Rating the Functional Emotional Developmental Levels Ratings

Ratings

M	*Mastered*	Has child reached expected age capacities with full range of affect states in a stable manner?
C	*Constricted*	Has the child reached age-expected capacities, but with constrictions?
NP	*Not Present*	Capacity is not yet present though expected for age.
NA	*Not Applicable*	Because the capacity is not yet expected for the child's age.

Functional Emotional Developmental Level	Rating Chart			
	M = Mastered	C = Constricted	NP = Not Present	NA = Not Applicable
Shared Attention and Regulation (0-3 months and beyond)				
Engagement and Relating (3-6 months and beyond)				
Purposeful Emotional Interactions (6-9 months and beyond)				
Shared Social Problem Solving (9-18 months and beyond)				
Creating Symbols and Ideas (18-30 months and beyond)				
Building Bridges between Ideas: Logical Thinking (30-48 months and beyond)				

NOTE: A reliable, validated parent questionnaire–*The Greenspan Social Emotional Growth Chart*–that assesses each functional emotional developmental capacity is available from http://www.harcourtassessment.com (Greenspan, 2004).

Axis III: Regulatory-Sensory Processing Capacities

There are a number of constitutional-maturational differences in the way in which infants and young children respond to and comprehend sensory experiences and plan actions. The different observed patterns exist on a continuum from relatively normal variations to disorders. Disorders occur when the variation or individual differences are sufficiently severe to interfere with age-expected emotional, social, cognitive, or learning capacities. The clinician should indicate in this axis the presence or absence of regulatory-sensory processing differences in the categories. It should be noted, however, that if the primary diagnosis is a regulatory-sensory processing disorder, these patterns are already described in the primary diagnosis and this axis need not be repeated. To summarize the range of these regulatory-sensory processing differences, the clinician may use the following demarcations to indicate the degree to which the pattern represents normal variations versus severe impairments. For each category, such as sensory over-responsiveness, the clinician can indicate:

- Not Present
- Present, but within a Range of Normal Variation
- Mild To Moderate Impairments (e.g., makes it difficult for the child to get dressed or remain calm in noisy settings), and
- Severe Impairments (makes it difficult for the child to engage in relationships, form basic patterns of communication, or learn to think).

Axis IV: Language Capacities

Children vary considerably in their ability to comprehend and express intentions and ideas. In the section on language disorders, a developmental classification approach is described to capture each child's unique language pattern in terms of its overall developmental level as well as different features characterizing language functioning at that level. The overall language stages parallel the functional emotional developmental stages because both are describing the presymbolic as well as the symbolic levels of the child's overall functioning and communication. The language capacities, however, focus on communication, particularly from the toddler through the preschool years.

The language axis is suggested as part of the overall developmental profile of the child because differences in language functioning, just as differences in regulatory-sensory functioning and family patterns, contribute to the primary symptom patterns of the child (i.e., the primary diagnosis). Therefore, even when the primary diagnosis may not directly involve language functioning per se (e.g., a disruptive behavior disorder), the child's language functioning may be important to consider. For example, confusion over shared meaning or an inability to "read" preverbal communicative gestures may heighten frustration, increase the likelihood of misperception, or both, and contribute to aggressive behavior.

In Axis I: Language Disorders, there are more detailed descriptions of all the different facets of language functioning that may be considered. Once the evaluation is completed, the clinician's narrative will describe the language profile of the child along with a clinical formulation of the different facets of language functioning. In this axis, the clinician can provide an overall rating of child's language functioning. The rating, however, is not a substitute for the clinical narrative. Note, however, that if the primary diagnosis is a language disorder, these patterns will already be described in Axis I: Language Disorders and this axis need not be repeated.

As with regulatory-sensory processing capacities, the age-expected language profile of the child can be characterized along the following demarcations:

- Within range of normal variation
- Mild to moderate impairment
- Severe impairment

Axis V: Visuospatial Capacities[1]

Axis V addresses visuospatial capacities and how these are integrated into cognitive and emotional functioning in order to evaluate their possible contribution to the various disorders described in this manual. The inclusion and assessment of visuospatial capacities have not been as systematic in literature on early development as other capacities, such as language and communication or movement, have been. We include it here since what a person can understand from a particular visuospatial experience and, eventually, coordinate with other aspects of body and sense thinking, as well as the development of self-awareness in relation to other people and objects, is essential for emotional development as well as cognition and learning. The child eventually coordinates with other aspects of body and sense thinking and the development of self-awareness in relation to other people and objects.

Each visuospatial capacity has a developmental sequence beginning at birth which continues to develop through childhood. Successive capacities develop as the child's nervous system matures, affect comes in, and the child's experience in the environment expands. Each capacity builds on earlier ones and functions simultaneously with prior capacities, as well as with all the other sensory systems. For conceptual purposes, we break down each capacity and describe its developmental sequence from birth through early childhood. However, different things occur at different times under different situations for individual children. The early capacities are first partially mastered and then further experience makes them complete as the child developmentally matures. The clinician should try to form a judgment about whether or not the child has mastered a particular capacity with respect to typical age expectations.

We outline the development of six visuospatial capacities during infancy and early childhood (pre-school years) which interact simultaneously with the other sensory processing capacities and support or impede emotional and cognitive development. Some examples are given to illustrate each capacity, but these are not all-inclusive. It is important to remember that all the described capacities overlap and that the clinician should keep the developmental continuum in mind, as opposed to just focusing on a chronology of milestones.

We present a summary table first to help illustrate the overall continuum and then we describe each capacity separately in more detail. The table can also be used to evaluate the overall visuospatial capacities by indicating whether the child has overall age-expected capacities, partially developed capacities, or has not yet developed age-expected levels. This can also be applied to the six specific capacities. However, these demarcations do not take the place of a clinical narrative that describes the individual capacities of the child on each level and relates it to his or her primary disorder and functional development on the other axes.

---

[1] In other books we discuss how to help a child with visual deficits master the important components of visuospatial thinking through the development of other sensory modalities (Furth & Wachs, 1974; Interdisciplinary Council on Developmental and Learning Disorders Clinical Practice Guidelines Workgroup, 2000; Greenspan, 2005)

Table 3: Summary of Visuospatial Capacities by Age

Visuospatial Capacities **Indicate the overall capacity for expected age levels** (Note that Year 1 is actually birth to first year, Year 2 is first birthday to second birthday, and so on)	1= Mastered at age expected level 2= Partially mastered at age expected level 3= Not yet mastered
1. Body Awareness and Sense Year 1: Purposeful, coordinated movement, guided by vision and sound. Year 2: Purposeful movement for interactive play (rolling a ball back and forth) Year 3: Awareness of body boundaries of self and others Year 4: Awareness of body affecting others in space and time Year 5: Awareness of body for coordinated actions	
2. Location of the Body in Space Involves location of own body parts in relationship to each other, location of body as a whole in its immediate surroundings; and location of the body in terms of the broader environment. Year 1: Beginning movement in space Year 2: Observes things move in space in relationship to self Year 3: Purposeful movement in relation to other moving objects Year 4: Planning and organization of movement prior to the action Year 5: Becoming a team player	
3. Relation of Objects to Self and Other Objects and People Year 1: Reciprocal interactions with people and things Year 2: Self-control in relation to other people and things Year 3: Development of symbols Year 4: Rules and expectations Year 5: Boundaries and Membership	
4. Conservation of Space Year 1: Space is uni-dimensional Year 2: Space is three-dimensional and movement in space is alterable Year 3: Relationship of object in three dimensional space Year 4: Relationship of object to object in space Year 5: Combining time and space	
5. Visual Logical Reasoning Year 1: Knowledge through sensorimotor action Year 2. Moving from action knowledge to planning the actions Year 3: Understanding the cause and effect of the action Year 4: Stability of early visuospatial thinking Year 5: Logical thinking to solve problems	
6. Representational Thought (Drawing, Thinking, Visualizing) Year 1: Direct representation Year 2: Words, pictures, gestures, and toys Year 3: Early imaginative play Year 4: More purposeful representations Year 5: Matching space to representational thought	

BODY AWARENESS AND SENSE

Year 1: Development of the knowledge of body parts and their coordination for purposeful movement guided by all the senses

Infants' lives begin with the process of finding the dimensions and structure of their bodies. First the infant becomes aware of her body parts and sensations in them through mouthing and touching. Within days and weeks after birth, infants put their fingers or toes in their mouths and soon explore the various orifices of their bodies. They begin to look at and identify the body parts they just experienced through touching or mouthing. They also look at faces and can mirror facial expressions associated with different emotions. Soon their hands make contact with each other and the realization that "both are a part of me" follows. However, the infants do not yet realize that the two hands belong to one person. They can even experience one hand at a time very early because of the Palmer Reflex. If a finger or small rattle comes into their hand, they grasp it reflexively and soon become aware that by moving a part of themselves such as their arms, they can move the rattle. The ability to isolate and move the body parts intentionally is to become aware that "I did that!"

At the same time they turn their heads to the sound to look at what they hear in a very purposeful way. Before long the infant can reach out with her hands and feet to make something happen as she learns to use her body for purposeful action. As the infant develops an interest in both sides of her body (i.e., tries to switch items from one hand to another), she is beginning to make a mental map of her body. The baby begins to move (e.g., roll, crawl and creep), as well as use hand-eye, hand-hand, and hand-foot interactions (e.g., picks up small objects she sees, claps her hands, holds on to pull up, stand, and cruise).

Some infants have difficulty using both hands at the midline at the same time so they reach for their parents' hands instead. Many infants initiate walking by the end of the first year, and thereby become capable of purposeful, coordinated movement, guided by vision, sound and gravity.

Year 2: Purposeful movement for interactive play and actions

By the end of the second year, the toddler uses his awareness of his body actions to interact with the actions of someone else's body or things. He can act upon the interactions of his caregiver when he cooperates with dressing and knows which part of the body to extend in response to the caregiver's actions. Using his body awareness, he can also imitate the actions of someone else's actions. He can also use purposeful movement for interactive play such as rolling a ball back and forth or pulling the scarf off and on his mother's head in an interactive peek-a-boo game and tug of war. He can also make his body cry or throw things to get someone to give him what he wants. His growing independence also extends to using his body awareness to act upon objects or things, such as stacking blocks high until they fall, stopping a ball rolling towards him with his hands so it doesn't hit his body, or scribbling with chalk and seeing what his hand did.

Year 3: Awareness of body boundaries of self and others

By 3 years of age, the young child's awareness of the boundaries between herself and others in space is used as part of social interactions, but the child isn't necessarily aware of, or respectful of, someone else's space. This is seen when the child bumps into someone, has difficulty keeping his place in line, or hits or pushes another person. In some cases caregivers may also fail to respect the child's space and boundaries, such as when they wipe the child's nose or face intrusively without signaling. The gradual development of body awareness as it influences other people's bodies and as it operates in the larger context of time and space prepares the child for location in space.

An indication of delayed development would be the child who cannot alternate his feet to walk steps. This child lacks spatial awareness of both his body and external space and does not have adequate depth perception, knowing where something is (his feet) in relation to other things (the stairs). Similarly, the child may be unaware when he bumps into someone or something and causes him or it to fall on the floor. He may similarly drop something and not look down to pick it up.

Year 4: Awareness of body affecting others in space and time

By the time the child reaches the fourth year, once the boundaries of her body are relatively defined, the child develops the awareness of her body affecting others in space and time. This is seen when the child moves over to make space for someone else to sit down or begins to play movement games (e.g., tag) and ball games. There is also growing awareness of how each side of her body performs different parts of the action in which the whole body is involved, such as riding a scooter or tricycle, or learning to hop on one foot by balancing the rest of her body. The child is now developing the capacity to interrelate all the body parts to coordinate actions.

The child who has difficulties may not be able to turn the scooter that she is riding around or stop the scooter to avoid crashing into a parked car. Similarly, the child who can't help knocking over the bottle as she reaches for a nearby cup does not have the body awareness to coordinate her arm going around the bottle and reaching for the cup. Without adequate awareness, the child does not realize what his arm is going to do and doesn't involve each side of the body in a bilateral activity. Another indicator might be if the child can't successfully carry something over to somewhere else in the room directly or immediately.

Year 5: Awareness of body for coordinated actions

By year 5 the child is able to coordinate her actions and develops the mastery of visuospatial capacities from the year before. The child's body awareness now allows her to isolate which body part is being touched without looking. She can hop, skip, and jump in all directions and is aware of her body in relation to things under, over, or to the side of her. She can catch a ball with two hands rather than against her body and also walk forward on a straight line in tandem or cross over bilaterally. This awareness now allows her to take turns while playing, and to share her body awareness or knowledge with peers for whom she observes and demonstrates how to coordinate actions to do things independently or with a group.

During the next year the child is able to consolidate her capacities for coordinated actions. It is also the period in which children often learn to do coordinated actions they did not master earlier, like skipping or riding a bike. While the continuum of body awareness described here is human specific, the chronology is cultural in that the culture shapes the actions expected of children at certain times. For example, Zulu children at age 3 can skip very well in Africa. In the Western world, it's age 6, while South American Indians can't skip at all and when jumping up in the air, don't land on two feet simultaneously.

LOCATION OF THE BODY IN SPACE

The development of this capacity involves several elements: location of one's own body parts in relationship to each other; location of body as a whole in its immediate surroundings; and location of the body in terms of the broader environment (e.g., location of objects, distance, etc.). Children are now continuously moving through space, across distances and climbing up and down. They can focus on an object in the distance and judge if they can reach it. They can search for an object they don't see. They can throw a ball across space in the direction they want and put out their hands to intercept it, but don't yet catch solely with hands. They can locate and regulate the proximity or distance they want from others, e.g., run faster to greet daddy or run faster to be chased by daddy.

Year One: Child begins to move in space

(1) Location of own body parts in relationship to each other

By age one, the foundation for this capacity is laid, using the early development of body awareness to construct location in space, and it develops with more experience moving through space. With awareness of his body's hands and feet, the infant starts to realize that one hand is on one side and the other is on the other side. He can locate his body parts and find his foot and put it into his mouth, can reach with his hand and touch his foot, and soon begins to transfer objects from hand to hand. The infant is starting to realize how all these parts work together in his endogenous (internal) space.

(2) Location of body as a whole in its immediate surroundings

During the first year, the infant is also encountering the world around him. For example, when he first thrusts his hand out and hits side of his crib, he is realizing something is over there on that side that will limit what he can do and how far he can go.

(3) Location of the body in terms of the broader environment (location of objects, distance, etc.)

The infant also becomes visually aware of spatial verticality looking up and down. For example, when mother picks her infant up, the infant sees the difference when being held vertically in mother's arms as opposed to lying in the crib. When an infant is immobile and not picked up sufficiently, he does not have adequate knowledge of being upright against gravity which is necessary later to operate in the mobile stage. As the infant develops mobility, he can relocate himself in space by rolling, crawling, and creeping. For example, when the infant begins to crawl towards his caregiver or a favorite toy, he also discovers new areas he can move towards. The infant is making the transition from an environment thrust upon him when he was immobile to where he himself can seek things in the environment. As he expands his sense of body in space to explore, he can purposefully manipulate objects below or above his location. He also begins to appreciate that he can crawl faster to get to his dad faster, which is the beginning of temporal exploration. The highlight at the end of the first year is making accurate visual judgments between things in space for mobility purposes, i.e., walking. The infant realizes he is responsible for his moving in space.

Year 2: Things move in space in relation to the child

By 2 years, the toddler has mastered his movement in space and becomes aware that other people and things move in space in relation to him. Toddlers are now continuously moving through space, across distances, and climbing up and down. They can focus on an object in the distance and judge if they can reach it. They can search for an object they don't see. They can throw a ball across space in the direction they want and put out their hands to intercept it, but they don't catch it yet with their hands. They can locate and regulate the proximity or distance they want from others, such as run faster toward daddy to greet him or run away faster to be chased by daddy. The toddler now comprehends space in all dimensions in relationship to where he is located, but does not as yet fully comprehend proximal-distal relationships. This is why a 2 year-old runs out in front of a car—he does not realize how far away it is and how fast it reaches him.

Year 3: Move purposefully in relation to other moving objects

By 3 years, the child can intervene purposefully with objects moving in space, e.g., move faster to keep up with Daddy or intercept the toy truck rushing towards him before it crashes.

He begins to tie together spatial and temporal dimensions and figures out what to do to keep up with someone or something else moving in space. This is the age where the child is becoming less egocentric and has a better understanding that what he does affects others, i.e., he is getting an appreciation of others and their space both physically and emotionally. He is also beginning to match his movement with other temporal demands such as matching the rhythm of beating drums or marching in place in his class parade. During this year, the child also enjoys obstacle courses of increasing challenge which require moving in space and moving on objects which move in space. He also notices where things fall when he drops them and picks them up. In addition, this is when the child demonstrates greater awareness of the influence of one's body on others in social interactions in the context of space and time as he and his friends become moving targets in their social interaction games and thematic play with toys, e.g., riding trikes, flying to space, playing "Duck, Duck Goose" or tag.

Year 4: Plans and organizes movement prior to the action

By 4 years, the child can organize his movement through space and time more systematically. He can learn the rules to ball games and throws and catches a ball. He can locate the direction to move on a board game or running bases. He also has greater awareness of his movement impact on others when he plays musical chairs, does relay races, or participates on a team. Difficulties in this area are manifest in the classroom if he can't find his seat in the circle, can't put materials back in bins on the shelf, or can't find his belongings in the cubby. He may prefer to always play with trains where the tracks show him where to move and he does not have to find his own destinations. At home he may have the right number of cups and plates to set the table but can't arrange them in space and locates them all near each other. When he undresses for a bath, his clothes may be scattered everywhere. He may have trouble finding them even when asked to put them in the hamper. Yet, he is very likely to know how to walk the six blocks to the ice cream store.

Year 5: Mastering the organization of self and objects in space

He can organize his actions to cooperate with the actions of others for a common goal, and, therefore, can now begin to play soccer, football and T ball. He has the basic ability to carry out tasks and helps to unpack the groceries. He can also carry out the totality of planned action such as setting the table from beginning to end with the appropriate number of utensils and place settings. Challenges are evident when the caregiver gets frustrated that the child cannot carry out a total task, e.g., finish what they start. At age 5, the child can also copy geometric shapes except diagonals and develops more graphic control to draw and begin printing.

RELATIONSHIP OF OBJECTS TO SELF, OTHER OBJECTS AND OTHER PEOPLE

Year One: Reciprocal interactions with people and things

From the start of life the newborn infant is relating to people and objects by looking out on the world. He follows a moving object such as mother's face or a bright red ball when moved side to side. Within the first 6 months, the infant begins to coordinate sight, gravity, and spatial localization. He begins to experiment with objects, such as dropping a toy on the floor or moving objects closer or further away. With movement, the infant further explores where something might be and sees what he can do with objects (e.g., he crawls over to mommy who is holding his favorite toy or bangs the spoon on the pot to make different sounds).

The infant also discovers what she can do to human objects or other people. She can bop daddy's nose and hear a funny sound, or open his hand to discover the Cheerio, or exchange bites of a donut. By one year the child also begins to develop rudimentary object constancy, i.e., the object remains constant even if she does not see it and it is no longer is "out of sight out of mind." This is evident when the infant continues to search for something he just saw which was suddenly covered up. For example, he picks up the cup covering the block or pulls off the scarf to find mommy. At this point, however, the infant is not able to search directly for the block; he may look under two cups and only look in one place for the block and give up.

Year 2: Exerts self-control over people and things spatially

The toddler is acting upon objects even more actively and exerting self-control over people and things spatially. She discovers she can roll the car harder and it moves faster. She can compare objects and know which one she prefers or tell whether they are the same. She also begins to stack blocks and build simple structures, or uses toys to express ideas such as feeding the baby doll or baby elephant. She can search for the toys she wants in different spaces and locate them now employing visual strategies. On an object permanence task hiding a block under one of two cups, she goes to the first cup and picks it up. If she's wrong, she'll put it down and then go to the second cup, thus indicating she's developed object permanence.

Year 3: Development of symbols

By 3 years, symbols are available for items of regard. The child realizes symbols can be used to take the place of things and people based on the child's object permanence and can expand symbolic play from toys that are miniatures of the real thing to toys or things they substitute or they use gestures to substitute. They also understand the definition of a symbol outside their real (direct) experience such as running with a piece of paper to represent the wind, or flying the pencil as an airplane. The symbol they choose usually is appropriate to some feature of the object (e.g., pencil has long shape of plane). The child also recognizes a graphic logo as a symbol of her favorite fast food place and becomes interested in the sound-symbol connection as she sees signs, recognizes their names, and looks at books. In addition, the child distinguishes what is the "same and not same," recognizing the visual components of objects and can discriminate shapes, block arrangements, size and patterns. On an object permanence task, he watches the switching of the cups and does not go to the first cup, but goes directly to the second cup and finds the block underneath.

Year 4: Conforming to rules and expectations of society

By age 4, children cooperate with the rules and begin realizing their role in the rules. They can understand taking turns in a simple game with rules such as Candyland. They cooperate with other people and recognize when they need to get out of the way in a running game. If they don't do their part in a relay race, their team does not win or if they don't help with clean up, recess is delayed. The child who can watch a soccer game, but not play it, can't follow the coach's direction because that child doesn't grasp the concept of the game. At home she can help unpack the groceries so dinner is ready faster. The child learns to do more things because she can copy complex gestural or social interactions such as help prepare sandwiches, bake cookies, or help wash daddy's car (e.g., imitating body actions of others to carry out necessary sequence). She can also classify, sequence, and place things she sees in a series according to multiple attributes and represent these relationships in space (e.g., arranging furniture in a play house or animals in a zoo, etc.). By getting order into their world, children are getting ready for academic teaching.

Year 5: Boundaries and Membership

By age 5, the child develops respect for the territory and rights of others. Children know what is theirs or not theirs, they accept sharing and dividing, and know they have to negotiate changes and make deals to belong to their society. They develop personal boundaries between themselves and others with the start of personal standards and consolidate earlier rules and expectations. Now they also realize they do not win just because they "said so," and also they do not have to win every game. They also begin to understand the difference when they win by chance or luck and when they win by skill, e.g., Candyland versus Connect Four.

CONSERVATION OF SPACE

As part of understanding the world around him, the child needs to know whether what he sees changes when he moves. For example, when he starts to walk and move in space, does he understand that space isn't moving, but he is? This capacity is called conservation of space and is the mental operation necessary for visuospatial capacities.

Year 1: Space is uni-dimensional

By 1 year, the infant experiences space as uni-dimensional, that is, he sees in a one way direction. If he drops a toy on the floor from the high chair, he looks at it in the direction of falling down. He would actually have to go down on the floor and look up to see it going back up. At this point, the way the infant sees is the only way and no other way exists. He cannot alter what he sees and thus lives essentially in a two-dimensional plane. As a child becomes mobile, (e.g., crawls, rolls, creeps), the child starts to construct three dimensionality.

Year 2: Space is three-dimensional and movement in space is alterable

By 2 years, we see the initiation of the concept of the world as three-dimensional. During the last year the toddler's mobility let him actively explore space. He moves in and around space, he climbs up the ladder to go down the slide, he enjoys obstacle courses, he plays chase and stays clear of things in his way, etc. The toddler who is afraid to go down the slide may be having a problem conserving space because it seems much higher from the top, and he is used to looking from down-up rather than up-down. The child who won't jump into the pool from the edge may have the same experience and prefers to have his daddy standing and reaching out to him. If the child is conserving space, it won't have that effect. He enjoys sliding down or jumping in. By 2 years, the child begins to realize that something moving in space can alter directions or move in reverse, e.g., batting a balloon up in the air and expecting it to come back down.

Year 3: Relationship of object in three dimensional space

By 3 years, the child knows he is living in a three-dimensional sphere and not a flat plane. He now not only realizes that a batted balloon comes down or bouncing a ball against a wall makes it come back, he begins to intercept it if it moves in another direction sideways. Before he would hold his hands out to catch the ball coming to him, but now he knows he may have to move to the side to catch it. By this time the child is also able to match three-dimensional items with two-dimensional pictures to play games or do parquetry.

Year 4: Relationship of object to object in space

By age 4, conservation of space allows the child to start intercepting a missile flying through the air. He can now try to catch a ball playing "monkey in the middle." This is when shooting baskets changes from turn taking to crudely playing basketball with blocking and intercepting the ball. He can do this because he is starting to integrate temporal dimensions with spatial dimensions of the environment and can anticipate where the ball is going to go and intercept it. Difficulties with this capacity can be observed when a child tries to play tag with other kids and runs towards the child, but can't slow down to touch the other kid so he shuts his eyes and collides. This is similar to a child who shuts his eyes as a ball flies towards him to catch or his opponent's sword comes too close and he is disarmed and cannot swing back.

Year 5: Combining time and space

By age 5, the child integrates the different dimensions of space more fluidly and successfully. He can now anticipate multiple senses of direction more fluidly and can turn around to catch a ball coming from different directions. He is starting to integrate temporal with spatial dimensions of the environment (e.g., beginning to anticipate where ball is and intercept it). He also knows if another child is running right to the left, you have to run to where the child is when he gets there and not to where he is when he first spots him (e.g., to play dodge ball). This is also necessary to catch a moving butterfly using a net and taking into account the distance of the net from the hand as well as the flight of the butterfly (visual knowledge of where the butterfly goes).

VISUAL LOGICAL REASONING

This capacity involves applying logic and reasoning to understand what one sees in the world. Visual thinking and logic is making sense of sight and together with verbal reasoning, shapes intelligence, and later academic performance. It is especially involved in mathematical thinking and science. Until the child develops object permanence, the world is too sporadic to become logical. He must be able to retain objects in his mind for mental operations in order to start thinking logically. Precursors of visual thinking are developed in the first few years of life during the sensorimotor period where children learn through their actions. First comes action knowledge, which leads into another action knowledge, until the child can use thinking. For example, the child first tries to place a shape in the shape sorter and if it doesn't fit, then tries another space until he finds the space it fits into and knows it is right. Later, he can look at the shape and look at the space and think through or abstract it correctly. The hierarchy of visual thinking starts at about 3 years of age until 7 when it is fully established. It is not taught or just picked up by watching others, but requires the development of conservation of visual constructs and emerges over time with experience. Keep in mind that development is on a continuum and the yearly ages provided vary for individual children.

Year 1: Knowledge through sensorimotor action

Between birth and one year, the infant is learning cause and effect by seeing what happens when he drops an object, pushes the button on a pop up toy, or spills his cereal on the tray. When she does something new, like rolling over the first time, she is quite amazed. She does not think it happens. Surprise is usually evident when she sees the result of her action as she did not anticipate (think of) the result. Similarly, when the baby discovers if he pulls the string it shakes the rattle, he tries to pull it a second time and a third time even when the rattle is no longer attached. He can do the action but not the thinking.

Year 2: Moving from action knowledge to planning the action

By the time the child reaches 2 years of age, he is moving on from action knowledge, from where he "knows" what he does to thinking. For example, to complete the shape sorter he first used trial and error to see what shapes fit in and relied on what he saw rather than thinking of the shape's dimensions. He arbitrarily tried to fit in pieces, tried to force a square peg into a round hole, tried another hole, then tried to rotate, and finally looked at it, matched it up, and fit it in. To complete the shape sorter by looking at the shape, he has to be able to form a pictorial image of the shape, recall it, and match it to the space. This process occurs roughly between 30 months on solid pieces and 40 months on split pieces. By the end of his second year he is also beginning to use language to describe the problem he sees, e.g. "That's too big!"

Year 3: Understanding the cause and effect of the action

By the time the child reaches 3 years, sensorimotor actions give way to elementary thinking. The child can recognize and imitate a pattern of inch cubes, e.g., red, yellow, green, red, yellow, green, etc. He can discriminate "same/not same" or find the same object from a group of objects. He also can classify attributes of shapes and begins to form conceptual groupings, e.g., find all the big yellow circles in a larger group of blocks. His early thinking now includes counting with 1:1 correspondence as he can put his finger on objects in space without skipping or missing one. During this time some children may try to put on the doll's bright red boots which are so similar to his, or go down a toy slide, or even sit on a small chair, without regard to size or shape, and try to make it fit. The younger child might just give up and walk away, but the older one is willing to see if the shoes fit the doll or use the doll to represent himself and his wish to go splashing in the puddles or down the slide. This process shows the child making the developmental transition from sensorimotor action to representational thinking fueled by his affect or desire to enjoy the action.

Year 4: Stability of early visual spatial thinking

Between 3 and 4 years of age, a whole host of logical visual thinking capacities develop. The earlier pattern of blocks in order can now be extended on either left or right sides, forward, away, and vertically. The child can also copy simple two- and three-block patterns from a sample. He can use trial and error efforts to complete part-whole puzzles where shape forms or things are cut into two or three separate parts and must be rearranged into a whole. By age 4, he is also conserving numbers (amount). Using 1:1 correspondence, he can count out two equal sets of marbles, put each set into two different clear beakers, and realize they have the same number even one looks high (a tall skinny beaker) and the other looks low (short fat beaker). While he thinks they are the same, he is not yet able to explain the logic of his thinking. Prior to age 4 he would think the marbles in the tall skinny beaker were "more" because they rise higher.

Year 5: Logical thinking to solve problems

By 5 years, the child sees everything faster and more complexly. Conservation of number becomes established. He also begins to understand simple Venn diagrams, matrices, and even early probability, e.g., he predicts whether the coin lands on heads or tails, or the likelihood he picks an orange from a basket of ten oranges and three lemons. He starts analogous thinking, e.g., a small square is to a big square, like a small circle is to a ____ (big) circle. He can expand the earlier pattern in different directions, not only going from side to side, but toward and away, as well as up from a designated spot. He can also indicate classification of attributes and series of number mentally (small to big), as well as sounds (low to high pitch), and speed (slow to fast). The child is no longer fooled by appearances and begins to think through what he sees. He is understanding rudimentary retention of reality. Visual logic moves forward with the further development of conservation, including linear length (e.g., a stick displaced in front and forward of an equal stick is not longer); mass (e.g., the amount of clay doesn't change if the clay ball is divided into parts); area (e.g., the amount of space doesn't change if same number of blocks cover different locations on the page, lined up along one edge of the paper versus scattered on the page); weight (e.g., a pound of feathers weigh the same as a pound of blocks); and volume (e.g., one cup of liquid in a tall or short beaker is the same).

REPRESENTATIONAL THOUGHT (DRAWING, THINKING, VISUALIZING)

The capacity to represent something one is thinking of in another form can be done pictorially (drawing) or visually, through gestures (movements) using one's body or with toys, through the rhythm of sounds (auditory), and through words. The capacity for representational thought where one form represents another is essential for higher level thinking and not being bound by just what you see in time and space in the immediate environment. As with all the capacities, representational thought starts to develop early in life and takes several forms, including visualization, the picture image of what you see; motor imagery, the imagination of movement; verbal or concept imagery to express thoughts; and signs or gestures when words are not available.

Year 1: Direct Representation

By the end of the first year, the infant can represent her thinking directly by using vocal gestures and reaching or pointing to the real thing she wants. The infant vocalizes, "Eh eh eh," to represent the juice she wants as she looks or reaches toward the counter.

Year 2: Use words, pictures, gestures and toys to represent the "real thing"

By the end of year 2, there is a dramatic leap in the ability to represent thoughts or desires. The infant can now use words and now says "Juice, juice, I want juice" even when he does not see it. He can use a picture to show you with whom and where he wants to go. He also begins to combine gestures, construction, and toys to represent reality-based experiences and, for example, feeds the baby dolls, pushes cars on the road, hammers the broken doll house, and pushes the toy swing. Sometimes, prior to this development, they try to use a toy as if it is real until they realize it is too small as they make the transition from direct experience to just pretending or representing what they wish to do. They do not yet account for space, and can put one thing on top of another, and not notice they put the gas station on the train track.

Year 3: Early Imaginative Play

By the end of year 3, the child is able to construct the total picture of his thoughts or ideas, but not the total action or consequence of his action. For example, the child runs around shooting his missiles into the air, but does not aim at his target or have the spaceship fall down. Similarly, he can leap his figure from the pirate ship at sea to the roof of the king's castle without representing how he got there. In other words, he does not have a visual or motor image of what precedes or follows his action although he has the global thought or intent to get the "bad guys." At this stage of development, the child does not represent the end result of his thoughts in that he doesn't anticipate where the things he throws land. He can see the parts of his thought and visualize, but can't translate a motor image to its actions, and inappropriately puts the gas station on the train tracks or leaps from the pirate ship to the castle.

Year 4: More Purposeful Representations

By the end of year 4, the child is both more accurate and purposeful in what he chooses to represent. In play, he does not just "knock the bad guys off," but considers how to use the cannon to reach the pirate ship. Sweeping motions and throwing are replaced with some beginning realistic visual strategy to move across space and get to the destination using motor imagery. However, the child is still unable to represent his body with the same orientation in space as someone opposite him. For example, he may not know his right hand is on the opposite side of his body if he is facing you. During this year, the child cannot yet draw in three dimensions. There is also evidence of early graphic intent to represent objects and the child scribbles on paper and tells you he has drawn a person, even pointing to body parts "in his mind" as he interprets the scribbles for you.

Year 5: Organizes space to match representational thought

By age 5, the child can initiate a thought intrinsically and represent it somehow in a logical visual sequence. He can visualize what must happen to organize space to match his representational thought For example, he has his train go into the tunnel and later can say it is still in there because he can represent or visualize that train in the tunnel even though he does not see it. He can pick up a pencil and make it into a train. This contrasts with the younger child who thinks the train has disappeared because he cannot see it and tells you the pencil is a pencil! Similarly, in contrast to a younger child who can respond to or solve a visuospatial problem to build a road to the next town when there is a mountain in the way, and can build the road around the tunnel, the 5 year-old not only visualizes the tunnel but also hauls out the dirt in trucks, builds the scaffolding to hold up the walls, etc. He both visualizes and uses motor images to make it happen, starting inside like the architect who has to design a building by starting inside.

By age 5, the child is also able to draw a simple drawing of a figure, but may not have visual stability which results in letter reversals or writing a word backwards and must wait for further development. By age 7 the child should be competent in all forms of representation of thought–graphic, construction, and language that represent ideas which develop to verbal and written expression. Not until age 9 does the child draw in three dimensions.

Axis VI: Caregiver and Family Patterns

Axis VI describes the overall functioning of the caregiver and tries to identify the degree to which the parent or other caregiver is able to support the child's negotiation of each developmental level. This axis complements Axis II which asks the clinician to describe the interactive patterns at each stage of the child's development and provides a profile of the child's functioning. Since caregiver and family patterns affect children in every group of disorders, and not just the interactive disorders, it is included here as a separate axis. The clinician needs to explore the issues that might be interfering with optimal support. These issues might stem from the nature of the child's specific difficulties, or from the feelings, wishes and conflicts the parent experiences (past and present), from stress of the disorder and/or the stress of the environment, and their interactions. This axis will help the clinician and parent reflect on where the challenges lie and where they stem from. This is essential for the caregiver's central role in the intervention. The family history and functioning can be described in the clinical narrative along with a clinical formulation of how they contribute to the current caregiver and family patterns.

Before considering the overall rating described below, it is important to use the following guidelines to observe each caregiver's interaction with the child:

1. **Caregiver tends to comfort the infant or child**, especially when he or she is upset (by relaxed, gentle, firm holding; rhythmic vocal or visual contact, etc.), rather than tending to make the child more tense (by being overly worried, tense, or anxious; or mechanical or anxiously over- or under-stimulating).
2. **Caregiver tends to find appropriate levels of stimulation to interest the infant or child** in the world (by being interesting, alert, and responsive, including offering appropriate levels of sound, sights, and touch–including the caregiver's face–and appropriate games and toys, etc.), rather than being over-stimulating and intrusive (e.g., picking at and poking or shaking the child excessively to gain his attention).
3. **Caregiver tends to pleasurably engage the infant or child** in a relationship (by looking, vocalizing, gentle touching, etc.), rather than tending to ignore the infant or child (by being depressed, aloof, preoccupied, withdrawn, indifferent, etc.).
4. **Caregiver tends to read and respond to the infant's or child's emotional signals and needs in most emotional areas** (e.g., responds to desire for closeness as well as need to be assertive, explorative, and independent), rather than either misreading signals or only responding to one emotional need. For example, caregiver can hug when baby reaches out, but hovers over baby and cannot encourage assertive exploration or vice versa.
5. **Caregiver tends to encourage the infant or child** to move forward in development, rather than to misread child's developmental needs and overprotect, "hold on," infantilize, be overpressured and/or punitive, be fragmented and/or disorganized, or overly concrete. For example:
   a. The caregiver helps the baby to crawl, vocalize, and gesture by actively responding to the infant's initiative and encouragement (rather than overanticipating the infant's needs and doing everything for him or her).

b. The caregiver helps the toddler make the shift from proximal, physical dependency (e.g., being held) to feeling more secure while being independent (e.g., keeps in verbal and visual contact with toddler as he or she builds a tower on the other side of the room).
c. The caregiver helps the 2 to 3 year-old child shift from motor discharge and gestural ways of relating to the use of "ideas" through encouraging pretend play (imagination) and language around emotional themes (e.g., gets down on the floor and plays out dolls hugging each other, separating from each other, or soldiers fighting with each other).
d. The caregiver helps the 3 to 4 year-old take responsibility for behavior and deal with reality, rather than "giving in all the time," infantilizing or being overly punitive.

The caregiver characteristics described above cover a number of developmentally-based adaptive patterns. If in considering these patterns there is an impression that the caregiver patterns are less than optimal, it may be useful to consider the characteristics described below.

Caregiver tends to be:
1. Overly stimulating.
2. Withdrawn or unavailable.
3. Lacking pleasure, enthusiasm or zest.
4. Random or chaotic in reading or responding to signals (e.g., vocalizes and interacts but without regard for infant's signals as in a pinching, poking, "rev-the-infant-up" type caregiver).
5. Fragmented and/or insensitive to context (e.g., responds to one part of an infant's communication but misses the "bigger pattern" as when a caregiver gets excessively upset and hugs her active toddler who accidentally banged his leg while trying to run and obviously wants to keep exploring the room).
6. Overly rigid and controlling. Trying to get the infant to conform to rigid agenda (e.g., making the toddler only play with a toy one way).
7. Concrete in reading or responding to communication (e.g., unable to tune in to symbolic level in pretend play or in dialogue and instead keeps communication at behavioral and gestural levels. For example, a child is pretending with a toy telephone that he won't talk to his mother. Mother perceives this as a literal sign of rejection and refuses to "play anymore").
8. Illogical in reading or responding to infant's communication (e.g., the caregiver is so flooded with emotion that he or she misreads what is communicated. A 3½ year-old says, "I am scared of the monster, but I know it is just make believe." The caregiver explains "monsters will never get in the room because the door has a big lock on it and monsters can be nice, too, you know. You shouldn't play with these toys anyhow and how did you get that scratch on your hand?").
9. Avoidant of selected emotional area(s) (e.g., in pretend play parent ignores the child's interest in aggression and always ignores separation themes).

Consider the following emotional areas:
a. Security and safety
b. Dependency
c. Pleasure and excitement
d. Assertiveness and exploration
e. Aggression
f. Love
g. Empathy
h. Limit setting

10. Unstable in the face of intense emotion (e.g., caregiver can support development only if emotions are not too intense; if emotions are strong, tends to become chaotic, unpredictable, withdrawn, or overly rigid).

The evaluation of the above features will allow the clinician to make an overall clinical formulation of the quality of the caregiver support. In many families there are a number of caregivers. As one becomes aware of which parent or nanny or daycare caregiver tends to do what, indicate the person and the amount of time he or she spends with the infant or child each day (e.g., Father/3 hrs). Just as the clinician can look at the key caregiver in terms of the parameters described above, he or she can also observe how the family functions as a unit along these same parameters. Both the impressions about individual caregivers and the family's functioning as a whole should inform the clinical narrative of caregiver and family, as well as the formulation the clinician uses to characterize the impressions. The following demarcations (ratings) can be used by the clinician to reflect caregiver and family functioning.

- Fully supporting the child's age-expected functional emotional developmental capacities
- Evidencing minor interferences such as difficulty in engaging a child in the specific area of emotional functioning while supporting others (e.g., family conflicts over aggression)
- Moderate interferences, such as when caregiver or family patterns are unable to support whole domains of functioning, such as assertiveness or autonomy
- Major impairments, such as when caregivers or family patterns undermine the fundamental foundation of healthy functioning, such as the capacity for intimacy and relating

Axis VII: STRESS

There is often the inclination to overlook or minimize the impact of psychosocial stress from the environment on the infant or young child, who cannot understand or won't remember the stress—and in this way is protected from these uncontrolled events. Yet, we know that various sources of psychosocial stress from the environment or personal stress certainly affect older children and adults and can also affect infants and young children. These stressors may be the cause of, contribute to, or exacerbate primary symptoms or difficulties in mastering developmental tasks.

It is not always possible to tease out the degree to which the infant's basic functional and developmental capacities may be affected by stress, but it is essential to assess the stress factors for the infant, the family and the environment. This assessment could lead to measures to alleviate the stress whenever possible and to offer some protective factors to support the infant's and young child's coping. Children who have been found to be more resilient in coping with stress have often had alternative relationships to support and secure their adaptation in addition to basic constitutional strengths.

The purpose of this axis is to identify and consider the possible contribution stress may be having on the presenting symptom patterns as part of the overall evaluation. This impact may range from none or minimal, such as moving to a new home where adjustment difficulties may be evidenced in some sleep disruption, especially if a new bed replaces the beloved crib. The impact may be moderate such as general anxiety in response to the felt impact of a diagnosis of a significant illness in a parent who is hospitalized. Or, the impact may be very severe, such as highly disruptive behavior and aggression when persistent unemployment creates tension and conflict in the home. Each of these stressors can vary considerably depending on what they mean to the child and family and the individual resources of the child and family to mobilize adequate support at the time of the stress.

While the impact of stress is most likely to be seen on the interactive disorders, it should not be minimized with respect to the other disorders where the biology of the child may be the primary factor contributing to the disorder. Psychosocial stress can exacerbate a significant neurodevelopmental disorder, further derailing the important interactive experiences necessary to develop functional emotional developmental capacities. For example, a parent worried about a spouse's illness or subsumed by grief may find it more difficult to engage or establish co-regulated affective interactions necessary for shared problem solving. In fact, having a child with a developmental, emotional or medical disorder is a source of stress for a family requiring attention. Assessing the impact of stressors is essential for mobilizing the full range of interventions necessary for the child and the family in a comprehensive program.

Use the following sequence to assess the impact of stress:

First, identify and list the possible sources of stress:

- Is the stress direct, e.g., pain, disability, sudden injury, illness, hospitalization, school change, neglect, abuse, witness of violence, removal to foster care, etc?
- Is the stress related to primary caregivers or siblings, e.g., illness in the caregiver, loss or death, birth of sibling, child's or sibling's disability, parent absence or conflict, etc.?
- Is the stress related to the stability of the family, e.g., unemployment, moving, poverty, poor health care, poor education, etc.?
- Is the stress in the general environment, e.g., war, terrorism, fires, natural disasters?

Second, determine the onset, severity and duration of the stressors identified.

Third, assess the changes in the child's functioning and mental health possibly influenced by the stressors. Consider the following.

- Child's age, developmental capacities, history, strengths (resiliency) and vulnerabilities
- Protective factors in the caregiving environment to help the child cope, e.g., grandparents or other family who can help nurture the children or provide housing
- Anticipated duration and ongoing severity of stressors
- Available resources in the community to support the child and/or family
- Cumulative impact of multiple stressors

The degree each component is contributing to the stress and the greater the number of stressors listed relative to the protective factors and community resources, the more likely the stress is having a significant impact on the disorder.

The clinical narrative can reflect the clinician's judgment of the relative contribution of various aspects of the stress and the resources for coping with it. Consider whether the impact is:

- No Impact,
- Mild to Moderate Impact,
- Severe Impact.

For example, the stress of sudden hospitalization on an infant with regulatory disorder and severe reflux who has dehydrated over a period of a week may be offset by the child's caregiver's sensitive nurturance and home visits by the visiting nurse resulting in an overall lower rating of the impact of that stress on the child. In contrast, the same infant in a distressed family (where parents are in conflict and unable to soothe and feed the baby, and where there are few outside supports) may be under severe stress reflected in the cumulative stressors involved.

Axis VIII: Other Medical and Neurological Disorders

Frequently, children with mental health, developmental, regulatory-sensory processing, language, and/or learning disorders evidence medical disorders that may contribute. For example, children with allergies may evidence behavioral, as well as respiratory or dermatological, reactions. Children with thyroid disorders may evidence over- or underresponsivity to their environments. Gastrointestinal disorders are not uncommon in children with pervasive developmental problems. Whether clearly contributing or not, it's important for the clinician to indicate medical disorders that are in evidence. Careful listing of medical disorders facilitates their thorough investigation and the exploration of possible relationships with the child's mental health, developmental, or learning challenges. Axis VIII is provided for this purpose.

References

References

REFERENCES IN THE INTRODUCTION

Committee on Educational Interventions for Children with Autism, N. R. C. (2001). *Educating children with autism Washington, DC*: National Academies Press.

Greenspan, S. I. (1979). Intelligence and adaptation: An integration of psychoanalytic and Piagetian developmental psychology. *Psychological Issues. (Monograph No. 47-48)*. New York, International Universities Press.

Greenspan, S. I. (1981). Psychopathology and adaptation in infancy and early childhood: Principles of clinical diagnosis and preventive intervention. *Clinical Infant Reports, No. 1*. New York, International Universities Press.

Greenspan, S. I. (1992). *Infancy and early childhood: The practice of clinical assessment and intervention with emotional and developmental challenges*. Madison, CT: International Universities Press.

Greenspan, S. I. & Lourie, R. S. (1981). Developmental structuralist approach to the classification of adaptive and pathologic personality organizations: infancy and early childhood. *American Journal of Psychiatry, 138*, 725-735.

Greenspan, S. I., Wieder, S., Lieberman, A., Nover, R., Lourie, R., & Robinson, M. (1987). Infants in multirisk families: Case studies in preventive intervention. *Clinical Infant Reports. (3)*. New York, International Universities Press.

Interdisciplinary Council on Developmental and Learning Disorders Clinical Practice Guidelines Workgroup, S. I. G. C. (2000). *Interdisciplinary Council on Developmental and Learning Disorders' Clinical practice guidelines: Redefining the standards of care for infants, children, and families with special needs*. Bethesda, MD: Interdisciplinary Council on Developmental and Learning Disorders.

Spievel, A. (2005). *The dictionary of disorder: How one man revolutionized psychiatry*. The New Yorker [On-line]. Available: http://www.newyorker.com/fact/content/?050103fa_fact

REFERENCES IN AXIS I: INTERACTIVE DISORDERS

Bowlby, J. (1944). Forty-four juvenile thieves: Their characters and home life. *International Journal of Psychoanalysis, 25*, 19-52-107-127.

Bowlby, J. & Robertson, J. (1953). A two-year old goes to hospital. *Proc R Soc Med, Jun; 46*, 425-427.

Carlson, G. A. & Weintraub, S. (1993). Childhood behavior problems and bipolar disorder: relationship or coincidence? *Journal of Affective Disorders, 28*, 143-153.

Castillo, M., Kwock, L., Courvorise, H., & Hooper, S. R. (2000). Proton MR spectroscopy in children with bipolar affective disorder: Preliminary observations. *American Journal of Neuroradiology, 21*, 832-838.

Coates, S., Friedman, R. C. & Wolfe, S. (1991) The aetiology of boyhood gender identity disorder: A model for integrating temperament, development and psychodynamics. *Psychoanalytic Dialogues, 1*, 481–523.

Cytryn, L. & McKnew, D. H. (1974). Factors influencing the changing clinical expression of depressive process in children. *American Journal of Psychiatry, 131*, 879-881.

Egland, J. A., Blumenthal, R. L., Nee, J., & Sharp, E. L. (1987). Reliability and relationship of various ages of onset criteria for major affective disorders. *Journal of Affective Disorders, 12*, 159-165.

Ferster, C. B. & Skinner, B. J. (1957). *Schedules of reinforcement.* B.F. Skinner Foundation.

Geller, B., Zimmerman, B., Williams, M., Bolhafner, K., & Craney, J. (2001). Bipolar disorder at prospective follow-up of adults who had prepubertal major depressive disorder. *American Journal of Psychiatry, 158*, 125-127.

Greenspan, S. I. (1975). A consideration of some learning variables in the context of psychoanalytic theory: Toward a psychoanalytic learning perspective. New York, International Universities Press. *Psychological Issues IX(1)*, Monograph 33.

Greenspan, S. I. (1992). *Infancy and early childhood: The practice of clinical assessment and intervention with emotional and developmental challenges.* Madison, CT: International Universities Press.

Greenspan, S. I. & Glovinsky, I. (2002). *Children with bipolar patterns of dysregulation: New perspectives on developmental pathways and a comprehensive approach to prevention and treatment.* Bethesda, MD: The Interdisciplinary Council on Developmental and Learning Disorders.

Greenspan, S. I., Wieder, S., Lieberman, A., Nover, R., Lourie, R., & Robinson, M. (1987). Infants in multirisk families: Case studies in preventive intervention. *Clinical Infant Reports. (3).* New York, International Universities Press.

Harrington, R., Fudge, H., Rutter, M., & Pickles, A. (1991). Adult outcomes of child and adolescent depression: II. Links with antisocial disorders. *Journal of the American Academy of Child & Adolescent Psychiatry, 30*, 434-439.

Lewis, D. O. (1992). From abuse to violence: psychophysiological consequences of maltreatment. *Journal of the American Academy of Child & Adolescent Psychiatry, 31*, 383-391.

Lish, J., Dime-Meenan, S., Whybrow, P., Arlen-Price, R., & Hirschfeld, R. (1994). The National Depressive and Manic-Depressive Association (DMDA) survey of bipolar members. *Journal of Affective Disorders, 31*, 281-294.

Radke-Yarrow, M., Nottelmann, E., Martinez, P., Fox, M. B., & Belmont, B. (1992). Young children of affectively ill parents: A longitudinal study of psychosocial development. *Journal of the American Academy of Child & Adolescent Psychiatry, 31*, 68-76.

Sigurdsson, E., Fombonne, E., Sayal, K., & Checley, S. (1999). Neurodevelopmental antecedents of early-onset bipolar affective disorder. *British Journal of Psychiatry, 174*, 121-127.

Spitz, R. A. (1945). Hospitalism: An inquiry into the genesis of psychiatric conditions in early childhood. *The Psychoanalytic Study of the Child, 1*, 53-74.

Strober, M., Morrell, W., Burroughs, J., Lampert, C., & Freeman, R. (1988). A family study of bipolar I disorder in adolescents: Early onset of symptoms linked to increased familial loading and lithium resistance. *Journal of Affective Disorders, 15*, 255-268.

Yeager, C. A. & Lewis, D. O. (2000). Mental illness, neuropsychologic deficits, child abuse, and violence. *Child & Adolescent Psychiatric Clinics of North America, 9*, 793-813.

REFERENCES IN AXIS I: REGULATORY-SENSORY PROCESSING DISORDERS

Adrien, J.L., Lenoir, P., Martineau, J., Perrot, A., Hameury, L., Larmande, C., & Sauvage, D. (1993). Blind ratings of early symptoms of autism based upon family home movies. *Journal of the American Academy of Child and Adolescent Psychiatry, 32*(3), 617-626.

Ahn, R.R., Miller, L.J., Milberger S., & McIntosh, D.N. (2004). Prevalence of parents' perceptions of sensory processing disorders among kindergarten children. *American Journal of Occupational Therapy. 58*(3), 287-93.

Ayres, J. (1964). Tactile functions: their relation to hyperactive and perceptual motor behavior. *The American Journal of Occupational Therapy, 18*, 6-11.

Ayres, A.J. (1966). Interactions among perceptual motor function in a group of normal children. *American Journal of Occupational Therapy, 20*, 288-292.

Ayres, A.J. (1972). *Sensory integration and learning disabilities.* Los Angeles: Western Psychological Services.

Ayres, A.J. (1989). *Sensory integration and praxis tests.* Los Angeles: Western Psychological Services.

Ayres, A. J., & Tickle, L. S. (1980). Hyper-responsivity to touch and vestibular stimuli as a predictor of positive response to sensory integration procedures by autistic children. *American Journal of Occupational Therapy, 34*, 375-381.

Bundy, A.C. (2002). Play theory and sensory integration. In A.C. Bundy, S.J. Lane & E.A. Murray (Eds.), *Sensory Integration: Theory and Practice* (2nd ed., pp. 227-240). Philadelphia, PA: F.A. Davis Company.

Dahlgren, S.O., & Gillberg, C. (1989). Symptoms in the first two years of life: a preliminary population study of infantile autism. *European Archives of Psychiatry and Neurological Science, 238*(3), 169-174.

DeGangi, G. (1991). Part 1: Assessment of sensory, emotional, and attentional problems in regulatory disordered infants. *Infants and Young Children, 3,* 1-8.

DeGangi, G. (2000). *Pediatric disorders of regulation in affect and behavior: A therapist's guide to assessment and treatment.* San Diego: Academic Press.

DeGangi, G. A., DiPietro, J. A., Greenspan, S. I., & Porges, S. W. (1991). Psychophysiological characteristics of the regulatory disordered infant. *Infant Behavior and Development, 14,* 37-50.

DeGangi, G. A. & Greenspan, S. I. (1988). The development of sensory functioning in infants. *Physical and Occupational Therapy in Pediatrics, 8*(3), 21-33.

DeGangi, G. A., & Greenspan, S. I. (1989). The development of sensory functions in infants. *Physical and Occupational Therapy in Pediatrics, 8*(4), 21-34.

DeGangi, G. A., Porges, S. W., Sickel, R. Z., & Greenspan, S. I. (1993). Four-year follow-up of a sample of regulatory disordered infants. *Infant Mental Health Journal, 14,* 330-343.

Doussard-Roosevelt, J. A., Walker, P. S., Portales, A., Greenspan, S. I., & Porges, S. W. (1990). Vagal tone and the fussy infant: atypical vagal reactivity in the difficult infant. *Infant Behavior and Development, 13,* 352 (abstract).

Dunn, W. (1994). Performance of typical children on the sensory profile: an item analysis. *American Journal of Occupational Therapy, 48,* 967-974.

Ermer, J., & Dunn, W. (1998). The sensory profile: a discriminant analysis of young children with and without disabilities. *American Journal of Occupational Therapy, 52*(4), 283-290.

Escalona, S. (1968). *The roots of individuality.* Chicago: Aldine.

Greenspan, S.I. (1981). Psychopathology and adaptation in infancy and early childhood: principles of clinical diagnosis and preventive intervention. *Clinical Infant Reports, 1,* 263.

Greenspan, S. I. (1992). *Infancy and early childhood: The practice of clinical assessment and intervention with emotional and developmental challenges.* Madison, CT: International Universities Press.

Greenspan, S. I. (2004). *Greenspan social-emotional growth chart.* Bulverde, TX: The Psychological Corporation.

Greenspan, S. I. & Wieder, S. (1997). Developmental patterns and outcomes in infants and children with disorders in relating and communicating: a chart review of 200 cases of children with autistic spectrum diagnoses. *Journal of Developmental and Learning Disorders, 1*, 87-141.

Greenspan, S. I., Wieder, S., Lieberman, A., Nover, R., Lourie, R., & Robinson, M. (1987). Infants in multirisk families: case studies in preventive intervention. *Clinical Infant Reports* (3). New York: International Universities Press.

Kagan, J., Reznick, J. S., & Snidman, N. (1988). Biological Bases of childhood shyness. *Science, 240*(4849), 167-171.

Kientz, M.A., & Dunn, W. (1997). A comparison of the performance of children with and without autism on the sensory profile. *American Journal of Occupational Therapy, 51*(7), 530-537.

Knickerbocker, B. (1980). *A holistic approach to learning disabilities.* Thorofare, NJ: Slack.

Mangeot, S.D., Miller, L.J., McIntosh, D.N., McGrath-Clarke, J., Simon, J., Hagerman, R.J., & Goldson, E. (2001). Sensory modulation dysfunction in children with attention deficit hyperactivity disorder. *Developmental Medicine and Child Neurology, 43*, 399-406.

McIntosh, D.N., Miller, L.J., Shyu, V., & Dunn, W. (1999). Overview of the short sensory profile (SSP). In W. Dunn (Ed.), *The Sensory Profile: Examiner's Manual* (pp. 59-73). San Antonio, TX: The Psychological Corporation.

McIntosh, D.N., Miller, L.J., Shyu, V., & Hagerman, R. (1999). Sensory-modulation disruption, electrodermal responses, and functional behaviors. *Developmental Medicine and Child Neurology, 41*, 608-615.

Miller, L.J., Cermak, S.A., Lane, S., Anzalone, M., & Koomar, J. (2004, Summer). Position statement on terminology related to sensory integration dysfunction. *S.I. Focus*, pp. 6-8.

Miller, L.J., McIntosh, D.N., McGrath, J., Shyu, V., Lampe, M., Taylor, A.K., Tassone, F., Neitzel, K., Stackhouse, T., & Hagerman, R. (1999). Electrodermal responses to sensory stimuli in individuals with Fragile X syndrome: A preliminary report. *American Journal of Medical Genetics, 83*(4), 268-279.

Miller, L. J., Robinson, J., & Moulton, D. (2004). Sensory modulation dysfunction: identification in early childhood. In R. DelCarmen-Wiggins & A. Wiggins (Eds.), *Handbook of Infant, Toddler and Preschool Mental Health Assessment* (pp. 247-270). New York: Oxford University Press.

Miller, L.J., & Summers, C. (2001). Clinical applications in sensory modulation dysfunction: assessment and intervention considerations. In S.S. Roley, E.I. Blanche & R.C. Schaaf (Eds.), *Understanding the Nature of Sensory Integration with Diverse Populations* (pp. 247-274). San Antonio, TX: Therapy Skill Builders.

Murphy, L. B. (1974). *The individual child.* Publication no. OCD 74-1032. Washington, DC, US Government Printing Office. Department of Health, Education and Welfare.

Ornitz, E.M., Guthrie, D., & Farley, A.H. (1977). The early development of autistic children. *Journal of Autism and Childhood Schizophrenia, 7*(3), 207-229.

Parham, L.D., & Fazio, L. (1996). *Play in occupational therapy for children.* Baltimore: CV Mosby.

Parham, L.D., & Mailloux, Z. (2001). Sensory integration. In J. Case-Smith (Ed.), *Occupational Therapy for Children* (4th ed., pp. 329-381). St. Louis, MO: Mosby, Inc.

Porges, S. W. & Greenspan, S. I. (1990). Regulatory disordered infants: A common theme. In *Presented at the National Institute on Drug Abuse RAUS Review Meeting on Methodological Issues in Controlled Studies on Effects of Prenatal Exposure to Drugs of Abuse, June 8-9* Richmond, VA.

Portales, A. W., Porges, S. W., & Greenspan, S. I. (1990). Parenthood and the difficult child. *Infant Behavior and Development, 13*, 573 (abstract).

Rothbart, M. K. (1981). Measurement of temperament in infancy. *Child Development, 52*, 569–578.

Rothbart, M. K., & Posner, M. I. (1985). Temperament and the development of self-regulation. In L. C. Hartlage & C. F. Telzrow (Eds.), *The Neuropsychology of Individual Differences: A Developmental Perspective* (pp. 93–123). New York: Plenum.

Royeen, C.B., & Lane, S.J. (1991). Tactile processing and sensory defensiveness. In A.G. Fisher, E.A. Murray, & A.C. Bundy (Eds.), *Sensory Integration Theory and Practice* (pp. 108-133). Philadelphia: FA Davis.

Schaaf R.C. Miller L.J. Seawell D., O'Keefe S. (2003). Children with disturbances in sensory processing: A pilot study examining the role of the parasympathetic nervous system. *American Journal of Occupational Therapy. 57*(4): 442-9.

Talay-Ongan, A., & Wood, K. (2000). Unusual sensory sensitivities in autism: A possible crossroads. *International Journal of Disability, Development and Education, 47*(2), 201-212.

Thomas, A., & Chess, S. (1985). The behavioral study of temperament. In J. Strelau, F. H. Farley, & A. Gale (Eds.), *The Biological Bases of Personality and Behavior, Vol. 1: Theories, Measurement Techniques, and Development.* New York: Hemisphere Publishing Corp/Harper & Row Publishers, Inc.

Wieder, S. & Greenspan, S. I. (2005). Can children with autism master the core deficits and become empathetic, creative, and reflective? A ten to fifteen year follow-up of a subgroup of children with autism spectrum disorders (ASD) who received a comprehensive developmental, individual-difference, relationship-based (DIR) Approach *Journal of Developmental and Learning Disorders, 9.*

Williamson, G.G., & Anzalone, M.E. (2001). *Sensory integration and self-regulation in infants and toddlers: helping very young children interact with their environment.* Washington, DC: Zero to Three.

REFERENCES IN AXIS I: NEURODEVELOPMENTAL DISORDERS OF RELATING AND COMMUNICATING

Diagnostic Classification Task Force (1994). *Diagnostic classification: 0-3: Diagnostic classification of mental health and developmental disorders of infancy and early childhood.* Arlington, VA: ZERO TO THREE: National Center for Clinical Infant Programs.

Greenspan, S. I. (1992). *Infancy and early childhood: The practice of clinical assessment and intervention with emotional and developmental challenges.* Madison, CT: International Universities Press.

Greenspan, S. I. & Shanker, S. (2004). *The first idea: how symbols, language and intelligence evolved from our primate ancestors to modern humans.* Reading, MA: Perseus Books.

Greenspan, S. I. & Wieder, S. (1997). Developmental patterns and outcomes in infants and children with disorders in relating and communicating: A chart review of 200 cases of children with autistic spectrum diagnoses. *Journal of Developmental and Learning Disorders, 1*, 87-141.

Greenspan, S. I. & Wieder, S. (1998). The child with special needs: *Encouraging intellectual and emotional growth.* Reading, MA: Perseus Books.

Greenspan, S. I. & Wieder, S. (1999). A functional developmental approach to autism spectrum disorders. *Journal of the Association for Persons with Severe Handicaps (JASH)*, 24, 147-161.

Interdisciplinary Council on Developmental and Learning Disorders Clinical Practice Guidelines Workgroup, S. I. G. C. (2000). *Interdisciplinary Council on Developmental and Learning Disorders' Clinical practice guidelines: redefining the standards of care for infants, children, and families with special needs.* Bethesda, MD: Interdisciplinary Council on Developmental and Learning Disorders.

REFERENCES IN AXIS I: LANGUAGE DISORDERS

Bates, E. (1976). *Language in context.* New York: Academic Press.

Bloom L. (1973). *Language development: Form and function in emerging grammars.* Cambridge, MA: MIT Press.

Bloom, L. & Lahey, M. (1978). *Language development and language disorders.* New York: Wiley.

Bloom, L. & Tinker, E. (2001). The intentionality model and language acquisition: Engagement, effort, and the essential tension. *Monographs of the Society for Research in Child Development. 66* (Serial No. 267).

Bruner, J. S. (1990). *Acts of meaning.* Cambridge, MA: Harvard University Press.

Greenspan, S. I. & Shanker, S. (2004). *The first idea: How symbols, language and intelligence evolved from our primate ancestors to modern humans.* Reading, MA: Perseus Books.

Tomasello, M. (2003). *Constructing a language: A usage-based theory of language acquisition .* Cambridge, MA: Harvard University Press.

Wetherby, A. M. & Prizant, B. M. (1993). Profiling communication and symbolic abilities in young children. *Journal of Childhood Communication Disorders, 15*: 23-32.

REFERENCES IN AXIS I: LEARNING CHALLENGES

Calfee, R., Lindamood, C., & Lindamood, P. (1973). Acoustic-phonetic skills and reading -kindergarten through twelfth grade. *Journal of Educational Psychology, 64*, 293-298.

Castro-Caldas A, Petersson KM, Reis A, Stone-Elander S, & Ingvar M (1998). The illiterate brain. Learning to read and write during childhood influences the functional organization of the adult brain. *Brain, 121*, 1053-1063.

Catts, H. (1991). Early identification of dyslexia: evidence of a follow-up study of speech-language impaired children. *Annals of Dyslexia, 41*, 163-177.

DeFries, J. C. & Light, J. G. (1996). Twin studies of reading disability. In J.H.Beitchman, N. J. Cohen, Konstantareas M.M., & R. Tannock (Eds.), *Language, Learning, and Behavior Disorders* (pp. 272-292). New York: Cambridge University Press.

DeFries, J. C., Olson, R. K., Pennington, B. F., & Smith, S. D. (1991). Colorado Reading Project: an update. In D.D.Duane & D. B. Gray (Eds.), *The Reading Brain. The Biological Basis of Dyslexia.* (pp. 53-87). Parkton, MD: York Press.

Gogtay N., Giedd J. N., Lusk L, Hayashi K. M., Greenstein D., Vaituzis, A. C. et al. (2004). Dynamic mapping of human cortical development during childhood through early adulthood. In Proceedings of the National Academy of Science of the United States of America. (Ed.), (pp. 8174-8179).

Heilman, K., Voeller, K., & Alexander, A. (1996). Developmental dyslexia: A motor-articulatory feedback hypothesis. *Annals of Neurology, 39*, 407-412.

Hinshelwood, J. (1907). Four cases of congenital word-blindness occurring in the same family. *British Medical Journal, 2*, 1229-1232.

Lindamood, P., & Lindamood, P.D. (2004). Lindamood ® auditory conceptualization (LAC-3) test. Austin, TX: PRO-ED. (Initially published 1971.)

Lyytinen, H. T., Ahonen, T., Eklund, K., Guttorm, T. K., Kulju, P., Laakso, M. L. et al. (2004). Early development of children at familial risk for dyslexia--follow-up from birth to school age. *Dyslexia, August, 10*, 146-178.

Lyytinen, H. T., Ahonen, T., Eklund, K., Guttorm, T. K., Laakso, M. L., Leinonen, S. et al. (2001). Developmental pathways of children with and without familial risk for dyslexia during the first years of life. *Developmental Neuropsychology, 20*, 535-554.

Maurer, U., Bucher, K., Brem, S., & Brandeis, D. (2003). Altered responses to tone and phoneme mismatch in kindergartners at familial dyslexia risk. *Neuroreport, 14*, 2245-2250.

Menyuk, P., Chesnick, M., Liebergott, J. W., Korngold, B., D'Agostino, R., & Belanger, A. (1991). Predicting reading problems in at-risk children. *Journal of Speech and Hearing Research, 34*, 893-903.

Molfese, D. L. (2000). Predicting dyslexia at 8 years of age using neonatal brain responses. *Brain and Language, 72*, 238-245.

Morgan, W. P. (1896). A case of congenital word blindness. *British Medical Journal, 2*, 1378.

Pennington, B. F. & Lefly, D. L. (2001). Early reading development in children at family risk for dyslexia. *Child Development, 72*, 816-833.

Richardson, U., Leppanen, P. H., Leiwo, M., & Lyytinen, H. T. (2003). Speech perception of infants with high familial risk for dyslexia differ at the age of 6 months. *Developmental Neuropsychology, 23*, 385-397.

Ruff, S., Marie, N., Celsis, N., Cardebat, D., & Demonet, J. F. (2003). Neural substrates of impaired categorical perception of phonemes in adult dyslexics: an fMRI study. *Brain and Cognition, 53*, 331-334.

Scarborough, H. S. (1984). Continuity between childhood dyslexia and adult reading. *British Journal of Psychology, 75*, 329-348.

Scarborough, H. S. (1991). Early syntactic development of dyslexic children. *Annals of Dyslexia, 41*, 207-220.

Shankweiler, D., & Liberman, I.Y. (1989). *Phonology and reading disability*. Ann Arbor: University of Michigan Press.

Snowling, M. J., Gallagher, A., & Frith, U. (2003). Family risk of dyslexia is continuous: individual differences in the precursors of reading skill. *Child Development, 74*, 358-373.

Stephenson, S. (1907). Six cases of congenital word-blindness affecting three generations of one family. *Ophalmoscope, 5*, 482-484.

Stevenson, J., Graham, A. A., Fredman, G., & McLoughlin, V. (1987). A twin study of genetic influences on reading and spelling ability and disability. *Journal of Child Psychology and Psychiatry, 28*, 229-247.

Tarkiainen A, Helenius P, & Salmelin R. (2003). Category-specific occipitotemporal activation during face perception in dyslexic individuals: an MEG study. *Neuroimage, 19*, 1194-1204.

Viholainen, H., Ahonen, T., Cantell, M., Lyytinen, P., & Lyytinen, H. T. (2002). Development of early motor skills and language in children at risk for familial dyslexia. *Developmental Medicine and Child Neurology, 44*, 761-769.

Willcutt, E. G., Pennington, B. F., Smith, S. D., Cardon, L. R., Gayan, J., Knopic, V. S. et al. (2002). Quantitative trait locus for reading disability on chromosome 6p is pleiotropic for attention-deficit/hyperactivity disorder. *American Journal of Medical Genetics (Neuropsychiatric Genetics), 114*, 260-268.

REFERENCES IN SECTION II

Axis II

Greenspan, S. I. (2004). *Greenspan social-emotional growth chart.* Bulverde, TX: The Psychological Corporation. (http://www.harcourtassessment.com - 1-800-211-8378)

Axis V

Furth, H. G. & Wachs, H. (1974). *Thinking goes to school: Piaget's theory in practice.* New York: Oxford University Press.

Greenspan, S. I. (2005). *Engaging autism.* Cambridge, MA: DaCapo Press/Perseus Books.

Interdisciplinary Council on Developmental and Learning Disorders Clinical Practice Guidelines Workgroup, S. I. G. C. (2000). *Interdisciplinary Council on Developmental and Learning Disorders' Clinical practice guidelines: Redefining the standards of care for infants, children, and families with special needs.* Bethesda, MD: Interdisciplinary Council on Developmental and Learning Disorders.

REFERENCES FOR APPENDIX I

DeGangi, G. and Greenspan, S.I. (1988). The development of sensory functioning in infants. *Journal of Physical and Occupational Therapy in Pediatrics, 8*(3).

DeGangi, G. and Greenspan, S.I. (1989a). The assessment of sensory functioning in infants. *Journal of Physical and Occupational Therapy in Pediatrics, 9*:21-33.

DeGangi, G. and Greenspan, S.I. (1989b). *Test of sensory functions in infants.* Los Angeles: Western Psychology Services.

DeGangi, G. and Greenspan, S.I. (in press, 2000). *The functional emotional assessment scale: Revised version and reliability studies.* Bethesda, MD: Interdisciplinary Council on Developmental and Learning Disorders.

Greenspan, S.I. (1979). Intelligence and adaptation: An integration of psychoanalytic and piagetian developmental psychology. *Psychological Issues, Monogr. 47/68*. New York: International Universities Press.

Greenspan, S. I. (2003). *The clinical interview of the child.* 3rd Edition, Arlington, VA: APPI

Greenspan, S.I. (1989). *The development of the ego: Implications for personality theory, psychopathology, and the psychotherapeutic process.* Madison, CT: International Universities Press.

Greenspan, S.I. (1992). *Infancy and early childhood: The practice of clinical assessment and intervention with emotional and developmental challenges.* Madison, CT: International Universities Press.

Greenspan, S. I. (1997). *The growth of the mind and the endangered origins of intelligence.* Reading, MA: Addison Wesley Longman.

Greenspan, S.I. & Wieder, S. (1998) *The child with special needs: Intellectual and emotional growth.* Reading, MA: Addison Wesley Longman,

Greenspan, S.I. & Wieder, S. (1999). The assessment and diagnosis of infant disorders: developmental level, individual differences and relationship based interactions. In J. Osofsky and H. Fitzgerald (Eds.), *World Association for Infant Mental Health Handbook of Infant Mental Health: Vol. 2: Intervention, Evaluation, and Treatment.* New York: Wiley & Sons.

REFERENCES IN APPENDIX II

Committee on Educational Interventions for Children with Autism, N. R. C. (2001). *Educating children with autism* Washington, DC: National Academies Press.

Greenspan, S. I. (1992). *Infancy and early childhood: The practice of clinical assessment and intervention with emotional and developmental challenges.* Madison, CT: International Universities Press.

Greenspan, S. I., DeGangi, G. A., & Wieder, S. (2001). *The functional emotional assessment scale (FEAS) for infancy and early childhood: Clinical & research applications.* Bethesda, MD: Interdisciplinary Council on Developmental and Learning Disorders.

Greenspan, S. I. & Shanker, S. (2004). *The first idea: How symbols, language and intelligence evolved from our primate ancestors to modern humans.* Reading, MA: Perseus Books.

Greenspan, S. I. & Wieder, S. (1997). Developmental patterns and outcomes in infants and children with disorders in relating and communicating: A chart review of 200 cases of children with autistic spectrum diagnoses. *Journal of Developmental and Learning Disorders, 1*, 87-141.

Interdisciplinary Council on Developmental and Learning Disorders Clinical Practice Guidelines Workgroup, S. I. G. C. (2000). *Interdisciplinary Council on Developmental and Learning Disorders' Clinical practice guidelines: Redefining the standards of care for infants, children, and families with special needs.* Bethesda, MD: Interdisciplinary Council on Developmental and Learning Disorders.

Rogers, S. J., Hall, T., Osaki, D., Reaven, J., & Herbison, J. (2000). The Denver model: A comprehensive, integrated educational approach to young children with autism and their families. In J. S. Handleman & S. L. Harris (Eds.), *Preschool Education Programs for Children with Autism* (2nd Ed.) (pp. 95-133). Austin, TX: Pro-Ed.

Shonkoff, J. P. & Phillips, D. A. (2000). *From neurons to neighborhoods: The science of early childhood development.* National Research Council, Committee on Integrating the Science of Early Childhood Development.

Smith, T., Groen, A. D., & Wynn, J. W. (2000). Randomized trial of intensive early intervention for children with pervasive developmental disorder. *American Journal on Mental Retardation, 105*, 269-285.

Solomon, R., Necheles, J., Ferch, D., & Bruckman, D. (2003). *Program evaluation of a pilot parent training program for young children with autism: The PLAY Project Home Consultation Program.* Presented at the 2004 ICDL Scientific Meetings, Bethesda, MD, Submitted for publication.

Sparrow, S., Balla, D. A., & Cicchetti, D. (1984). *Vineland Adaptive Behavior Scales.* American Guidance Service.

Tsakiris, E. (2000). Evaluating effective interventions for children with autism and related disorders: Widening the view and changing the perspective. In ICDL Clinical Practice Guidelines Workgroup (Ed.), *Clinical Practice Guidelines: Redefining the Standards of Care for Infants, Children, and Families with Special Needs* (pp. 725-820). Bethesda, MD: Interdisciplinary Council on Development and Learning Disorders.

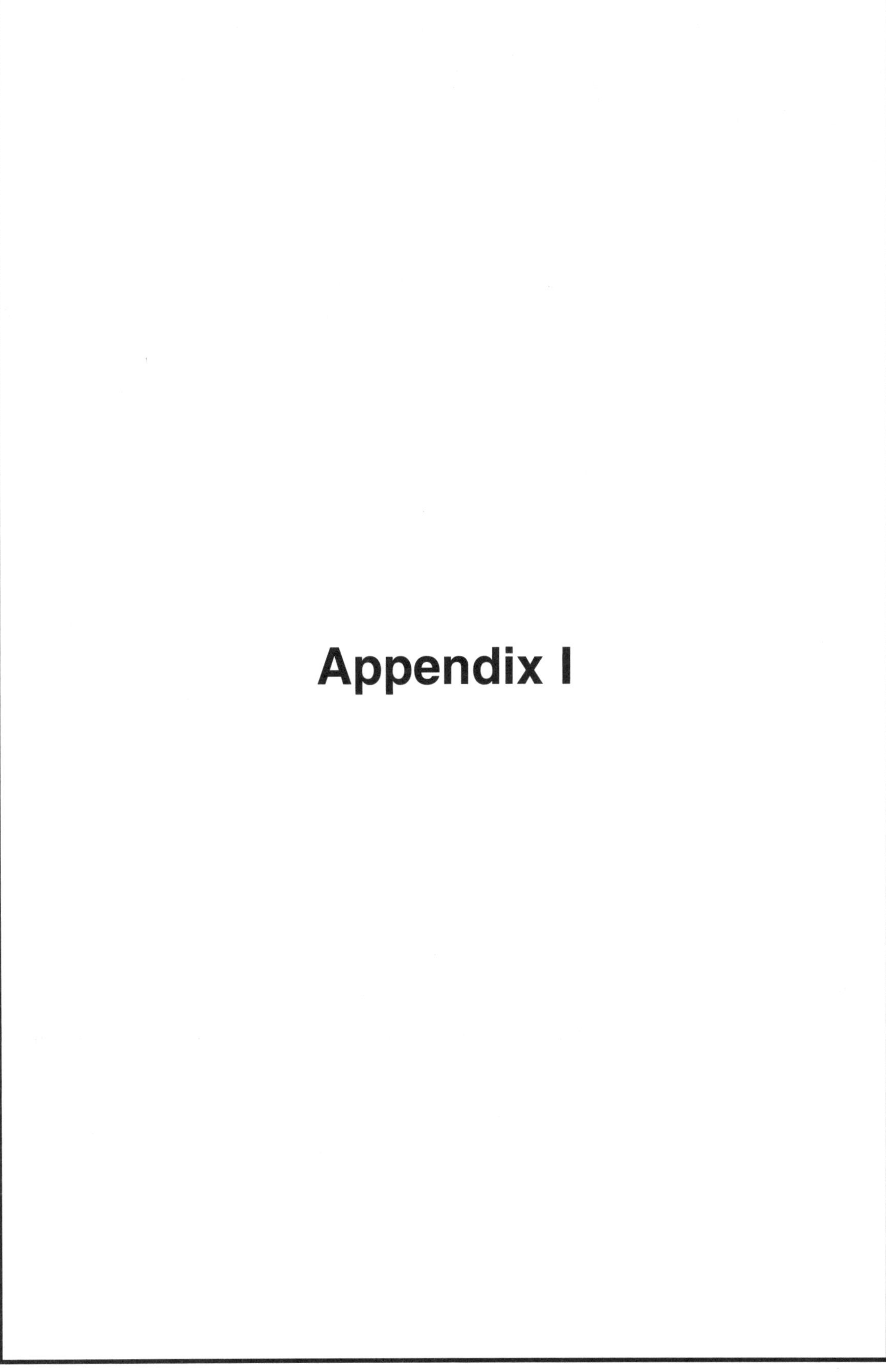

Appendix I

Appendix I: A Comprehensive Approach to Clinical Evaluation

In order to obtain the information required for a developmentally based diagnosis, it is vital to conduct a comprehensive clinical assessment. Often, there's a tendency to focus only on the areas of functioning relevant to the presenting problem or the potential intervention. However, a developmental approach to classification requires observing all the relevant areas of functioning in order to understand how the different facets in development influence and contribute to one another. The classification approach involves multiple axes that capture different facets of development. This, in turn, enables the clinician to formulate a developmental profile that includes various contributions to the child's challenges.

The following section describes the principles and practices of a comprehensive evaluation. There are specific recommendations for assessment procedures in the descriptions of some of the diagnostic categories (e.g., regulatory-sensory processing disorders). These specific recommendations should always be part of a comprehensive evaluation as described below.

BASIC PRINCIPLES: THE DEVELOPMENTAL, INDIVIDUAL-DIFFERENCE, RELATIONSHIP-BASED (DIR) APPROACH

Most non-progressive developmental and learning disorders are nonspecific with regard to their etiology and pathophysiology. Non-progressive developmental disorders are, therefore, best characterized in terms of types and degrees of functional limitations and processing differences (as well as symptoms that are often only one expression of a functional limitation, e.g., echolalia is a symptom; pragmatic language is the functional limitation).

Yet, as indicated, both historically and recently, we have focused on symptoms and groups of symptoms comprising syndromes with only partial emphasis on a broad range of important functional capacities and their related processing differences. For example, a mother was recently told by the senior clinician overseeing an evaluation team that because her child was "autistic," he couldn't interact with purpose and meaning and, therefore, intensive intervention would not be helpful and the therapeutic effort should be modest. Among other things, this clinician did not assess the relative strengths and weaknesses of all the child's areas of functioning and underlying processing capacities to see which ones required work and which ones could be harnessed immediately for interacting and learning. For example, was this child's lack of purposeful interaction related to auditory processing and motor problems? Did he have some relative strengths in visuospatial processing that could be harnessed partially to enable him to interact with others more purposefully? Would working with him around activities which were associated with high motivation (e.g., to go outside) help him become more purposeful? Or, was his lack of purposeful interaction part of a biologically-based CNS impairment which, by definition, would remain chronic and relatively untreatable?

The evidence is mounting that (1) that most complex non-progressive developmental and learning disorders involve processing dysfunctions (each with its own natural history and complex, poorly-understood etiology and neurobiology; (2) that key functional capacities, as well as related symptoms, learning problems, adaptive capacities, and a variety of surface behaviors, in turn, are often the result of the interaction between early and ongoing interactive experiences and these biologically-based processing dysfunctions; and (3) the resulting functional capacities, symptoms, or behaviors are not tied to these underlying processes in a rigid, fixed manner. For example, a child who cannot use words to symbolize a desire for juice may well be able to learn to use a sign or a picture to symbolize his desire, suggesting many roads rather than one road to symbolization.

Observed behavior is, therefore, often the result of dynamic interactions between the environment and genetic, prenatal, perinatal, and maturational variations. For example, genetic expression is influenced by a number of cellular and extra-cellular biological processes, including different hormones and toxic substances. Resultant physiologic levels are modified by different levels of interaction with the physical, cognitive, and social environment. Resultant functional capacities and behaviors are further influenced by interactions with different aspects of the environment.

Many practitioners, especially in speech and language pathology, occupational therapy, physical therapy, education, and psychology have been expanding a dynamic functional approach that takes these considerations of the dynamic relationship between behavior and the central nervous system into account. They are demonstrating that interactions that are geared to individual differences can facilitate important functional capacities such as relating, thinking, and communicating. For example, motor planning, including oral-motor exercises, can help with learning preverbal vocal, motor, and affective gesturing, imitation, and language development; visuospatial problem-solving approaches can help with logical thinking and abstract academic challenges; sensory modulation work can help with learning to relate to others and receptive language; and auditory discrimination work can facilitate phonemic awareness as a basis for reading.

Yet, in spite of an expanding functional approach, there is a tendency to continue to focus predominantly on symptoms and only a few of the functional areas (e.g., more on verbal development and less on intimacy, relating, and preverbal affect gesturing). Similarly, there is a tendency to focus only on a few of the critical underlying processing differences (e.g., more on auditory processing and less on motor planning and sequencing which is essential for imitation, social interaction, play, and language; more on rote cognitive and social skills and less on affective processing through promoting spontaneous interaction).

Therefore, it is important to further systematize and expand a functional approach. In this approach, assessments and interventions must include all the contributions of relevant areas of functioning, processing differences, and interactive relationships are summarized below.

Table 1: Relevant Areas to Consider

The Functional Developmental Level of the Child's Communicative, Cognitive, and Emotional Capacities (i.e., how the child integrates all his capacities to meet emotionally meaningful goals, such as using a continuous flow of social problem-solving gestures to get Daddy to reach for and get him a desired toy). **These include the capacities for:** 1. Shared attention and regulation, 2. Engagement, 3. Purposeful preverbal/gestural and affective communication, 4. Complex social problem-solving interactions, 5. The creative and meaningful use of ideas, and 6. Building logical connections between ideas or symbols (Greenspan, 1992).
Individual Differences in the Functioning of the Child's Motor, Sensory, and Affective Patterns **This includes:** 1. Sensory modulation (e.g., the degree to which the infant or child is over- or under-responsive to sensations in each sensory modality such as touch, movement, sound, sight, etc.), 2. Auditory processing, visuospatial processing, and 3. Motor planning and sequencing, and affective processing (i.e., the connection between affect, motor planning, other processing capacities, and emerging symbols).
Relationship and Affective Interaction Patterns, Including Developmentally Appropriate (which utilize understanding of the child's functional developmental level and individual differences), or Inappropriate, Interactions **This includes** 1. Existing caregiver, parent, family patterns 2. Educational patterns, and 3. Peer patterns.

The Functional Developmental Approach to Assessment

To implement an appropriate assessment of all the relevant functional areas requires a number of sessions with the child and family. These sessions must begin with discussions and observations. Structured tests, if indicated, should be implemented at a later point to further understand specific functional areas. The sessions include:

1. Review of current functioning with parents and other caregivers, looking at both problems and adaptive capacities
2. Review of prenatal, perinatal, and postnatal developmental history, including development in all the functional areas

3. Observations of caregiver/child interactions for 45 or more minutes, including coaching or interactions with the clinician to elicit the child's highest adaptive level. There should be at least two observation sessions and more if there is a discrepancy between parental reports and observed functioning. These dynamic, interactive sessions should serve (along with history and review of current functioning) as a partial basis for a preliminary impression of the child's functional developmental capacities, individual processing differences, including often-unemphasized ones such as motor planning, visuospatial processing and affective processing, and current as well as potentially optimal child-caregiver interactive patterns.
4. Discussion of caregiver personality patterns and child-caregiver interactions, including identification of strengths and vulnerabilities, as well as family and cultural patterns.
5. Review of all current interventions, educational programs, daily activities, behaviors and interaction patterns. Review of current understanding of "developmentally appropriate" interaction patterns and practices at home, in school, including with peers and in different interventions. Consideration of these hypothesized developmentally appropriate interactions and practices in relationship to their capacity to foster the next level in child's functional abilities.
6. Review and assessment to rule out concurrent and/or contributing medical disorders including conducting appropriate biomedical assessments. Appropriate biological assessments should be carried out to help understand the causes of the functional impairments, including related or contributing medical problems. Appropriate biological assessments are also essential to identify biological interventions that may contribute to the clinical management (e.g., an extended sleep EEG may reveal the potential usefulness of Depakote or other anti-seizure medications).
7. Additional developmental and learning assessments, such as speech and language functioning, motor and sensory functioning, specific aspects of cognitive functioning, should be conducted as needed to answer specific questions (as opposed to routinely). For example, a child with a circumscribed receptive language difficulty may benefit from structured language assessments to tease out more precisely the nature of the deficit. A child with a circumscribed learning problem may benefit from specific structured tasks to tease out areas of strength and weakness (such as visuospatial processing or motor planning [e.g., a neuropsychological battery]). Specific assessments, however, must always build on a basic evaluation because even circumscribed processing difficulties often make it more difficult for a child to process and understand important functions of social relationships and, therefore, may be associated with emotional, behavioral, and/or family challenges. In contrast, a child who is only fleetingly engaged and purposeful with his receptive as well as expressive language problems may be best understood from ongoing interactive observation and the response to a comprehensive intervention program. Structured assessments are conducted routinely at great expense and time even when the best the assessor may be able to do is describe the child's behavior around the structured tasks. In such circumstances, clinical observation of caregiver and clinician-child interactions to observe functional

capacities coupled with a review of current and past functioning provides an initial picture of strengths and challenges. Further profiling is then best done as part of the intervention process.

The Functional Profile

The functional assessment leads to an individualized functional profile which captures each child's unique developmental features and serves as a basis for creating individually-tailored intervention programs (i.e., tailoring the program to the child rather than fitting the child to a general program). The profile describes the child's functional developmental capacities and contributing biological processing differences and environmental interactive patterns, including the different interaction patterns available to the child at home, at school, with peers, and in other settings. The profile should include all areas of functioning, not simply the ones that are more obviously associated with pathologic symptoms. For example, the preschooler's lack of ability to symbolize a broad range of emotional interests and themes in either pretend play or talk is just as important, if not more important, than that same preschooler's tendency to be perseverative or self-stimulatory. In fact, clinically we have often seen that as the child's range of symbolic expression broadens, perseverative and self-stimulatory tendencies decrease. Similarly, areas of special strength may also be critical to the intervention program. Visuospatial thinking capacities may enable a child with severe language problems to interact with others, learn, and reason.

Because the profile captures the child's individual variations, children with the same diagnosis (i.e., Pervasive Developmental Disorder) may have very different profiles and children with different diagnoses may have similar profiles. The functional profile is updated in an ongoing manner with continuing clinical observations as part of the intervention. These ongoing observations and updated profiles then serve as a basis for revising the child's intervention program.

Developmentally Based Approach to the Evaluation Process[1]

Now, it may be useful to look at the evaluation process in more detail.

The Basic Model

The basic developmental model guiding the evaluation process needs to be re-emphasized in the context of the evaluation process. It can be visualized with the infant's or child's constitutional-maturational patterns on one side and the infant's or child's environment, including caregivers, family, community, and culture, on the other side. Both of these sets of factors operate through the infant-caregiver relationship which can be pictured in the middle. These factors and the infant-caregiver relationship, in turn, con-

[1] Adapted from The assessment and diagnosis of infant disorders: developmental level, individual differences and relationship based interactions (Greenspan & Wieder, 1999), Infancy and Early Childhood: The Practice of Clinical Assessment and Intervention with Emotional and Developmental Challenges (Greenspan, 1992), The Child with Special Needs: Intellectual and Emotional Growth (Greenspan, & Wieder, 1998), and The Clinical Interview of the Child. (Greenspan, 2003).

tribute to the organization of experience at each of six different developmental levels, which may be pictured just beneath the infant-caregiver relationship.

Each developmental level involves different tasks or goals. The relative effect of the constitutional-maturational, environmental, or interactive variables, therefore, depends on and can only be understood in the context of the developmental level they relate to. The influencing variables, therefore, are best understood, not as they might be traditionally, as general influences on development or behavior, but as distinct and different influences on the six distinct developmental and experiential levels. For example, as a child is negotiating the formation of a relationship (engaging), his mother's tendency to be very intellectual and prefer talking over holding may make it relatively harder for him to become deeply engaged in emotional terms. If constitutionally he has slightly lower than average muscle tone and is under-responsive with regard to touch and sound, his mother's intellectual and slightly aloof style may be doubly difficult for him, as neither she nor the child is able to take the initiative in engaging the other.

Functional Developmental Levels

In this model, there are six functional developmental levels. They include the infant-child's ability to accomplish the following:

1. Attend to multisensory affective experience and at the same time organize a calm, regulated state and experience pleasure.
2. Engage with and evidence affective preference and pleasure for a caregiver.
3. Initiate and respond to two-way pre-symbolic gestural communication.
4. Organize chains of two-way communication (opening and closing many circles of communication in a row), maintain communication across space, integrate affective polarities, and synthesize an emerging pre-representational organization of self and other.
5. Represent (symbolize) affective experience (e.g., pretend play, functional use of language). It should be noted that this ability calls for higher level auditory and verbal sequencing ability.
6. Create representational (symbolic) categories and gradually build conceptual bridges between these categories. This ability creates the foundation for such basic personality functions as reality testing, impulse control, self-other representational differentiation, affect labeling and discrimination, stable mood, and a sense of time and space that allows for logical planning. It should be noted that this ability rests not only on complex auditory and verbal processing abilities, but visuospatial abstracting capacities as well.

The theoretical, clinical, and empirical rationale for these developmental levels is discussed in *The Development of the Ego* (Greenspan, 1989) and *Intelligence and Adaptation* (Greenspan 1979), *The Growth of the Mind* (Greenspan 1997), and *The First Idea: How Symbols, Language and Intelligence Evolved from Our Primate Ancestors to Modern Humans* (Greenspan & Shanker, 2004).

To make a developmental assessment of the functional level, the clinician should make a determination regarding each of the six developmental levels in terms of whether they have been successfully negotiated or not, and whether there is a deficit at any level that has not been successfully negotiated. Sometimes these levels have been successfully negotiated, but are not applied to the full range of emotional themes. For example, a toddler may use two-way gestural communication to negotiate assertiveness and exploration by, for example, pointing at a certain toy and vocalizing for his parent to play with him. The same child may either withdraw or cry in a disorganized way when he wishes for increased closeness and dependency instead of, for example, reaching out to be picked up or coming over and initiating a cuddle. This would indicate a constriction at that level.

Sometimes children are able to negotiate a level with one parent and not the other, with one sibling and not another, or with one substitute caregiver but not another. If it should reasonably be expected that a particular relationship is secure and stable enough to support a certain developmental level, but that level is not evident in that relationship, then there is a constriction at that level as well.

It is useful to indicate which areas or relationships are not incorporated into the developmental level. Consider the following areas of expected emotional range: dependency (closeness, pleasure, assertiveness [exploration], curiosity, anger, empathy [for children over 3½ years]); stable forms of love, self-limit-setting (for children over 18 months); interest and collaboration with peers (for children over 2 years); participation in a peer group (for children over 2½ years); and the ability to deal with competition and rivalry (for children over 3½ years).

If the child has reached a developmental level, but the slightest stress, such as being tired, having a mild illness (e.g., a cold), or playing with a new peer leads to a loss of that level, then there is an instability at that level.

A child may have a defect, constriction, or instability at more than one level. Also, a child may have a defect at one level and a constriction or instability at another. Therefore, the clinician should make a developmental judgment based on the following developmental levels. The Functional Emotional Assessment Scale has been developed for research purposes and include reliability and validity studies (DeGangi & Greenspan, 2000).

Developmental Level	**Defect Constriction**	**Instability**
1. Regulation and interest in the world		
2. Attachment		
3. Intentional communication		
4. Behavioral organization (complex sense of self)		
5. Representational elaboration		
6. Representational differentiation		

Constitutional-Maturational Patterns

Constitutional-maturational characteristics are the result of genetic, prenatal, perinatal, and maturational variations and/or deficits. They can be observed as part of the following patterns:

1. Sensory responsiveness, including under- and over-responsivity in each sensory modality (tactile, auditory, visual, vestibular, olfactory)
2. Regulatory-sensory processing in each sensory modality (e.g., the capacity to decode sequences, configurations, or abstract patterns)
3. Sensory affective reactivity and processing in each modality (e.g., the ability to process and react to degrees of affective intensity in a stable manner)
4. Motor tone
5. Motor planning and sequencing

An instrument to clinically assess aspects of sensory functions in a reliable manner has been developed and is available (DeGangi and Greenspan, 1988, 1989a,b). The following section describes the constitutional and maturational patterns.

Sensory responsiveness (under- or over-) and regulatory-sensory processing can be observed clinically. Is the child over- or under-responsive to touch or sound? The same question must be asked in terms of vision and movement in space. In each sensory modality, does the four-month-old process a complicated pattern of information input or only a simple one? Does the four-and-a-half-year-old have a receptive language problem and is, therefore, unable to sequence words he hears together or follow complex directions? Is the three-year-old an early comprehender and talker, but slower in visuospatial processing? If spatial patterns are poorly comprehended, a child may be facile with words, sensitive to every emotional nuance, but have no context, never see the big picture (the "forest"); such children get lost in the "trees." In the clinician's office, they may forget where the door is or have a hard time picturing that mother is only a few feet away in the waiting room.

In addition to straightforward pictures of spatial relationship (e.g., how to get to the playground), they may also have difficulty with seeing the emotional big picture. If the mother is angry, the child may think the earth is opening up and he is falling in because he cannot comprehend that she was nice before and she will probably be nice again. Such a child may be strong on the auditory processing side, but weak on the visuospatial processing side.

Our impression is that children with a lag in the visuospatial area can become overwhelmed by the affect of the moment. This is often intensified by precocious auditory-verbal skills. The child, in a sense, overloads himself and does not have the ability to see how it all fits together. Thus, at a minimum, it is necessary to have a sense of how the child reacts in each sensory modality, how he or she processes information in each modality, and particularly, as the child gets older, a sense of the auditory-verbal processing skills in comparison to visuospatial processing skills.

It is also necessary to look at the motor system, including motor tone, motor planning (fine and gross), and postural control. Observing how a child sits, crawls, or runs; maintains posture; holds a crayon; hops, scribbles, or draws; and makes rapid alternating movements provides a picture of the child's motor system. His security in regulating and controlling his body plays an important role in how he uses gestures to communicate his ability to regulate dependency (being close or far away); his confidence in regulating aggression ("Can I control my hand that wants to hit?"); and his overall physical sense of self.

Other constitutional and maturational variables have to do with movement in space, attention, and dealing with transitions.

Parent and Family Contributions

In addition to constitutional and maturational factors, it is important to describe the family contribution with regard to each developmental level. If a family system is aloof, it may not negotiate engagement well; if a family system is intrusive, it may overwhelm or overstimulate a baby. Obviously, if a baby is already overly responsive to touch or sound, the caregiver's intrusiveness is all the more difficult for the child to handle. We see, therefore, the interaction between the maturational pattern and the family pattern.

A family system may throw so many meanings at a child that he or she is unable to organize a sense of reality. Categories of me/not-me may become confused, because one day a feeling is yours, the next day it is the mother's, next day it is the father's, the day after it is little brother's; anger may turn into dependency, and vice versa. If meanings shift too quickly, a child may be unable to reach the fourth level–emotional thinking. A child with difficulties in auditory-verbal sequencing has an especially difficult time (Greenspan, 1989).

The couple is a unit in itself. How do husband and wife operate, not only with each other, but how do they negotiate on behalf of the children, in terms of the developmental processes? A couple with marital problems could still successfully negotiate shared attention, engagement, two-way communication, shared meanings, and emotional thinking with their children. But the marital difficulties could disrupt any one or a number of these developmental processes.

Each parent is also an individual. How does each personality operate vis-à-vis these processes? While it may be desirable to have a general mental health diagnosis for each caregiver, one also needs to functionally observe which of these levels each caregiver can naturally and easily support. Is the parent engaged, warm, and interactive (a good reader of cues)? Is he or she oriented toward symbolic meanings (verbalizing meanings), and engaging in pretend play, and can the caregiver organize feelings and thoughts, or does one or the other get lost between reality and fantasy? Are there limitations, in terms of these levels, and if so, what are they?

Each parent also has specific fantasies that may be projected onto the children and interfere with any of the levels. Does a mother see her motorically active, distractible, labile baby as a menace and therefore overcontrol, overintrude, or withdraw? Her fantasy may govern her behavior. Does a father, whose son has low motor tone, see his boy as passive and inept, and therefore pull away from him or impatiently "rev" him up?

In working only with the parent-child interaction, and not the parent's fantasy, one may be dealing with only the tip of the iceberg. The father may be worried that he has a overly passive son, or the mother may be worried that she has a monster for a daughter (who reminds her of her retarded sister). All these feelings may be present, and they can drive the parent-child interactions.

Infant-Caregiver Relationship Patterns

It is the caregiver-infant relationship that mediates these other variables and, in addition, determines how each of the developmental processes is successfully or unsuccessfully negotiated.

Often, parents bring a baby in, and we watch the parent-infant interaction in the first session, while we are hearing about their concerns. With an older child, a four-year-old, for example, we have them wait to bring the child in, because we want them to talk freely at the outset.

Usually, we let each parent play with the child for at least fifteen or twenty minutes, and then we play with the child for about the same amount of time. We look for a pattern of interaction in the context of the developmental processes. We observe which levels are present and not present, and also look for the range of emotional themes in each of the core processes and the stability of these processes. For example, a four-year-old may be playing out wonderful fantasies of fairy princesses going off to a castle and being tied up by an evil witch and then being saved by the hero. While we are interested in the content, we first keep an eye on how the child is relating with his caregiver (and later on with us), as well as the breadth of emotion and the stability of the relatedness.

Therefore, for each of the developmental levels, or core processes, it is necessary to look at the child's constitutional and maturational status, the family/parent/couple patterns, and the actual caregiver/parent-infant interaction (See Figure 1 which follows). For each level one must look at what is influencing the successful or compromised negotiation at that level. Therefore, a therapist tries to reach a conclusion about a child 3 years and older on all levels, and for the child less than 3 years, on the levels they should have attained (e.g., for a $2^{1}/_{2}$-year-old, through the first three levels; for a 14-month-old, the first two levels–attention and engagement, and two-way communication).

Figure 1

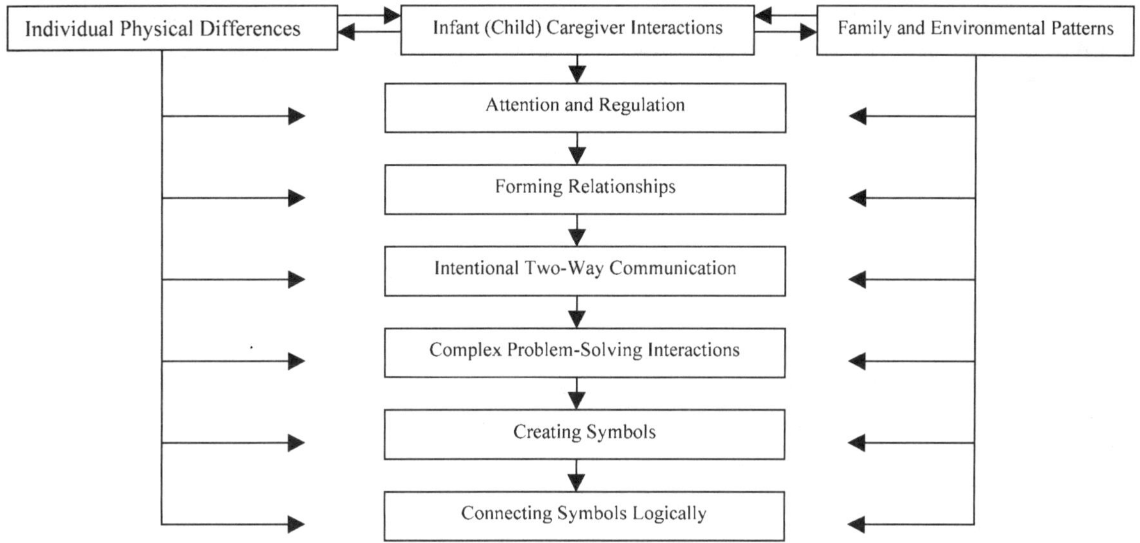

The Process Of Clinical Assessment

Each clinician may develop his own way of doing an evaluation. However, any assessment should (1) encompass certain baseline data; (2) organize data by indicating how each factor contributes to the baby's ability to develop; and (3) suggest methods of treatment. A comprehensive assessment usually involves the following elements: presenting complaints, developmental history, family patterns, child and parent sessions, additional consultations, and formulation. Table 3 below presents a brief outline, followed by a discussion of selected elements.

Table 3: Formal Assessment

I.	**Review of current challenges and functioning, including** • Each functional developmental capacity (e.g., from attention and engagement to thinking) • Each processing capacity (e.g., auditory, motor planning and sequencing, visuospatial, sensory modulation) • In relevant contexts (e.g., at home with caregivers and siblings, with peers, in educational settings)
II.	**History, including history of the above, beginning with prenatal development.**
III.	**Two or more observational sessions of child-caregiver interactions** with coaching and/or interactions with clinician (each sessions should be 45 minutes or more). These observational sessions should provide the basis for forming a hypothesis about the child's functional emotional developmental capacities, individual processing and motor planning differences, and interactive and family patterns.
IV.	**Exploration of caregiver(s) personalities, marital and family patterns, and siblings.** This exploration should focus on the caregiver/family/sibling patterns in their own right and in relationship to their role in enabling the child to negotiate the functional developmental milestones (minimum of one 45 minute session).

Table 3: Formal Assessment *(continued)*

V.	**Biomedical evaluations** (e.g., extended sleep EEG, metabolic work-up, genetic studies, and nutrition)
VI.	**Speech and language evaluation.**
VII.	**Evaluation of motor and regulatory-sensory processing, including** • Motor planning • Sensory modulation • Perceptual motor capacities • Visuospatial capacities
VIII.	**Evaluation of cognitive functions, including neuro-psychological and educational assessments.**
IX.	**Mental health evaluations of family members, family patterns, and family needs.**

NOTE: The evaluations listed in number V – IX should only be carried out to answer specific questions which arise from the history, review of challenges, and current functioning and observations of the child-caregiver interactions patterns and family functioning.

Presenting Complaints (Overall Picture)

We frequently spend a whole session on the presenting complaints or picture, which includes the development of the problems, the infant's or child's and family's current functioning, and preliminary observation of the infant or child both with the caregiver(s), or, in the case of a child over three, without them as well.

We usually suggest that the parents bring the baby or young child with them to the first session. Even though we spend most of the time talking to the parents, we have our eyes on the baby or young child and we watch what is going on spontaneously between parents and child. If an older child (three or four years of age) is involved, we have the parents leave the child at home the first time, if possible, so the parents can talk more freely.

We begin by asking the parents, "How can I help?" and we try to listen to their responses. We encourage the parents to elaborate about the child's problem, whether it has to do with sleeping, eating, or being too aggressive or too withdrawn. If we ask a question, it is usually to clarify something they have said, such as, "Can you give me some examples of that?" "How is this different now from what it was six months ago, and when wasn't it a problem?" We try to find out when the problem started, how it evolved, and its nature and scope. For example, if a two-and-a-half-year-old is aggressive with peers, we want to know whether it is with all peers or only certain children. We are interested in what precipitated the problem and what may be contributing to it. Was there a change within the family, such as the father getting a new job? Was there marital tension? Were new developmental abilities emerging which paradoxically were stressful to the child?

When the parents say, "Well, I think we have told you everything about the problem," then we ask, "Is there more to tell about Johnny or Susie that would help fill out the picture?" It is much more helpful to ask open-ended questions than to ask specific questions about cognitive, language, or motor development at this point. One gathers together more relevant information when the parents elaborate spontaneously. Parents also reveal their own feelings and private family matters if the therapist is empathetic as he or she helps them describe their child. Therefore, a clinician should strive to be unstructured; ask facilitating, elaborative questions rather than yes or no or defining questions; and never be in a hurry to fill out a checklist.

The initial session also should establish rapport with the family and child in order to begin a collaborative process. The developmental process discussed earlier in relation to the child—mutual attention, engagement, gestural communication, shared meanings, and the categorizing and connecting of meanings—may occur between an empathetic clinician and the parents. How the clinician relates to the parents reflects how they are encouraged to relate to their baby. If the therapist asks hurried questions, with yes or no answers, he or she sets up an untherapeutic model. It usually takes parents a long time to decide to come for help. They should be able to tell their story without being hurried or criticized.

As part of this presenting picture it is important to learn about all the areas of the child's current functioning. If the primary focus is initially on aggression and distractibility, one wants to know the child's other age-expected capacities. One considers if the child is at the age-appropriate developmental level and if so, the full range of emotional inclinations. Is the eight-month-old capable of reciprocal cause-and-effect interchanges? Is a four-month-old wooing and engaging? Is a two-and-a-half-year-old exhibiting symbolic or representational capacities? Does he do pretend play? Does he use language functionally? How does he negotiate his needs? At each of these levels, how is he dealing with dependency, pleasure, assertiveness, anger, and so forth?

Toward the end of the first session, we may fill in more gaps by asking questions about sensory, language, cognitive, and fine and gross motor functioning. Usually, we have a sense of these capacities and patterns from anecdotes and more general descriptions of behavior. We listen for indications of the child's ability to retain information; how he does or does not follow commands; word retrieval skills; word association skills; and fine and gross motor and motor planning skills.

Some clinicians write down what parents say right after the session; others write during the session. Taking notes need not be an interference if one stops throughout to make good contact. We take detailed notes during the first fifteen or twenty minutes because we want as much information as we can get in the parents' words.

By the end of the first session, clinicians have a sense of where the child is developmentally. They have a sense of the range of emotional themes the child can deal with at his developmental level. They have an awareness of the support, or lack of support, the child gets from his fine and gross motor, speech and language, and cognitive abilities. Clinicians also form an impression of the support the child gets from his parents. They observe how the parents communicate and organize their thinking, the quality of their engagement, their emotional availability, their interest in the child. They have a good sense of their relative comfort or discomfort with each emotional theme. In general, the therapist observes how the parents attend, engage, intentionally communicate, construct and organize ideas, and are able or not able to incorporate range of emotional themes into their ideas as they relate to the therapist.

Developmental History

In the second session, we construct a developmental history for the child. (However, sometimes martial or other family problems burst out during the first session. The parents may be at each other's throats; the mother and/or the father may be extremely depressed. In such cases, in the second session we will focus on the individual parent problems, as well as family functioning.)

We usually start the session in an unstructured manner. We want to hear how development unfolded and what the parents thought was important. We encourage them to alternate between what the baby or child was like at different stages and what they felt was going on as a family and as individuals in each of those stages. We try to start with the planning for the child and progress through the pregnancy and delivery. Next, we cover the six developmental stages, outlined earlier, in order to organize the developmental history.

Family Patterns

The next session focuses in greater depth on the functioning of the caregiver and family at each developmental phase. For example, the mother may say that she was a little depressed or angry, or that there were marital problems at different stages in the child's development.

Sometimes clinicians who are only beginning to work with infants and family feel reluctant to talk to the parents about any difficulties in the marriage. However, an open and supportive approach can elicit relevant information. One might ask, "What can you tell me about yourselves as people, as a married couple, as a family?" We are also interested in concrete details of a history of mental illness, learning disabilities, or special developmental patterns in either of the parents' families.

Some families do not hesitate to discuss marital difficulties or other problems. Sometimes there is a discussion of how the "problem child" relates to the father and mother in terms of power struggles. If they describe a pattern, for example, between mother and child or father and child, we are likely to ask, "Does that same pattern operate in other family relationships-between mother and father, for example?" Is the pattern a carryover from a parent's own family? By following the couple's lead, we try to develop a picture of the marriage, careers of one or both parents, relationship with other children and between all the children, the parents' relationship with their own families of origin, as well as friendships and community ties.

Sometimes the family as a whole functions in a very fragmented, presymbolic way. They gesture, "behave at" each other, overwhelm each other, withdraw from one another, but they don't share any meanings with one another. Nothing is negotiated at a symbolic level. Even though each individual may be capable of functioning on a symbolic level, something about the family dynamics cancels out that ability. In this context, we want to know how the family handles dependency, excitement, and sexuality, as well as anger, assertiveness, empathy, and love.

For each unit of the family—the parents, each parent-child relationship, as well as the family as a whole—we want to find out how the different emotional themes were dealt with at different developmental levels.

Child (or Infant) and Parent Sessions

We spend the next two sessions with a focus on the child or infant. We conduct the session differently with an older child (a three- or four-year-old, for example) than with an infant. With an infant, we may ask the parent to play with the baby to "show me how you like to be with or play with your baby or child." The parents may ask, "What do you want me to do?" "Anything you like," is our response. We offer the use of the toys in the office or tell them they may bring a special toy from home.

We watch each parent with the child, playing in an unstructured way, for about fifteen or twenty minutes We are looking for the developmental level, the range of emotional themes at each level, and the use of and support that the child is able to derive from motor, language, sensory, and cognitive skills. We are also watching for the parents' ability to support or undermine the developmental level, range in that level, and use of sensory, language, and motor systems. After we watch the mother and father separately, we watch the three of them together to see how they interact as a group, because sometimes the group situation is more challenging. Later, we join them do some coaching and/or start to play with the child (briefly in the first session and for a longer period in the second session).

During this time, we want to see the child interacting at his or her highest developmental level, as well as how he relates to a new person whom he knows only slightly. In addition, we want to determine how to bring out the highest developmental level at which the child can function. For example, if a child is withdrawn or self-absorbed and repetitively moving a truck, we suggest joining his play, trying to move the truck together, put up a fence (one's hands) or take another car and, with great joy and enthusiasm, announce "Here I come" to entice the child into interaction. Sometimes marching or jumping with an aimless child or lying next to a passive, withdrawn child and offering a back rub or tickle draws him in. If a child shows signs of symbolic functioning and the parents do not support symbolic functioning in their 3-year-old, we will try, through coaching or directing, to get pretend play going. If an 8-month-old is being overstimulated, we try to get cause-and-effect interactions going. If a 4-month-old looks withdrawn, we try to flirt to pull him in. We try to calm down a fussy five-month-old with visual or vocal support, gentle tactile pressure, and a change of positions. We work hands-on with an infant to explore his tactile sensitivity, motor tone, motor planning, and preference for patterns of movement in space.

Therapists can learn a great deal through observation. By way of example, they could offer a doll to a child moving a train to see if he gives it a ride, suggesting symbolic capacities, or playfully obstruct the path of a child aimlessly wandering around the room to see if he ducks under their arms or smiles or simply turns and wanders away. They could also say to a child who is moving a train, "Oh boy, I can see that you know how to make this train go." The child may put a doll on the train, make the doll a conductor, and add a passenger. The passenger may have a baby while the train is going through a tunnel, and at the same time a doctor makes sure the baby is all right. A 3-year-old who generates such a "drama" is sophisticated cognitively and evidences a rich fantasy life.

With children who can connect ideas together (e.g., hold a back-and-forth conversation), depending on the child's comfort in being separated from his caregiver, we may reverse the sequence. We may have the first session with the child alone to explore how he or she engages, attends, initiates intentional two-way communication, problem-solves, and shares and categorizes meanings.

During this time alone, a three-and-a-half-year-old may stand in the middle of the room and look the clinician over, while we look at him. If we don't try to control the situation too quickly and can tolerate ten or fifteen seconds of ambiguity, the child may start to play, ask us a question about the toys, or talk about his family. What the child has to say, without us saying, "Tell me what your mother told you about why you are here" or "Do you want to play with the toys?" can be very valuable. A child may look around and say, "I heard there were toys here. Where are they?" Such a statement indicates an organized, intentional child who has figured out why he is there and acts on his understanding. Another child may look puzzled and, after a silence, ask in a formal manner, "Can I sit down?"

Some 4-year-olds talk to us through the session. We can have an almost adult-to-adult kind of dialogue about school or home, nightmares or worries, or just a chat about anything, as one might have with a neighbor. Other children behave aggressively and want to jump on us or wrestle. They become too familiar too quickly.

We observe the way the child relates to us, that is, the quality of engagement–overly familiar, overly cautious, or warm. We look for how intentional he is in the use of gestures and how well he sizes up the situation and us (without words). We try to determine his emotional range and his way of dealing with anxiety (e.g., does he become aggressive or withdrawn?). We also note, during interaction with a child, the child's physical status, his speech, receptive language, visuospatial problem-solving skills (e.g., can he search for a toy), gross and fine motor skills, and general state of health and mood.

In general, we want to systematically describe the child's ability to attend, engage, initiate and be purposeful with affects and motor gestures, open and close many communication circles to problem solve, create ideas (pretend play), and converse and think logically.

The next step is to learn what is on the child's mind. If the child is symbolic, we look at the content of the play and dialogue, as well as the sequence of themes that emerge from them. Often, observing how a child shifts from one activity or theme to another (e.g., aggression to protectiveness or exploration to repetition provides some initial hypotheses). The therapist's job is to be reasonably warm, supportive, and skillful in engaging the child and helping him evidence his capacities and elaborate.

Formulation

After learning about the child's current functioning and history and observing the child and family first hand, there should be a convergence of impressions. If a picture is not emerging, one may need to spend another session or two developing the history or observing further.

We then asks ourselves a number of questions. How high up in the developmental progression has the child gone, in terms of (1) attending, (2) regulating and engaging; (3) establishing two-way intentional communication; (4) engaging in preverbal problem-solving chains; (5) sharing meanings; and (6) emotional thinking? How well are the earlier phases mastered and, if not fully mastered, what are the unresolved issues? For example, does a child still have challenges in terms of his attentional capacities, the quality of engagement, and/or his intentional abilities?

Determining the developmental level tells us how the child organizes experience. To use a metaphor, it provides a picture of the "stage" upon which a child plays out his "drama." The presenting symptoms—nightmares, waking up at night, refusal to eat, as well as other concerns and inclinations—make up the "drama." The "stage" may be age-appropriate. For example, a 4-year-old, who can categorize representational experience, has a drama of being aggressive to other children, but this drama is being played out on a stage that is age-appropriate. This child has the capacity to comprehend the nature of his aggression and use "ideas" to figure out his behavior. On the other hand, there may be major deficits in the stage (e.g., attending, being intentional, representing experience, or differentiating experience). If there are flaws in the stage, we want to pinpoint the nature of those flaws.

For example, if a child is not engaged with other people, he may be perseverative and self-stimulatory because he can't interact or he may be aggressive because he basically has no sense of other people's feelings. He may not even see people as human. Alternatively, another child may be aggressive because he cannot represent feelings and therefore acts them out. Still another child may represent and differentiate his feelings, but have conflicts about his dependency needs.

One also looks at the range of experience organized at a particular developmental level. If a child is at an age-appropriate developmental level, does she accommodate such things as dependency, assertiveness, curiosity, sexuality, and aggression at that level? On the other hand, even if a child is at the right developmental level, the stage may be narrow. In other words, he might be only at that developmental stage when it comes to assertiveness, but when it comes to dependency, he is not quite there, and when it comes to excitement, he functions at a much lower level. In other words, if he dances the wrong step, he could fall off the stage. One also looks at the stability of the developmental organization. Does even a little stress lead to a loss of function or are the functions stable?

Therefore, if the stage has cracks or holes in it because there are major problems from earlier developmental issues, we say there are defects in the stage. If the stage is solid (no defects), it is either very flexible and wide or very narrow and constricted (e.g., it tolerates a drama of assertiveness but it does not tolerate a drama of intimacy or excitement). In addition, it is stable or unstable.

Next, we want to know about the contributing factors. One set of factors relates to observations about family functioning; the other set of factors relates to the assessment of the child's individual differences. The parent-child interactions are the mediating factors. The developmental formulation or profile describes (1) the child's functional developmental level; (2) the contributing processing profile (e.g., over-responsivity to sound, auditory and visuospatial and motor planning difficulties; and (3) the contributing family patterns (e.g., high energy, overloading, confusing family pattern, as well as the observed interaction patterns of each of the significant caregivers and the types of interactions that would be hypothesized to enable the child to move up the developmental ladder and improve his processing difficulties.

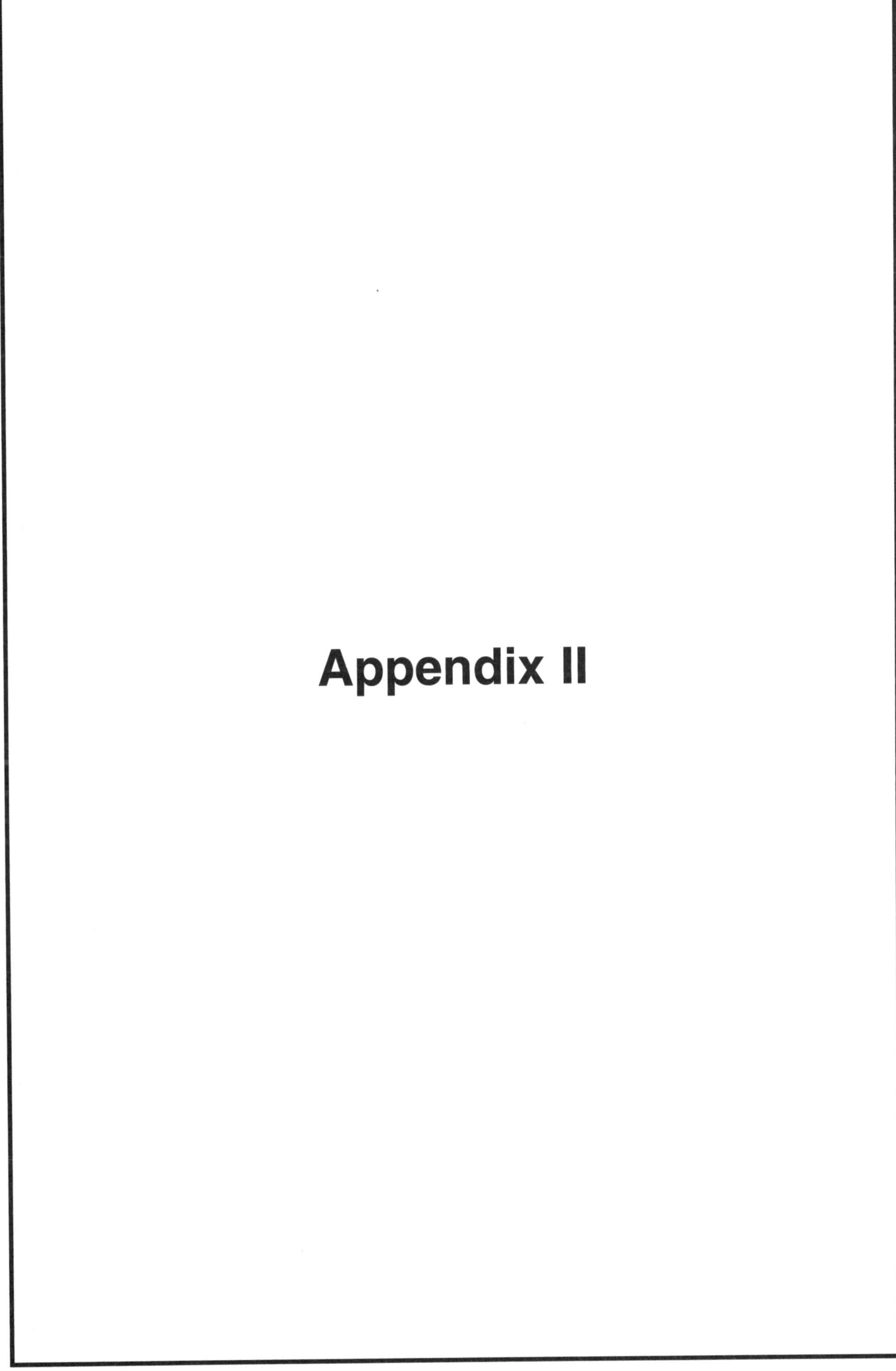

Appendix II

Appendix II: Implications of the ICDL Classification System for a Comprehensive, Developmentally-Based Approach to Intervention

A developmentally-based approach to classification reveals the developmental pathways involved in the child's challenges. As such, it provides a framework to guide the formulation of a comprehensive, developmentally based approach to intervention. The following sections describe the general principles involved in such an approach. It does not, however, attempt to specify in detail the technical strategies that may be employed to help the child master each of his challenges. The intention of this appendix is to discuss the implications of a comprehensive classification model for planning a developmentally-based intervention approach. Future volumes address approaches to intervention in more detail. The principles discussed attempt to deal with the challenges of a child with multiple special needs (e.g., a child with autism). Many children with more circumscribed challenges already have or are mastering a number of basic capacities or processes and may require less intensive or comprehensive interventions.

For more information, also see the *ICDL Clinical Practice Guidelines*, related books, such as *The Child with Special Needs* and *The Challenging Child* , and the ICDL Training Videotape Series.[1]

A COMPREHENSIVE DEVELOPMENTALLY BASED APPROACH TO INTERVENTION

A functional approach to assessment leads to a comprehensive approach to intervention, which deals with all the relevant functional areas in an integrated manner. In addition, a periodic review of the child's functional developmental profile, based on assessments of the child's functional developmental level and capacities, individual processing differences and the different interaction patterns available to the child at home, at school, with peers, and in other settings is essential. The functional assessment is updated in an ongoing manner with continuing clinical observations as part of the intervention. Ongoing observations serve as a basis for revising the child's intervention program.

A comprehensive intervention program–the Developmental-Individual Difference-Relationship-Based (DIR) approach–can be conceptualized as a pyramid. Each of the components of the pyramid builds on each other and is briefly described below.

[1] Interdisciplinary Council on Developmental and Learning Disorders Clinical Practice Guidelines Workgroup, S. I. G. C. (2000). *Interdisciplinary Council on Developmental and Learning Disorders' Clinical Practice Guidelines: Redefining the standards of care for infants, children, and families with special needs.* Bethesda, MD: Interdisciplinary Council on Developmental and Learning Disorders; Greenspan, S. I. & Wieder, S. (2001). ICDL video training tapes on the DIR and Floortime techniques. Bethesda, MD, ICDL; Greenspan, S. I. (1995). *The challenging child: Understanding, raising, and enjoying the five "difficult" types of children.* Reading, MA: Addison Wesley; Greenspan, S. I. & Wieder, S. (1998). *The child with special needs: Encouraging intellectual and emotional growth.* Reading, MA: Perseus Books.

Figure 1: Intervention Pyramid For Children With Special Needs

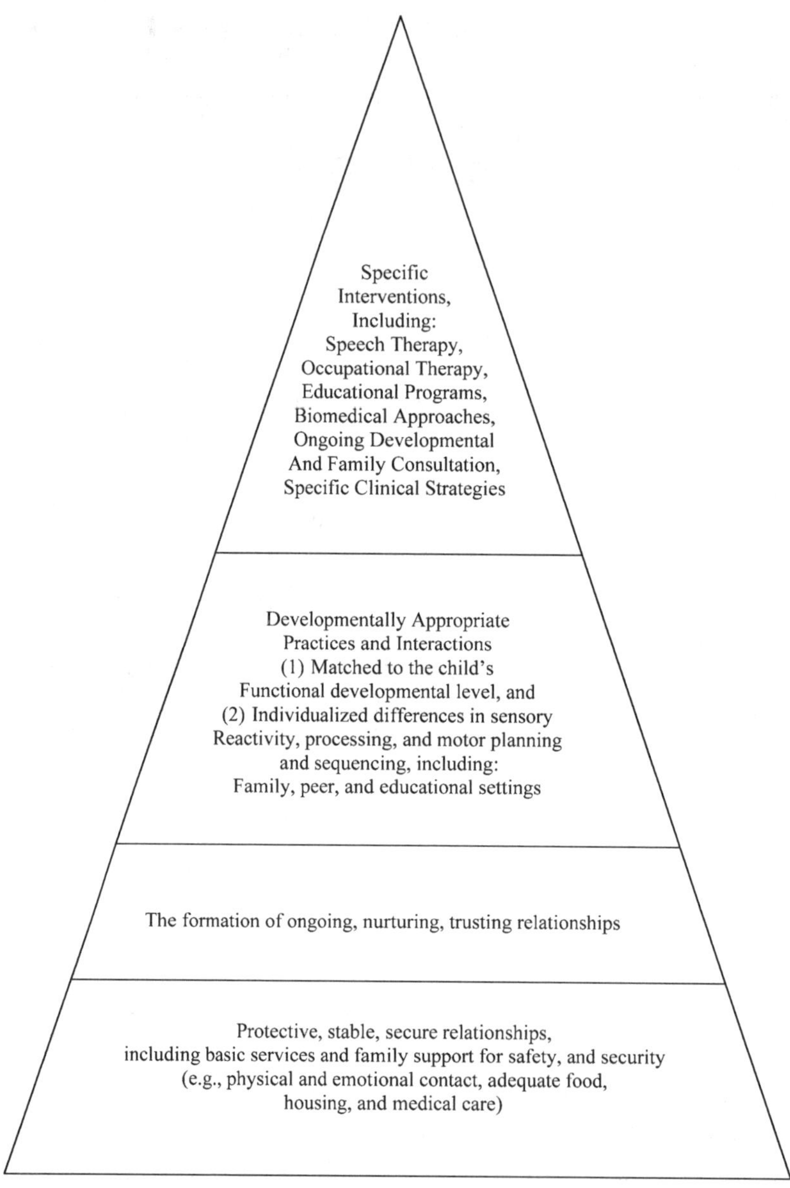

Stable, Secure, and Protective Relationships

At the foundation of the intervention pyramid are the protective, stable, developmentally supportive relationships and family patterns that all children require, especially children with developmental challenges. This foundation includes physical protection and safety and an ongoing sense of security. Some families require a great deal of support and/or therapy in order to stabilize and organize these basic family functions. The family may be dealing with extreme poverty and chronic states of fearfulness. Relationships within the family may be abusive, neglectful, or fragmented. Some families require counseling to explore family patterns and relationships, particularly in connection to the challenges of coping with a child with special needs and the changing family relationships between spouses and siblings that that entails.

Intervention programs need staff trained to assess family needs, develop alliances, problem-solve, advocate (including for social and economic support) and provide family counseling, and family or personal therapy where indicated (Barber, et al., 1988; Bronfenbrenner, 1986; Dunst & Trivette, 1988; Powell, et. al., 1992; Robbins, et al., 1991; Turnbull, et al., 1986).

Ongoing, Nurturing, Trusting Relationships

At the second level of our pyramid are the ongoing and consistent relationships that every child requires. Typically developing children require nurturing relationships to have any chance for emotional and cognitive competency. Children with special needs, who often already have compromises in their capacities to relate, are in even greater need of warm, consistent caregiving. Their caregivers, however, often face challenges to sustaining intimate relationships because it is so easy to misperceive their child's intentions. Understanding their children's behavior as attempts to cope with their difficulties or as being overwhelmed by their difficulties can often help caregivers over these misperceptions and towards more creative and empathetic ways of relating to their children. For example, children who are over-responsive to touch may not be rejecting the parents' comfort and care when they cry. For such a child it may be important to avoid light touch and to use deep pressure to help the child feel more comfortable. Or, the child who jumps on a toddler who is crying may not be primarily aggressive, but so responsive to the sounds of the cry that he panics and wants the noise stopped. Similarly, the child who has difficulty comprehending words may become confused and avoid communication. He may benefit from pictures or gestural signs to understand his environment and predict what will happen next in his interactions with caregivers. The child who is generally avoidant or self-absorbed and appears to prefer to play alone can be giving a signal. He may be under-responsive to sensations, with low muscle tone, needing greater wooing to get beyond his self-absorption.

The importance of interactive relationships cannot be underestimated. Almost all human learning occurs in relationships, whether these are relationships in the classroom, family, or therapeutic sessions. No one would deny that the ability to enjoy and participate in relationships is pivotal for learning to relate to others, experiencing intimacy and positive self-esteem, and developing healthy coping strategies. In addition, however, we suggest that most cognitive or intellectual capacities learned in the first four to five years of life are also based on emotions and relationships (Greenspan, 1997a). For example, infants first learn initial concepts of causality primarily in early relationships (where crying leads to comfort or reaching out leads to being picked up and smiles or frowns lead to caregivers' return emotional responses), rather than in activities such as banging objects on the floor (which leads to learning that this action makes a sound). Similarly, the meaning of words and gestures, the sense of time, and concepts of quantity are also learned as part of interactive, affective relationships early in life (Greenspan, 1997a). For example, for a toddler "a lot" is more than he expects or needs. "A little" is less than she wants. Words are connected to the emotional experiences that define them, and gestures become organized into patterns associated with emotions and expectations (for example, Dad's smile leading to a hug and tickle).

Relationships serve a number of functions for young children. Most importantly, a relationship must foster warmth, intimacy, and pleasure. In addition, relationships must provide the context in which children experience security, physical safety, protection from illness and injury, and get their basic needs for nutrition, housing and the like met. The regulatory aspects of relationships (for example, protection of the child from over- or under-stimulation) help the child maintain pleasure in intimacy and a secure, alert, attentive state that permits new learning and development to occur.

Relationships provide the basis for communication. Initially, the infant's communication system is nonverbal. It involves affect cueing (smiles, assertive glances, frowns), contingent behavioral interactions (pointing, taking and giving back, negotiating), and the like. From the earliest reciprocal smiles to a child taking mother's hand, walking to the refrigerator and pointing to a favorite food, there emerges a complex system of affect, gestural, and behavior interactions which continues throughout the life of the individual. Even though this nonverbal system eventually works in conjunction with symbolic-verbal modes of communication, it remains more fundamental. (For example, adults tend to trust someone's nonverbal nod or look of approval more than words of praise, which, at times, can be misleading). For relationships to take on the communicative intent that promotes development, therefore, the complex nonverbal aspects of relationships must be operating.

Relationships are the context for learning which behaviors are appropriate and which are inappropriate (Greenspan, 1974, 1975). As children's behavioral repertoires become more complex in the second year of life, discriminative and reinforcing properties of relationships define which behaviors increase and which behaviors decrease. Repertoires are built up through the give-and-take between children and caregivers (i.e., discriminative learning). Importantly, along with behaviors, however, affects, wishes, emerging self-perceptions, and a sense of self are also being organized. The emotional tone and subtle affective interactions of relationships are, therefore, just as important as more easily observable behaviors.

Relationships enable a child to learn to symbolize experience. The first objects with which the child has a highly emotional experience are not playthings, but rather the human "objects" he or she interacts with. In his interactions, the child goes from acting out his desires or wishes to picturing them in his mind and labeling them with a word. He goes from desiring Mom and grabbing her to saying "Mom" and looking lovingly. This transformation heralds symbolic awareness.

The ability to picture an object when it is displaced in both time and space is a much-used marker for the child's achievement of object permanence and the emergence of symbolic capacities. Yet pretend or imaginative play involving emotional human dramas (e.g., the dolls hugging or fighting) helps the child learn the types of affective-based symbolization that enable him to connect an image to a wish or intent and then use this image to think, "If I'm nice to Mom, she will let me stay up late." Figuring out the motives of a character in a story as well as the difference between ten cookies and three cookies depends on the capacity for affective symbolization (Greenspan, 1997a).

The child's ability to create mental pictures of relationship and, later, other objects, forms the basis for more advanced symbolic thinking (Greenspan, 1997a & b). For example, a key element essential for future learning and coping is the child's ability for self-observation, problem-solving, and creative thought. The ability to self-observe is essential for self-monitoring of activities as simple as coloring inside or outside the lines, or matching pictures with words or numbers. Self-observation also helps a person label rather than act out feelings. It helps him to empathize with others and match behavior to the expectations of the environment.

Self-observation is essential for advanced learning and social negotiation. The ability for self-observation emerges from the ability to observe one's self and another in a relationship, and is a product of the same emotional interactive relationships as earlier abilities. Similarly, advanced cognitive skills, involving working with numbers, reading, and analytic thinking, build on fundamental relationship-based capacities. For example, as relationships embrace symbolic capacities, language flowers with words, sentences, and concepts derived from daily affective experiences. Similarly, cognitive capacities involving time and space emerge out of the day-to-day negotiation of waiting or not waiting, or of having a little more or less of this or that. Even reading comprehension abilities blossom from the natural ebb and flow of dialogue with parents. The child can only understand the meaning of the words or pictures in a book in the context of his daily real emotional experiences with others. Without emotional experience to abstract from, there would be no symbolic meaning.

To support the child's ability to relate requires lots of time, consistency and understanding. Family difficulties or frequent turnovers among child care staff or teachers may compromise the requirement for consistency in a child who is just learning how to relate to others.

Developmentally Appropriate Practices and Interactions: Interventions Based on Individual Differences and Functional Developmental Capacities

At the third level of our pyramid lie consistent relationships and interactions that have been adapted to the individual differences and functional developmental needs of each child, which can be thought of as *developmentally appropriate practices and interactions* for the child with special needs.

In terms of processing differences, caregivers need to learn a variety of strategies, including wooing the low-tone, under-responsive child; protecting and soothing the over-responsive, easily fragmented child; and slowing down and making auditory communication more deliberate and visuospatial communication more clear to a child with severe auditory processing difficulties.

In terms of functional developmental levels, relationships and the emotional interactions which flow from them need to be geared to the current level of the child as a starting point for mobilizing growth. Children vary—some are unrelated and unpurposeful and require work on engaging and intentional communication, while others are purposeful but require extra help in using symbols. Still others are using symbols or ideas in a fragmented way and need to learn how to be logical and more abstract. For each developmental level, special types of interactions help a child to master that level and its related capacities.

Developmentally appropriate practices must characterize family and all interactions including home and educational programs. They should also be integrated into the different therapies. Developmentally appropriate interactions and practices, however, are not always easy for caregivers, educators, and therapists to make available. The child's tendency for self-absorption, perseveration, self-stimulation, impulsive actions, and/or avoidance often elicits counter-reactions which attempt to alter the immediate behavior rather than build interactions that both promote growth and alter the immediate behavior.

Children who do not have special needs often involve themselves in what the National Association of Education for Young Children has described as developmentally appropriate practices–playing on their own (part of the time) or with peers, siblings, or parents interactively with developmentally appropriate toys, games, puzzles, etc. in a constructive, growth-facilitating manner. The challenge is to help children with special needs, who because of their processing difficulties may find it very hard to interact with people or toys in a way that facilitates their development, become involved in their own special types of developmentally appropriate practices and interactions.

How can we construct developmentally appropriate interactions and practices for the child with special needs throughout his day? Such practices for the child with special needs involves using the profile of the child's functional developmental level, individual differences in regulatory-sensory processing, sensory modulation, motor planning and sequencing, and caregiver and family interaction patterns to construct interactions that will be pleasurable, and developmentally meaningful and facilitating.

For example, a 4-year-old may only have intermittent functional capacities of a two-year-old and understand visuospatial experiences more than auditory ones, and be over-responsive to sensations. The focus, therefore, involves working on engaging, gesturing, and the very beginning of elaborating symbols with lots of visual support and with pretend play in the context of being very soothing and regulating.

Developmentally Appropriate Interactions and Practices in the Home-Based Component of the Intervention Program

In developing intervention programs for children, we tend to underestimate the importance of family and other relationships as a vehicle for learning. Children spend many hours at home. When there are severe processing difficulties, activities chosen by the child may not be developmentally appropriate or facilitating. This includes hours of TV watching, perseverative behavior, repetitive computer games, and the like. Children generally are happier, more productive, less stressed, and make more progress when involved in developmentally appropriate interactions and practices. In fact, these interactions at home can become the most important factor in their growth.

Developmentally appropriate practices at home often require one-on-one work with the child. Parents must decide how much they can do on their own and how much to elicit from the help of volunteers, hired students or others, or, as is available in some states, home visitors through community, state, or county-supported intervention programs (e.g., wrap-around services in the state of Pennsylvania provide a very useful model where bachelor's and master's level professionals often spend over 20 hours a week supporting the program at home).

The home-based component of developmentally appropriate interactions and practices can be divided into two parts. One involves developmentally appropriate interactions based on following the child's natural interests and emotional inclinations. The other focuses on semi-structured problem-solving interactions which also harness the child's affect, but involve semi-structured created situations to facilitate mastery of specific processing capacities, emotional and cognitive, and language and motor skills. These two components of the home-based program are described below.

1. Developmentally Appropriate Practices Based on Following the Child's Natural Interests and Lead in Order to Mobilize Attention, Engagement, Interaction, Communication, and Thinking

The caregiver follows the child's emotional interests to engage with him at his functional developmental level and challenge him to move to the next level—gradually attempting to negotiate the six levels outlined earlier. For example, the caregiver hands the child a block to help him build a tower or jumps with him to turn a self-stimulatory activity into a dance. If the child is very perseverative, opening and closing doors, for example, the caregiver gets "stuck" behind the door. This leads to the child focusing on the caregiver as he's trying to push her away from the door, giggling as he succeeds only to have the caregiver run back to the door again to resume the game. In this way, focus and engagement may be facilitated. As the child purposefully tries to engineer moving the caregiver away from the door, intentional, two-way communication is facilitated. Eventually, complex problem-solving behaviors and even the use of words, such as "go" or "away" can be elaborated from the child's spontaneous, emotional interest in the door.

These spontaneous interactions in which one follows the child's lead often take on two qualities. First, parents and other caregivers help the child move in the direction that interests him, for example, putting the ball on their heads. The child may then take the ball off the caregiver's head, being drawn into focusing on the caregiver, engaging in pleasurable relating and purposeful, two-way communication. Second, the parents or other caregivers can become playfully obstructive, as described above, getting "stuck" behind the door. The strategies for the spontaneous use of developmentally appropriate interactions to help the child master each of the six necessary core functional emotional capacities is described in detail in the ICDL *Clinical Practice Guidelines* in the chapter on developmentally appropriate practices.

2. Developmentally Appropriate Practices Based on Problem-Solving Interactions

Another aspect of developmentally appropriate practices at home involves semi-structured problem-solving activities. The caregiver creates learning challenges for the child to master. These may involve social, motor, sensory, spatial reasoning, language, and additional cognitive skills. For example, if the goal were to help a child learn a new word, such as "open," we would put the child's favorite toy outside the door so he would want to open the door and then help him imitate the word "open." The child, in this way, is practicing gesturing, preverbal problem-solving. Semi-structured learning situations can include learning imitative skills, new words and concepts, motor planning and sequencing, as well as spatial reasoning. The child is also, at the same time, practicing focusing, engaging, and imitating words in a functional problem-solving context. Imitating the sounds ("ope" for "open," for example) while opening the door provides the child with immediate meaning. *Tying the word to affect (and meaning) facilitates generalization, in comparison to, for example, the child's saying the word "open" cued by a picture card and later trying to use it in real life in a functional way.*

An important component of the semi-structured problem-solving interactions is activities that enable the child to engage in (1) sensory modulation and motor planning exercises, such as jumping (on a trampoline or mattress), running, spinning, appropriate roughhousing with deep tactile pressure, and obstacle courses; (2) perceptual-motor exercises, looking and doing games, such as throwing and catching a big Nerf ball, kicking, reaching for moving objects; and (3) visuospatial exercises, such as treasure hunt games, hide and seek, and building complex structures from visual cues.

In general, it is most effective for the child's therapeutic team, including parents, educators, speech pathologists and occupational therapists, to meet weekly to design the functional goals for the semi-structured aspect of developmentally appropriate practices at home. At least a third to half the child's available time at home should be spent on spontaneous interactions (following the child's lead and working off of natural affect and inclination to foster the six functional levels described earlier) and the remaining half to two-thirds divided between developmentally appropriate semi-structured problem-solving activities.

Semi-structured problem-solving activities also need to be geared to each child's unique profile. When put into a problem-solving context with emotional intent, however, the following types of activities often have a place in this aspect of the program.

- Imitating new words and using concepts that help the child solve a problem he wants to solve (e.g., "open," "up there," "go," etc.)

- Motor-based challenges–gross motor movement, balance, movement in space, running, jumping, spinning, perceptual motor activities (involving looking and doing and crossing the midline)

- Spatial problem-solving, for example, treasure hunt games, where the child is given clues about how to find his favorite toy, first in the box in front of him and eventually in the box upstairs near another box behind the blue chair

- Motor imitation exercises (such as touching eyes, ears, nose) and eventually vocal (sound) imitations leading and then words

- Spatial and quantity concepts, such as "here," there," "big," "little," and including, eventually "more" or "less," and numbers, time, or distance, associated (e.g., finding Mommy in different parts of the house or negotiating one versus three cookies or showing with hands the difference between a little and a lot)

- As a child becomes ready for recognizing letters and words, conceptual understanding can be facilitated through semi-structured learning opportunities, where the word is under the picture and is used get the juice or a favorite toy, or as a cue for pretending what the word or sentence conveys

- As the child becomes older, visualization exercises can be added, where the child pictures in his mind words, sentences, or quantities (2 + 2 = 4) to facilitate a deeper conceptual understanding of concepts. These concepts may be acted out (dramatized) as well

Specific therapies often work in a semi-structured manner on these types of important capacities. Team meetings should suggest the goals of this part of the home program.

Peer Interaction

As part of developmentally appropriate practices at home it is also important for children to practice interactions with peers. Peer play is especially important once the child masters preverbal problem-solving skills and is moving into the early stages of using ideas in a functional and spontaneous manner. The now-engaged, intentional, partially-verbal, and imaginative child needs to practice his emerging skills not only with adults but with other children at a similar or higher developmental age (i.e., the other children need to be interactive, somewhat verbal and imaginative). However, the playmates need not be the same age as the child. For example, if the child is four and a half years old, but with a functional emotional developmental capacity of three years, he might enjoy the company (and vice versa) of three-year-olds, who may be closer to his functional developmental capacities.

At this point, individual one-on-one play dates should occur four or more times a week for one hour or more. Initially, an adult may have to facilitate the interactions; as the children may drift into parallel play. The adult may create a game where the children will work together, such as making something or having both children hide together while the adult tries to find them. While the caretaker follows the children's lead, he is also free to create games that facilitate interactions among the children. The goal is to help them to rub shoulders with each other, communicate with gestures and words.

The need for peer play occurs at about the same time that it is essential for children to be integrated, often with an aide, into a regular preschool program or to be part of an ongoing inclusion or integrated program.

SPECIFIC THERAPIES AND EDUCATIONAL STRATEGIES

At the apex of the pyramid are specific therapeutic or educational techniques to overcome particular challenges. These strategies, however, must build on and also facilitate the basic capacities for attention, engagement, intentional two-way communication, and the creative use of symbols. In this way, new capacities are tied to the child's sense of purpose and self (i.e., his affects). Integrating therapeutic strategies into the child's naturally-occurring interests and activities can be very helpful in simultaneously fostering his capacities to initiate, engage, communicate, problem-solve, and think, as well as learn new functional skills. As new skills are on the ascendancy, perhaps related to maturational shifts, it is an optimal time to intensify a particular therapy that supports that skill, such as physical therapy to facilitate walking.

A variety of strategies have been advocated. Some attempt to offer a comprehensive approach while others focus on specific issues. However, an approach cannot be truly comprehensive unless it works with all the levels of the pyramid. Both focused and partially comprehensive approaches must build on the foundation described above. These include educational approaches (e.g., Bailey & Wolery, 1992), cognitive, language, sensory, and motor processing approaches (e.g., Prizant & Wetherby, 1988; Bricker, 1993), peer models (Odom & Strain, 1986; Strain, et al., 1977), behavioral approaches (Lovaas, 1980, 1987; Durand, et al., 1993; Haring & Lovinger, 1989; Odom & Haring, 1993), work with family patterns (e.g., Barber, et al., 1988; Bronfenbrenner, 1986; Dunst & Trivette, 1988; Powell, et. al., 1992; Robbins, et al., 1991; Turnbull, et al., 1986), interactive Floortime dynamics (Greenspan, 1992), and the social milieu (e.g., Ostrosky, et al., 1993; Wolfberg & Schuler 1993).

Speech and Language Therapy

Speech and language therapy is especially helpful for preverbal, as well as all types of symbolic, communication (verbal, pictures, signs, etc.). It can also be especially valuable for oral-motor work and related expressive language. Three or more individual sessions per week of 30 to 60 minutes each is often required, in addition to consultation to and integration in the home and educational program. Many programs do not provide an adequate level of intensity.

Occupational and/or Physical Therapy

Occupational and/or physical therapy is especially helpful for motor problems, motor planning and sequencing difficulties and sensory modulation and processing challenges (e.g., over- or under-responsiveness to sensation). Two to three individual sessions per week of 30 to 60 minutes each are often required, in addition to consultation to and integration in the home and school programs. Many programs do not provide an adequate level of intensity.

There is often confusion between very helpful clinical strategies to foster sensory modulation, muscle tone, and motor planning and debates about the explanatory value of sensory integration theory. Like all broad theories, time and continuing research are needed for further refinement of sensory integration theory. In the meantime, clinical techniques that enable children to master functional developmental capacities should be employed based on their clinical usefulness.

Educational Program

An educational program should be geared to a child's functional developmental capacities and processing profile and must involve developmentally appropriate practices for children with special needs. For example, some programs attempt to have a child learn in a group when his or her profile is quite unique and requires a highly individualized approach. Often, only after children have advanced to the point of mastering individual relationships, preverbal problem-solving interactions and are already beginning to use their words are they able to learn in groups. Nonetheless, school settings with other children can be a very enriching environment, even if initially most of the work is happening on an individual basis. Gradually, learning can move more towards group interactions.

A child who is not yet engaged or purposeful needs to be involved in one-on-one interactions with a teacher, aide, or volunteer throughout most of the school day. The aide's role is not to sit behind the child or help the child conform to non-interactive routines, but rather to woo the child into learning interactions (i.e., two-way purposeful interactions and a constant flow of back and forth communication). Once a child progresses to purposeful gestural communication, complex imitation and, over time, to using symbols (e.g., words, pictures, signs, etc.) and is able to relate to and communicate logically with peers, two-way symbolic interactions need to be facilitated to promote logical thinking. As children become more logical and abstract, learning in groups and routine academic activities can provide constructive learning opportunities (but this stage is the culmination of a long learning process).

Many programs, however, find it especially challenging to provide the needed one-on-one interaction (for most of the school day) required by the child who has not yet fully learned to engage with peers and adults or communicate and problem-solve with gestures.

In addition, education for children with special needs can take many forms. Often, goals are derived from academic objectives of older children. When this occurs, there is often little attention to the sequence by which young children acquire the core functional abilities that enable them to relate, communicate, think, and learn (including mastering traditional academic tasks). Typically, for example, there is over-focus on compliance in a group situation before a child has learned to negotiate one-on-one relationships or even understand simple expectations. A child is taught in a rote manner to match shapes before he can engage in basic multi-step preverbal problem-solving interaction sequences, such as getting a toy out of a box, bringing it over, and motioning for us to play.

The child who is already attentive, engaged, purposefully interactive, involved in complex ongoing preverbal problem-solving communication (e.g., gesturing), and is beginning to use words, presents special opportunities. He needs to learn to elaborate and build bridges between ideas in a variety of contexts. To meet this goal, this child requires opportunities to interact with peers (one-on-one and in small groups) who are related, interactive, and verbal (often with an adult mediating). He requires an integrated setting or an aide in a mainstream setting.

It is important to emphasize that educational programs for a child with special needs should not be comprised of a series of disconnected cognitive learning opportunities. The important academic goals stated above do not emerge as isolated cognitive skills by simply practicing them. Having a child sit and look does not mean he understands or that he can learn from listening. Nor does having a child memorize a passage mean he understands it. These skills are part of a progression where each step builds on another. Comprehension, relating, communicating, and reading, math, writing, and engaging in high-level problem-solving must build on the six functional capacities described earlier. Education programs should identify where each child is on his or her unique progression, meet the child at his or her level, and work on the next steps. *Only this type of logical progression constitutes developmentally appropriate practices for a child in school.*

For example, to read with meaning or to understand math, a child must learn how to:

1. Want to attend and engage with others (first one person at a time and then a few) in order to be part of experiences that enable him to discriminate sounds and sights necessary for reading and math and eventually give words and quantity concepts meaning

2. Communicate logically with simple gestures and affect cues and then complex problem-solving behaviors in order to understand cause and effect, logic and patterns, both essential for any type of academic work

3. Represent or symbolize emotional experiences and build logical bridges between them so that what she knows from preverbal experience as well as new verbal experience can be understood and communicated and thought about logically with words, pictures, or other symbols (necessary for creative and logical thought, abstract thinking, and all academic tasks requiring the comprehension of words and reasoning with symbols)

In addition to difficulties in providing one-on-one interaction, most educational programs, due to administrative practice, change intervention teams for a child and his/her family when the child is three years old. For a child with autistic patterns who is learning to relate to and trust others, sudden change can undermine educational progress. Continuity of staff and program is needed during the infancy and preschool years.

Developing the most appropriate educational program for children with special needs is extremely challenging. We, therefore, must bring in more aides, or better yet, allow parents to volunteer, like in cooperative preschools, and increase one-on-one learning opportunities that enable children to climb the developmental ladder and eventually learn and communicate in groups.

Educational Programs for Learning and Attention Problems

Children who progress and master their basic challenges in relating and communication (as well as children who present with these skills already mastered), but have problems with attention and/or learning require an educational program that provides opportunities to resolve specific processing challenges and progress to high levels of abstract thinking and academic proficiency. Promising techniques to strengthen processing capacities such as visuospatial, auditory, and motor planning are being developed and are available in innovative schools and programs, but are not yet sufficiently available in all education and special education programs.

In addition, many intelligent children with moderate to severe circumscribed learning and/or attention problems who are fully capable of being mainstreamed often require both participation in regular classes and one-on-one and very small group (two to four children) learning opportunities to master specific processing challenges. Many require special learning opportunities for as much as half their day, where they can work on their processing challenges with the most up-to-date techniques. At present, unfortunately, many children with learning and attention problems do not get the adequate time or techniques they require.

As part of the home-based, semi-structured learning and educational programs are a number of innovative programs that focus on cognitive development, visuospatial thinking, perceptual motor development, and motor planning.

Exploration of Biomedical Interventions

Selected children with special needs benefit from biomedical interventions, including the use of medications. For example, medications, such as Prozac and others in the Selective Serotonin Reuptake Inhibitor group, may facilitate motor planning, sequencing, and attention, and reduce perseverative or repetitive behavior. In order to determine if a biomedical intervention should be a part of the therapeutic regimen, a basic biomedical assessment needs to be implemented. For example, an extended sleep EEG can often detect subtle differences in EEG patterns which may indicate the usefulness of a trial of one of the anti-seizure medications such as Depakote.

In exploring a trial of medication, it is essential to look carefully at the side effects and weigh the benefits and risks. Medications are not designed as precisely as we would wish and often affect non-targeted areas. In addition, exceptional caution and close monitoring is required if more than one medication at a time is being considered.

Consultation with Developmental Specialists Who Focus on Interactions with Child, Caregiver, and Family Patterns

In addition to conducting the initial diagnostic evaluation and monitoring progress, developmental specialists (e.g., psychologist, behavioral or developmental pediatrician, child psychiatrist) may be helpful in facilitating (e.g., coaching) developmentally appropriate interactions at home and/or school and working with the family. This consultation can take a number of forms. For some families, the form is regular meetings ranging from one or more times a week to once every one to six months, working with the parents and other caregivers on their interactions with the child, and, if needed, direct work with the child. Consultations may also involve periodic home visits. In addition, intensive family work with supports and coordination from community agencies will be necessary for some families. The form the consultation takes vary depending on the needs of the child and the family (see Greenspan, 1992 for detailed discussion).

SPECIFIC CLINICAL TECHNIQUES

Specific clinical techniques to deal with difficult symptoms or behaviors are often needed as part of an overall program. Perseveration, self-stimulation, avoidance of eye contact, and aggression or impulsivity are typical challenges. There are two broad philosophies that tend to guide parents, educators, and clinicians.

The more behavioral philosophy attempts to decrease the target behavior directly by ignoring it and/or with negative consequences, as well as attempting to replace it with another behavior supported by positive consequences (e.g., interrupting perseverative behavior and insisting on and reinforcing another activity).

The more functional, developmental philosophy attempts to understand the broad category of functioning that the worrisome behavior is part of, the broad functional category that may be missing. "Functional" in this context means a broad developmental capacity essential for the child's progress, such as purposeful gesturing or using ideas. It does not refer to a narrow functional behavior, like dressing. Developmentally appropriate interactions and practices are used to help the child master new functional capacities. For example, opening and closing a door is part of the larger category of repetitive and rigid ways of dealing with the world. The missing functional category is the developmentally more advanced capacity for flexible, creative interactions in the world. In this model, the worrisome, repetitive behavior serves as a window of opportunity for progressing to higher functional developmental levels of flexible, creative interactions. A perseverative behavior, like opening and closing a door is turned into a purposeful interaction. The clinician may get stuck behind the door and playfully entice the child to push or pull the clinician away or say, "GO." If successful, the aimless, repetitive behavior becomes purposeful, creative, and interactive, and more importantly, the child becomes more engaged, interactive, and problem-solving.

We recommend the functional developmental philosophy because it keeps the larger therapeutic goal of higher level functional capacities in the forefront. For example, simply directing a child from the door to a toy may or may not promote interaction. Using the child's interest in the door to get a peek-a-boo game going often leads to gleeful interactions. At times, both philosophies can be used in an integrated manner. For example, the child's self-injurious behavior is interrupted, but the child is simultaneously drawn into interactions that serve a similar sensory need, such as deep tactile pressure coupled with warm engagement and two-way intentional communication. The functional developmental approach guides the clinician to entice the child toward behaviors that are part of a needed new developmental capacity, rather than just an alternative behavior, such as being compliant.

Setting Limits and Meeting Clinical and Educational Goals

Developmentally appropriate practices used to foster new functional capacities can help parents, clinicians, and special education programs with one of their most difficult challenges—how to integrate the process of following limits and compliance with other clinical and educational goals. Following rules and maintaining safety are understandable goals. Not infrequently, however, the need for compliance and control takes the form of strapping a child into a chair, physically forcing him to walk to the bathroom, or other types of restraint.

The key to teaching a child to follow rules is the basic principle of providing developmentally appropriate practices and interactions (i.e., meeting the child at his or her functional developmental level in the context of his or her individual differences). For example, for a child who is impulsive and is not yet capable of logical, verbal thinking and conversation, developmentally appropriate interactions mean a one-on-one aide working with the child on the basics as relating and purposeful interaction. The back-and-forth signaling, which includes limits, however, is of the type one would implement with a one- to two-year-old child. Through this type of one-on-one interaction, the child gradually learns how to be a purposeful, preverbal communicator. Gradually, responding to limits becomes a part of this purposeful communication. Expecting a child who can not yet negotiate basic needs with a series of back and forth signals to follow group-oriented rules often results in frustration, anger, impulsive behavior, and, more importantly, slower progress.

Developmentally appropriate practices are more likely to tap into potential plasticity from within the individual child's own brain than externally-imposed structured techniques (i.e., too complex or restrictive) that bypass neural networks already in place.

As a child makes progress and is purposefully interactive, both encouragement and sensitive limits can help him work with groups of children and follow expectations. Dangerous, as opposed to non-compliant, behavior needs to be dealt with immediately with firm but gentle limits. These should be based on the child's functional developmental capacities, not actual age or expectations for the other children in a group. Just as we are appropriately mandated to provide each child with the least restrictive environment, we should use the *least restrictive, developmentally appropriate* tactics to teach each child to control his behavior and be sensitive to the needs of others.

Family Support and Dynamic Family Processes

In addition to being at the base of the intervention pyramid, often special clinical techniques are needed to support families. There is a long tradition of family-based programs for children with special needs, yet many programs only offer minimal help to the whole family, including siblings. Marital conflicts, misperceptions of the special needs child or siblings, and higher levels of stress can characterize families' functioning. It is also difficult for families to orchestrate an entire intervention program. Often, various levels of support are needed.

BRIEF SUMMARY OF RESEARCH ON THE DIR/FLOORTIME MODEL[2]

The DIR/Floortime model is based on a number of areas of research. The conceptual framework is supported by a large number of studies documenting the role of each of the elements of the DIR/Floortime model for healthy and disordered development. These elements include the functional emotional developmental capacities (D), individual motor and sensory processing and language differences (I), and relationship patterns—caregiver, child and family (R) (Greenspan, 1992; Greenspan & Shanker, 2004; Interdisciplinary Council on Developmental and Learning Disorders Clinical Practice Guidelines Workgroup, 2000; Shonkoff & Phillips, 2000; also see the section on Regulatory-Sensory Processing Disorders in this manual (ICDL-DMIC).

The cornerstones of the DIR/Floortime model—the functional emotional developmental capacitates and the individual processing differences—are further supported by a recent study on a representative population of infants and children conducted by the Psychological Corporation as part of their field trials of the newly revised Bayley Infant Assessment scales. The functional emotional developmental capacities and individual processing differences are included in the new Bayley kit and is also available as a separate instrument (i.e., The Greenspan Social Emotional Growth Chart). The study found that the functional emotional developmental capacities occurred at the predicted ages and discriminated children developing normally from those with developmental and emotional disorders. Individual processing differences also discriminated between children developing normally and those with disorders. The disorders included Down Syndrome, Pervasive Developmental Disorder, At-Risk Populations, Asphyxia, Cerebral Palsy, Fetal Alcohol Exposure, Language Impairment, Prematurity/Low Birth Weight, and Small for Gestational Age.

In addition, there were strong correlations between the early functional emotional developmental capacities (presymbolic capacities) and higher level (symbolic capacities) as hypothesized in the DIR/Floortime model.

Interventions focusing on each of the components of the DIR/Floortime model have been shown to improve outcomes for children with autism spectrum disorder (ASD) and other special needs conditions. These include interventions for social-emotional functioning, language capacities, motor and sensory processing differences, and family patterns (Tsakiris, 2000).

[2] See http://www.icdl.com for an article on Research Support for DIR Model.

In a chart review of 200 children receiving a comprehensive DIR/Floortime intervention approach, the children evidenced significant gains in the areas of functioning most undermined in autism spectrum disorders—relating, communicating, and thinking (Greenspan & Wieder, 1997) (a more definitive clinical trial outcome study is being planned). Over 50% of the children in the 200 cases reviewed evidenced gains in creative and reflective thinking, empathy (theory of mind), reading and responding to social cues, and social relationships thought to be beyond the reach of children with ASD. An in-depth study of 20 of these children demonstrated that they were indistinguishable from age-matched peers (with no history of developmental challenges) on assessments of emotional functioning using the Functional Emotional Assessment Scale (Greenspan, DeGangi, & Wieder, 2001) and the Vineland Adaptive Scales (Sparrow, Balla, & Cicchetti, 1984). A recent follow-up of sixteen of these children ten to fifteen years after the initiation of their DIR/Floortime intervention program demonstrated that these gains have continued significantly after the formal intervention programs were completed. All sixteen were functioning well in challenging mainstream academic programs and enjoying friendships. While a few of the children were evidencing expectable levels of anxiety and depression, none were evidencing autism spectrum symptoms or patterns.

In a recent community-based application of the DIR/Floortime approach with community agencies delivering the DIR/Floortime services free of charge to families—the Michigan PLAY Project—gains were demonstrated in relating, communicating, and thinking, along with a reduction ASD symptoms (Solomon, Necheles, Ferch, & Bruckman, 2003). In addition, research on other developmental models (as compared to behavioral models) has demonstrated positive gains in social, language, and cognitive functioning in children with ASD (Rogers, Hall, Osaki, Reaven, & Herbison, 2000).

The National Academy of Sciences, in their report on interventions for autism spectrum disorders (Committee on Educational Interventions for Children with Autism, 2001), cited the DIR/Floortime model as one of the models with some evidence supporting it. The Academy emphasized that, at present, no intervention model, including behavioral models, had definitive clinical trial research support. The only clinical trial study of intensive ABA-Discrete Trial behavioral approaches for children with ASD showed only modest educational gains and no emotional and social differences (Smith, Groen, & Wynn, 2000). The National Academy of Sciences emphasized the need for comparative clinical trial intervention research on the most widely used approaches, such as the DIR/Floortime developmental model and the behavioral models. They also stressed the importance of tailoring the intervention approach to the child's unique developmental profile.

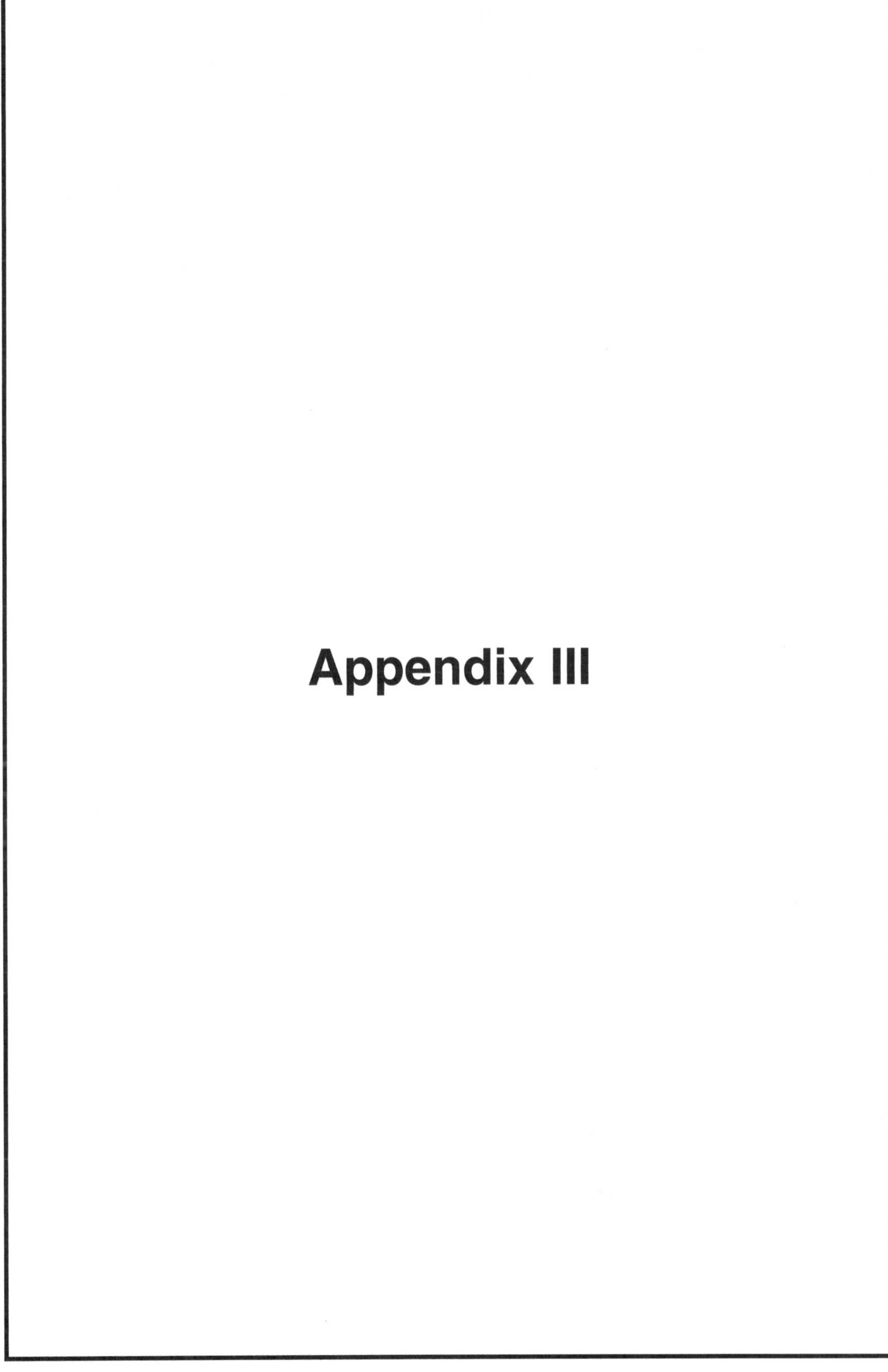

Appendix III

Guide for Observations During Clinical Evaluation of Regulatory-Sensory Processing Disorders: Version 1.0

Miller L.J., Lane S.J., Cermak S., Anzalone M., Osten E., and Greenspan S..: March, 2005

INTRODUCTION

Purpose of this Guide

The *Guide for Clinical Observation of Regulatory Sensory Processing Disorders* is designed to provide clinicians with suggestions for observing children for signs and symptoms of Regulatory-Sensory Processing Disorders (RSPD). To be designated as a disorder, symptoms must impact significantly on daily living abilities, otherwise they are associated or correlated symptoms and do not constitute a disorder.

As with all clinical guides, supplementing these observations with caregiver interview including developmental history and/or other screening or standardized evaluation tools is recommended to validate findings and interpret behaviors observed.

This guide has been designed to accompany the definitions of RSPD found in Axis I: Regulatory-Sensory Processing Disorders in the *Interdisciplinary Council on Developmental and Learning Disorders Diagnostic Manual for Infancy and Early Childhood* (ICDL-DMIC). It focuses on the major areas of sensory processing challenges that contribute to the specific RSPDs. This observation guide is revised as it is used by clinicians over time.

Related Developmental Sensory Principles

As the observations take place, it is important to keep some principles of sensory functioning in mind. First, sensory functions can be influenced by developmental level. Younger children typically show less ability to independently self-regulate (e.g., they may at times demonstrate wide emotional swings, such as going from contentment to temper tantrums). Further, with very young children, behavior is often generalized to the whole child; thus, it is often not feasible to distinguish between functioning of the various sensory systems. Throughout the observation, it is essential that clinicians are aware of age-appropriate behavior so that differences in the child being observed from behaviors expected by children who are typically developing can be identified. The large range of normal individual differences from a developmental perspective must be considered before labeling a child as dysfunctional in sensory and/or regulatory functioning.

A second consideration is the observation environment (e.g., physical and social context), and the child's expected behavior within any given environment. A potentially sensory-seeking child may appear a little rambunctious if observed on a playground, but when observed in a quiet office space, the need for sensation may be played out very differently. Likewise, a child avoidant of sensory stimuli may not demonstrate overly problematic behavior in the confines of an office with only the clinician and caregiver present, but observed in the classroom or on the playground, this child's withdrawal/ behavior (or aggressive responses) are more apparent.

Third, responses to sensory stimuli are also influenced by who is creating the stimulus (e.g., the clinician or the caregiver), as well as the child's arousal state (e.g., what has happened in the child's day prior to the observation period and the child's reaction to the evaluation session). Verifying behavioral observations by asking caregivers whether the behavior you see is typical helps to address this variability. Emotional and physiologic states affect sensory responsivity, so if a child is stressed, tired, hungry, angry, etc. when he comes to the evaluation, his symptoms may appear to be RSPD. However, you may, in fact, be seeing evidence of an emotional or physiologic state not representative of this child's behavior in general.

The Nature of the Test Session

During an observation, every effort should be made to design activities that are really **fun** for the child. This entails knowledge of typical development, and some knowledge of what this particular child enjoys doing. In addition, it is crucial to establish a positive relationship with the child and engage him in play. Efforts made by the clinician to design both a welcoming and a fun environment for the child create an optimal perspective on the child's ability to process sensory stimuli from the environment.

Each characteristic intended for evaluation should be tested within the context of a play-based approach. The availability of specialized equipment such as that found in a typical occupational therapy intervention facility is extremely helpful, but is not required. What is required is a playful interaction with the child, reliance on parent participation (especially with young children), and an interview with the caretaker regarding whether what you are observing is typical. As with other assessments, the observer should look for a collection of behaviors indicative of a problem, not a single behavior.

RSPD as a Diagnosis

This guide can be used to diagnose RSPD as a primary diagnosis, or to identify associated RSP symptoms in children with other primary diagnoses. In using the guide for diagnostic assessment, the clinician should carefully consider the limits of the tool. This tool is not designed to differentiate RSPD from autism or any other disability. It is only designed to determine if the child has symptoms of RSPD. Other, broader diagnoses, if present, should be considered primary and RSPD used as a diagnosis only if other broader diagnoses do not fit. Thus, in the absence of another primary diagnosis, one of the classic patterns of RSPD may become a primary diagnosis.

This guide can also be used as a supplement to standardized evaluations tools, for identification of regulatory-sensory processing as a disorder, or identification of associated symptoms of regulatory and sensory processing problems if the child has another diagnosis. The observation of these problems should, when possible, be a part of a comprehensive multidisciplinary evaluation, so that the potential role regulatory and sensory processing difficulties play in the overall diagnosis of the child can be determined.

Qualifications Needed to Diagnose RSPD

Diagnosis of RSPD should only be made by an expert clinician with advanced knowledge and training in regulation and sensory processing. Entry-level education plus specialized courses in regulation or sensory processing and/or an extensive mentored experience working with children with similar difficulties are required to be qualified to make a diagnosis of RSPD. In general, professionals with the training to diagnose this disorder are occupational therapists, child psychiatrists, some physical therapists, some psychologists, and a few other interventionists with specialized training.

Age of Detection

A diagnosis of RSPD is often made in early childhood, but can also be made at later ages, including adulthood. Developmental differences exist in the manifestation of RSPD with maturation. Many of the observations described below target the infant-toddler-preschool aged child and may be applicable to older children with developmental disabilities. The symptoms below may also apply to older children, but the toys/objects used to stimulate the response must vary with age.

As children get older they have increasing abilities to self-regulate in the presence of discomforting stimulation and the clinician must be attuned to subtle signs. Also, it is critical to avoid over-diagnosing RSPD. Not every child who is fussy or has temper tantrums has RSPD. Diagnosis depends on carefully considering the criteria provided below, determining that the cause of the dysregulation is sensory, and making sure that other diagnoses are first ruled out.

Psychometric Data

Currently no reliability and validity data exist on this suggested observational method, although authors intend to collect data in the future. Studies will evaluate the stability and validity of the observations suggested in this guide. These studies over time will illuminate the psychometric properties of this scale. In the absence of empirical data, observations based on this guide must be considered clinical. The overall clinical impression of the examiner is much more important in this scale than a score.

RSPD Patterns

There are three classic patterns of challenges that characterize RSPD and two of them include subtypes. The criteria for each primary pattern of challenges and subtype noted below should be carefully considered. Note that children commonly have more than one subtype. The sensory domains include the five well-known sensory domains (i.e., sound, sight, touch, smell and taste) plus vestibular and proprioceptive functioning, for a total of seven sensory domains.

INTRODUCTION TO THE ASSESSMENT PROCESS

This tool is designed to provide guidance for observation of, and caregiver queries about, regulation and sensory processing, particularly in young children. Clinicians are urged to direct their observation and caregiver questions toward the *quality* of the child's response, not the basic skills displayed. As with any assessment or observation, no clinical decisions should be based on performance on a single item (e.g., a young child may dislike having his face and hair washed, but this alone does not indicate Sensory Over-Responsivity to touch.) In addition, if at all possible, multiple observations in more than one setting are recommended to provide the most complete picture of the child. Useful information can be obtained observing the child in the waiting room, an office, on a playground, in a classroom, in a cafeteria, and/or in the home. Noting the interaction between caregiver and child in the waiting room or other environment can add additional information. Observations of sensory responsivity can also be made during administration of other standardized tests. Using information from a combination of contexts provides the most complete picture of sensory processing.

This guide is formatted to include brief descriptions of the sensory processing categories, general observation questions, and questions specific to discriminating classic patterns of challenges and subtypes. Suggested activities and/or materials clinicians may use to address the areas in the observation guide are noted on the record form with additional ideas in the Appendix. In working to answer the questions provided here, it is important that the examiner work at the pace of the child, and keep the assessment process child-directed, play-based, and flexible. Spontaneous play can and often does yield the richest information about sensory processing. If the child is reluctant to play or reluctant to engage with the examiner, the caregiver can be used to facilitate play and interaction. It is important to be able to observe both spontaneous play and adult-facilitated play to obtain the most complete picture of the child.

This observation guide is accompanied by a record form that facilitates the examiner's ability to administer each item. In addition, a summary table is provided to note overall clinical conclusions regarding each classic patterns of challenges and subtypes. The overall guide is rated with a Likert Scale and then a visual analogue scale. Sensory Responsivity in each category is first scored using a Likert score of:

4 = no indication, never or rarely a problem
3 = mild problem, or only occasionally a problem
2 = moderate problem, or frequently a problem
1 = severe problem, or almost always a problem

Thus the examiner determines first if there is a problem (scores of 1 or 2) or there is not a problem (scores of 3 or 4). Higher scores indicate better performance. Within each of the Likert scores is a visual analogue scale that allows the rater to indicate the extent to which that score reflects the child's sensory responsivity. Examiners consider where on the visual analogue line they would place the child's responsivity. The line has 10 dots, with the far left side indicating the child's responsivity is very strongly within this score, and the far right indicating that the child's responsivity may be edging toward more of a problem. Examiners should put a hatch mark "/ on the line where they feel the child's responsivity is best represented. (Each line has a midpoint period noted for reference.)

GUIDE FOR THE CLINICAL ASSESSMENT OF THE THREE CLASSIC RSPD PATTERNS

I. Pattern One: Sensory Modulation Challenges

The observations/questions below are designed to structure both clinical observations of the child and caregiver questions about aspects of functioning related to Sensory Modulation Challenges. This section is separated into content targeted at each of the three subtypes of sensory modulation dificulties: Sensory Under-Responsivity, Sensory Over-Responsivity, and Sensory Seeking.

Subtest 1. Sensory Over-Responsivity

General

- Is the child initially avoidant of specific sensory qualities associated with toys and play materials?
- Does the child avoid exploring the environment?
- Does the child have overt obvious signs of "fight, flight, or freeze" when presented with particular sensory stimuli?
- Does the child want to withdraw from or escape the toy or sensory input?
- Does the child have subtle signs of an aversive response such as irritability or wanting to do something else instead (e.g., get a drink, go to the bathroom)?

Visual Domain

- Do complex, moving, novel, flashing lights, and/or high intensity visual stimuli over-excite, anger, or overwhelm the child?
- Does the child seem to become overwhelmed or avoidant in visually cluttered spaces, e.g., waiting room? (The examiner can let toys build up in evaluation room and see how they respond.)
- Does the child wear sunglasses or caps all the time?

Tactile Domain

- Does the child have a consistent over-responsive pattern as in consistently pulls body part away when touched (e.g. shrugs shoulder, removes hand, pulls head away) to touch stimuli?
- Does child have discomfort with proximity of other people?
- Is the child particularly over-sensitive to certain types of clothing (e.g., labels, long/short sleeves, certain fabrics) or activities of daily living (e.g., hair washing, bathing)?
- Does child have an aversion to using soap and moving his hands around in hand washing?

Vestibular Domain

- Does the child avoid or become upset when put in certain positions (e.g., intolerance of prone or upside down)?
- Does the child seem fearful or upset when walking on uneven or not flat surfaces, (e.g., climbing up a slide)?
- Does the child seem uncomfortable or insecure when walking with others who may touch or push them?

Visceral Responses

- Do activities tend to make the child's "insides" feel bad (e.g., does the child get nauseated or throw up)?
- Does the child need to go to the bathroom frequently?
- Does the child's body go still or seem to shut down when he has an emotional reaction?
- Is affect in general seen in the body instead of in the face or verbalized (e.g., when the child is nervous or angry she/he seem to shut down, looking like responses well up inside body)?
- Does child have somatic symptoms indicating physiological over-reactivity, which may include irritable bowel syndrome, migraines, and constant stomach aches?

Subtest 2. Sensory Under-Responsivity

- Does the child attend or orient to salient stimuli?
- When the child is involved in play, does he/she still respond to name being called and other attempts to interact or is he/she overly absorbed?
- Does the child seem shut down instead of interacting with toys that are usually intriguing to his age group?
- Does the child pay too much attention to, or become overly focused on, certain stimuli such as blinking lights, moving wheels?
- Does the child try to investigate the object briefly, but can't seem to really engage with new toy?
- Is the child aware of or has appropriate responses to an obnoxious sounding toy such as a thunder spring? (Make the sound over and over and see if child indicates you should stop it.)
- Does the child orient to other sounds that children would orient to? (Make a tape of screeching tires, fire engine, etc., and see if child looks up when hearing these sounds while tape is playing)
- Does the child have a lack of awareness of bodily sensations (e.g. frequent accidents and delayed toilet training; not aware of being full or hungry; unaware of pain such as that associated with ear infection)?
- Does the child explore the environment without becoming so absorbed that he cannot be drawn back into play with the parent and/or examiner?

Subtest 3. Sensory Seeking

- Is the child immediately drawn to specific sensory qualities associated with toys, play materials, or the environment?
- Does the child seek high intensity of sensory input within an activity and appear unable to get enough input to feel satiated?
- Does the child crave high intensity input and resist moving on from the task, or resist increasing complexity of the task?
- Does the child seem unaware of potential danger or pain, or the consequences of his actions?
- As the child gets increasing sensory input, does he exhibit increasing impulsivity and behavioral disorganization?
- Do the child's responses tend to escalate as he becomes over-aroused, resulting in out of control behavior?

II. Pattern Two: Sensory Discrimination Challenges

Discrimination is different than modulation. Modulation is a screening, grading and regulating function, whereas discrimination is interpreting the stimulation. Discrimination requires higher level cognitive functions than modulation and is not automatic.

The following observations are aspects of functioning that you can observe or question related to Sensory Discrimination Challenges. All sensory systems are included below, first with observations/ questions that relate to children with all types of discrimination difficulties, followed by observations targeted specifically for each of the five discrimination subtypes: tactile, auditory, visual, taste/smell, vestibular/proprioceptive discrimination disorder. Please note that we have not attempted to comprehensively describe visual and auditory discrimination since they are covered elsewhere in this observational guide. Some examples of stimuli that may be used to administer these observations are provided in materials column of Record Form and in the Additional Materials section that follows.

General Observations

- Can the child differentiate similar types of objects with vision, with touch, by sound?
- Do children notice the salient aspects that differentiate one object from others (e.g., a circle from an oval or the word "cap from cab")?
- Can children translate information received through one sense into information received by another sense (e.g., haptic visual matching where they match a shape they feel, but don't see to a picture of the shape; match a picture of a train to a sound of a train)?
- Does the child investigate or seem aware of the specific characteristics and complexity of the way toys/objects feel?
- When more than one type of sensory stimuli is required for a task, does this seem to confuse or overwhelm the child and/or is he able to attend to only one of the types or modalities of stimuli at a time?

Auditory

- Does the child orient to sounds that most children orient to, both at the very loud and very soft end of the spectrum?
- Does the child orient to sharp, novel, dysrythmic sounds while engaged in another task such as coloring, sand or water play?
- Does the child discriminate his name from background noise (while child is engaged in task either use a taped version or use your voice: start with low volume and see how high you must raise the db level for the child to orient)?

Visual

- Does the child demonstrate a visual sensory processing challenge? (Differentiate visual sensory processing symptoms from both a motor problem and a visual-motor problem—which does the child have?

Note that many standardized tests are available to test motor free visual perception and visual motor functions: e.g., the Motor Free Visual Perception Test, the Beery Developmental Test of Visual Motor Integration, and others. We recommend using these when possible for standardized age comparisons.

The following aspects of visual perception and visual motor skills can be evaluated through standardized assessments as well as functional observations:

Figure Ground	Find a stimulus that can be separated from a background
Form and Space Perception	Find a form that fits in a specific space
Form Constancy	Know what an object is when it is seen from a rotated angle
Visual Discrimination	Match objects by specific criteria
Spatial Relations	See the distance between and among objects
Visual-Motor Integration	Reproduce shapes and forms using a pencil, crayon or pen; build with blocks and other skills that require use of the visual system and the fine motor system together
Motor Accuracy	Indicates the precision with which the child completes fine motor tasks requiring dexterous hand and arm movements

The following questions can guide your observation of visual perception as integrated into functional activities:

- Does the child enjoy and explore interesting, unusual, and novel visual stimuli?
- How far in his periphery of vision can child discriminate an object?
- Does the child get stuck in two-dimensional space (e.g. staring at picture book, TV screen, computer screen)? Look for perseverative behavior.
- Does the child have anticipatory visual skills?

- When you bring the child into a functional context – e.g., the OT room or playground, does the child notice objects in that space? (The child may look everywhere but not really "tune in" to anything or they may shut down and not orient to anything.)
- Does the child notice details in the environment, such as the presence of an obstacle in his or her pathway?
- Can the child sort out a specific figure from a background?
- Is the child able to shift visual attention (e.g., near to far, different targets around room)?
- Does the child visually reference (e.g., look at) the speaker in a conversation?
- Can the child visually organize stimuli (e.g., can he go into a room full of toys and selectively go to point A or point B or selectively find a certain object)?
- Can the child maintain eye contact or joint attention when moving?

Vestibular

- Can the child tell if he is up off the floor (e.g., when placed into loft, onto ladder, rope, standing on child-size chair)?
- Can the child feel where he is moving in space (e.g., differentiate falling forward from falling backward)?
- Does the child have such poor discrimination of movement through space that safety issues are a concern?
- Can the child discriminate movement of the body with eyes closed?
- Does the child change planes of movement in play (e.g., roll, somersault, look under things with head tipped down, etc.)?
- When the child receives vestibular stimulation, how does it influence his muscle control? Does she evidence appropriate postural and balance reactions (e.g., reactions on a swing set or moving equipment in OT room)?

Tactile/Kinesthetic

- Does the child show different exploratory patterns for different object tactile properties e.g., shape/contour, hardness, textures?
- Can the child identify objects in hand without seeing the object (stereognosis)?
- Can the child identify a finger lightly touching without watching where you touch them (finger localization, or gnosis)?
- Is the child aware of where her body is touched, specifically the localization of touch, (e.g., if he gets a scrape or cut, can he localize where the pain is)?
- Can the child tell the difference between hot water bottle with cold and hot water in it?
- Does child notice placement of socks and shoes? Does he notice when his socks slide down and is not overly aware of every little seam, but is aware if his socks are not on correctly or his shoe is on wrong foot)?
- Is child aware of hair care or notice when hair is uncombed and try to fix it?
- Does child seem aware of all fingers and thumbs (e.g., can he or she put all five fingers into gloves; can she or he isolate finger movements: play piano keys or play finger games like "Itsy Bitsy Spider")?

Olfactory and Gustatory

These behaviors are better studied in home kitchen and cafeteria than through standardized testing. However, examiners can use a contact lens case to hold cotton balls with smells on them and test in the clinic that way. In addition to real foods and smells you can look at:

- Can the child discriminate basic smells?
- Does the child have a preference for spicy foods?
- Does the child feel any unusual sensation with odd foods such as Pop Rocks, Sour Spray, and War Heads?
- Does the child refuse any foods? If so, could it be because of the texture?

Proprioceptive

- Is the child able to investigate objects with hand manipulation adjusting to the qualities of the materials? For example, does he know how to explore objects moving from palm to finger tips? Move objects around in hands to gather information? Does he have correct hand placement for use of a tool such as a pencil?
- Does the child have difficulty grading her movements and applying appropriate force (e.g., breaks things, spills things, throws too hard, or touches too hard)?
- Is the child surprised by the intensity of his actions as if he did not really mean to move or touch so forcefully?
- Can the child feel where his feet are without looking (e.g., climbing stairs - does he miss any steps; need to watch his feet go up and down each step)?
- Can the child tell the difference in weights held in the hand?
- Can the child feel where his body is in space?
- Can the child push and pull many different ways?
- Can the child pull himself up with rope or pull an object up with rope?
- Does the child get fatigued easily? (This may be related to muscle strength and tension.)
- Can the child repeat activities several times without becoming more tired than other children of his age?

III. Sensory-Based Motor Challenges

Subtest 1. Dyspraxia

The following observations are aspects of performance you should observe when looking at praxis. Look at the quality of the child's performance as it flexibly enables interaction with the environment. Look specifically at the complexity of the child's ideation (idea creation) and motor planning, not just at task mastery as reflected in motor execution. See the Appendix for sample items to administer in this section.

- Does the child have difficulty with action-based problem solving (e.g., does he look for a new strategy to try if what he is doing does not work)?
- Can the child figure out what to do but has trouble with how to do it (e.g., can he develop a plan of action but have difficultly enacting it)?

- Does the child appear to be clumsy and awkward in gross and/or fine motor tasks?
- Does the child have difficulty with motor imitation (e.g. postures, hand or mouth movements, rhythms)?
- Is the child able to form and use gestures to communicate?
- Can the child manipulate objects in space to achieve a goal?
- Is the child able to take small parts to make a whole (e.g., use a construction task)
- Does the child accurately perceive and replicate space and form in two- and three-dimensional constructions (e.g., block building or figure drawing)?
- Can the child perform functional activities requiring gross motor movement of her body in space?
- Does the child show joy in success? Is he motivated to persist with somewhat difficult activities requiring mastery motivation and active problem solving?
- Does the child persist, or instead refuse before trying, or give up after trying to use crash solutions when faced with a challenge?
- Does the child initiate activities? If so, what type of activity does child initiate spontaneously? Does the child initiate only when an activity is familiar, or is he/she able to initiate creative and novel play?
- As the child is completing activities, observe whether the goal is accomplished and also the quality with which it is attained. How effectively and efficiently does the child work towards accomplishing goals?
- What is the pace or rate at which the child does things? Is it age-appropriate?
- Once the child is engaged and the examiner either changes the activity or adds another element, can the child adapt to the new task demand or the novel situation?
- Can the child sequence in an age-appropriate manner (e.g., can the child put several steps together to achieve a goal)?
- Does the child talk his way through motor sequences or try to get out of doing something by talking?

Postural Challenges

The key to the following observations for postural problems is to determine whether the child is able to integrate sensory information from multiple systems, particularly visual, vestibular, and proprioceptive, into static (stationary) and dynamic (moving) reactions within the body.

- Can the child stabilize his posture while moving on stable or dynamic (unstable) surfaces? (Can he contract his muscles to hold still if you try to push on his arms, legs, neck, or trunk?)
- Is the child able to maintain appropriate postural alignment and stability during when standing and/or sitting at a desk or in a chair completing table top tasks? Specifically, is his bottom on the chair? Does he hook his feet around the chair legs? Does he rest his head on the table? Does he slump forward or have an overextended back?
- Does the child automatically use one hand to stabilize the paper while writing with the other or does he have to be reminded?

- Can the child maintain postural alignment and balance while moving her body in all planes of movement? Can she use trunk flexion/extension, lateral flexion, rotation during movement? Can she sit with crossed legs and reach to both sides for an object or stand and reach for object to both sides?
- Can the child balance while adapting his posture to interact with the environmental demands (e.g., can the child balance while throwing and catching or kicking a small ball)?
- Can the child adapt her posture on a moving surface (e.g., can she sit on a swing and adjust to the movement of the swing)?
- Can the child complete bilateral symmetrical activities (e.g. clapping or jumping with two feet)?
- Can the child complete bilateral reciprocal movements (e.g. play clapping games in which the hands take turns moving or ride a trike or bike)?
- Is the child's basic muscle tone and strength sufficient to accomplish antigravity activities and functional movement (e.g. as age appropriate, can he sit up from lying on his back on the floor)?
- How differentiated are the child's facial expressions during posturally challenging activities? (In the presence of postural difficulties, many children exhibit fixation and have a fixed facial expression.)
- Can the child shift his gaze across space – (e.g., look at his mom and back to a toy or switch from looking at paper on a desk to the blackboard in front of room)?
- Does the child have the motor control to automatically complete actions requiring visual attention and scanning as well as postural shifts (e.g., being able to follow the actions of children moving on the playground while climbing up the slide)?
- Does child have developmentally expected physical fitness as evidenced by endurance, strength measures?

Summary Sheet

RECORDING PERFORMANCE ON THE OBSERVATIONAL GUIDE

We recommend that materials for each type of stimuli be gathered together before testing begins. A method that works well is to accumulate materials in baskets such as a visual basket, a tactile basket, an auditory basket, etc. Suggestions for baskets appear after the Record Forms.

The Observation Guide has record forms for each of the three classic patterns, with one for each of the three subtests in Sensory Modulation Challenges, one for Sensory Discrimination Challenges and two in Sensory-Based Motor Challenges, a total of six record forms, plus a summary form. For each of the six primary record forms read each item in the left column under "Suggested Observation."

For each item place a check mark in the one box that describes the child's typical performance: not a problem (Not Prob); possible problem (Poss Prob); or yes a problem (Yes Prob). Suggested materials for administering the item are presented in the fifth column for most items. Some items say "query" meaning ask the child's caretaker. Some items say "Query/observe," which means the item can be recorded based on the caretaker's response to your query or observation made at any time during the session. Record general comments in the blank space to the right of materials column as needed.

Remember these record forms are for recording your observations during the assessment but are not based on standardized instructions for administration or scoring. Use your best clinical judgment to administer the scale and to score your observations. At the conclusion of your test administration, circle all behavioral indicators that apply to the child; there is no limit on the number of behavioral indicators you can circle. Circle behavioral indicators from any record form if they apply to the child.

Record scores (Not Prob, Poss Prob, or Yes Prob) for all items you want to observe during the test session. If the child is over-responsive, you may decide not to give the child the same materials as you would if the child is a sensory seeker. You can use your judgment to decide which test materials are appropriate for each child. Only record checkmarks if the appropriate items to observe that performance are administered. For example, if no motor planning materials are given to the child, do not score the dyspraxia record form.

When all item record forms are completed to your satisfaction, go on to summary scores described below.

SCORING AND SUMMARIZING

Higher scores indicate better performance. Decide first if the RSPD category is generally OK or functional (> 50% of the time the child has little or no difficulty in this area). If the child is OK the majority of time, he/she receives a score of 3 or 4. If the child is dysfunctional (>50% of the time the child has moderate or severe problems in this area), then he/she receives a score of 2 or 1. If you choose functional, then decide if this problem is never or rarely observed (4) or occasionally observed (3). If you choose dysfunctional (> 50% of the time), then decide if the dysfunction is frequently a problem (2) or almost always a problem (1).

Draw a hatch mark on the dotted line on the visual analogue scale where you would subjectively score the child's performance. The hatch mark can be anywhere on the line between whole numbers. For example, a mark at 3.5 is fine. These subjective holistic scores can be compared when the child is retested or between children tested by the same examiner. The scores present a subjective representation of the examiner's clinical opinion of the child's performance compared to other children the clinician has tested.

Table 1

Category	*Subtest*		Challenge in this area		
		4 = No indication never or rarely a problem	3 = Mild problem or only occasionally a problem	2 = Moderate problem or frequently a problem	1 = Severe problem or almost always a problem
Sensory Modulation	*Sensory Under-Responsive*	4 .-----.-----.	3 .-----.-----.	2 .-----.-----.	1 .-----.-----.
	Sensory Over-Responsive	4 .-----.-----.	3 .-----.-----.	2 .-----.-----.	1 .-----.-----.
	Sensory Seeking	4 .-----.-----.	3 .-----.-----.	2 .-----.-----.	1 .-----.-----.
Sensory Discrimination	*Tactile*	4 .-----.-----.	3 .-----.-----.	2 .-----.-----.	1 .-----.-----.
	Auditory	4 .-----.-----.	3 .-----.-----.	2 .-----.-----.	1 .-----.-----.
	Visual	4 .-----.-----.	3 .-----.-----.	2 .-----.-----.	1 .-----.-----.
	Taste/Smell	4 .-----.-----.	3 .-----.-----.	2 .-----.-----.	1 .-----.-----.
	Vestibular/ Propriocep.	4 .-----.-----.	3 .-----.-----.	2 .-----.-----.	1 .-----.-----.
Sensory-Based Motor Functioning	*Postural Challenges*	4 .-----.-----.	3 .-----.-----.	2 .-----.-----.	1 .-----.-----.
	Dyspraxic Challenges	4 .-----.-----.	3 .-----.-----.	2 .-----.-----.	1 .-----.-----.

Sensory Over-Responsivity

Suggested Observation	Check box that applies			Suggested Material	Comments
	No Prob.	Poss. Prob.	Yes Prob.		
Visual Domain					
Complex, cluttered, moving, novel, and/or high intensity visual stimuli over-excite, anger, or overwhelm				Flashlight with optic strands, disc that makes patterns when it moves	
Wears sunglasses or caps all the time				Sparkle wheel, light show, strobe toy	
Tactile Domain					
Consistently over-responsive to touch (pulls body part away when touched); discomfort when people too close				Gak, slime, boa, porcupine toy, Koosh balls	
Over-sensitive to certain types of clothing (e.g. labels, long/short sleeves, certain fabrics) or activities of daily living (e.g. hair or hand-washing, bathing)				Lotion, roll up in blanket, barefoot on surfaces, hand washing	
Vestibular/Proprioceptive Domain					
Avoids/becomes upset in certain positions (e.g., prone, upside down) or uneven surfaces				Playground slides, monkey bars	
Uncomfortable/insecure when walking with others who may push them				Query	
Visceral Responses					
Does the child need to go to the bathroom frequently?				Query/observe	
Does the child's body go still or seem to shut down when he has an emotional reaction?				Query/observe	
Shows somatic symptoms indicating physiological over-reactivity (e.g., irritable bowel syndrome, migraines, constant stomach aches)				Query/observe	
General					
Shows overt signs of "fight, flight or freeze" when presented with particular sensory stimuli; may seem irritable, avoidant				Query/observe	
Withdraws from/tries to escape a toy or sensory input				Query/observe	

BEHAVIORAL INDICATORS

Check all that apply

Negative and Stubborn:

- ☐ Aggressive or impulsive when overloaded by sensory stimuli or when stimuli unexpected
- ☐ "Difficult" and hard to soothe; irritable, fussy, moody; not adaptable, unsociable
- ☐ Defiant, controlling

Withdrawn and Avoidant:

- ☐ Avoids group activities; often plays alone
- ☐ Excessively cautious and afraid to try new things
- ☐ Frightened, clinging, worried or shy in new situations
- ☐ Prefers uniformity in the environment, repetition, absence of change; difficulty with transition
- ☐ May have difficulty forming peer relationships or engaging with new adults
- ☐ "Shuts down" to cope with over-arousal; may appear under-responsive
- ☐ Affect seen in the body; responses seem to "well up" inside the body

Sensory Under-Responsivity

Suggested Observations	Check box that applies			Suggested Materials	Comments
	No Prob.	Poss. Prob.	Yes Prob.		
Fails to attends or orient to salient stimuli.				Light show, Koosh balls, sparkle wheel, follow rolling ball down a ramp.	
Fails to responds to name when occupied; overly absorbed.				Call name during task such as coloring.	
Shuts down; stops interacting				Observe	
Overly focused to some stimuli (e.g., blinking lights, moving wheels).				Observe with toy with flashing light, moving parts.	
Investigates new object only briefly; fails to engage.				Fiber optic flashlight or other cool toy.	
Shows no or limited response to an obnoxious sounding toy.				Thunder-spring sound repeatedly—does child want to stop it?	
Fails to orient to sounds as expected.				Tape of screeching tires, fire engine; thunder-spring.	
Lacks awareness of bodily sensations.				Query; frequent accidents; delayed toilet training; not aware of being full or hungry; unaware of pain (e.g., ear infections).	

BEHAVIORAL INDICATORS

Check all that apply

Unaware; Disengaged/ Withdrawn Type:
- ☐ Passive and withdrawn.
- ☐ Good baby/easy child.
- ☐ Disinterested in exploring games or objects.
- ☐ Apathetic, easily exhausted.
- ☐ Lacking in motor exploration and social overtures.
- ☐ Difficult to engage.

Over-Focused/Self-Absorbed:
- ☐ Intelligent children who are in their own world.
- ☐ Out of touch with actions around them.
- ☐ Preference for solitary activities.
- ☐ May be difficult to engage; deeply self-involved.

Sensory Seeking

Suggested Observations	Check box that applies			Suggested Materials	Comments
	No Prob.	Poss. Prob.	Yes Prob.		
Seeks high intensity input in activity; appears unable to get enough; engages with high energy.				Free play in sensory rich environment.	
Resists moving from high intensity activity; resists increasing complexity of activity.				Experiment with getting child off of swing or other high intensity vestibular equipment and onto other less stimulating task.	
Child seems unaware of potential danger or pain, or the consequences of their actions.				Observe for lack of awareness of heights, etc.	
Increasing sensory input results in increasing impulsivity, behavioral disorganization.				Query; observe what happens if over active and add vestibular stimulation.	
Responses to input escalate, behavior gets out of control.				Observation. Query: What causes out of control behavior; what can break the cycle of escalation?	

BEHAVIORAL INDICATORS

Check all that apply

- ☐ Energetically engage in activities or actions providing intense sensation.
- ☐ Crave sensory input in one or more sensory channels (e.g., constantly moving, crashing, bumping, jumping; playing music/TV very loud; staring at visually stimulating scenarios; seeking intense smell or taste).
- ☐ Very active; difficulty sitting quietly; can disrupt other children's ability to maintain attention.
- ☐ May be restless, impulsive, aggressive, explosive in seeking sensation; out of control.
- ☐ May get in trouble or create situations others perceive as bad or dangerous.
- ☐ Increased arousal with input; gets wound up with increasing amounts of stimulation.
- ☐ May become demanding and insistent on getting their own way.

Sensory Discrimination Disorder

Suggested Observations	Check box that applies			Suggested Materials	Comments
	No Prob.	Poss. Prob.	Yes Prob.		
Auditory					
Fails to orients to most sounds (loud/soft) when otherwise engaged.				Novel sounds; soft, mid-range, loud.	
Does not discriminates name from background noise.				Background: music/conversation; call name.	
Visual					
Shows inadequate eye-hand coordination; ability to visually anticipate object movement.				Hitting balloon when moving.	
Fails to scan environment and spot what looking for in near or far space.				Partly hide toys/objects, ask to find.	
Fails to show age-appropriate figure-ground skills.				"Where is Waldo;" find spoon in box of utensils.	
Vestibular/Proprioception					
Cannot sense direction of movement in space, eyes open and closed.				Differentiate falling/moving forward from backward.	
Does not change planes of movement in play.				Stand, sit, look under objects, etc.	
Shows inappropriate postural and balance reactions in response to movement.				Swing set, moving equipment in OT room.	
Poor awareness of movement makes safety a concern.				Balance on a piece of foam eyes open/closed.	
Tactile/Kinesthetic					
Cannot identify objects by feel.				Find specific object in bin without vision.	
Unaware of location of bump/bruise; identifies finger touched, vision occluded.				Identify finger touched, vision occluded.	
Senses if socks twisted, shoes on wrong foot, hair needs combing, fingers in wrong place in gloves				Miscellaneous activities of daily living.	

BEHAVIORAL INDICATORS

Check all that apply

Auditory:
- ☐ Difficulty identifying/distinguishing sounds ("t" and "p" as in cat and cap; "b" and "k" in bag and back).
- ☐ Has trouble following directions, needing them repeated; processes slowly.
- ☐ Difficulty discriminating salient features of the sounds from noise in the milieu.

Visual:
- ☐ Difficulty with spatially guided movement; discrimination of the spatial characteristics of objects and letters.
- ☐ Difficulty with figure ground, spatial rotation of objects (find a puzzle piece; fit it into space).
- ☐ Trouble with anticipatory actions (e.g. catching, batting a ball, or throwing to a target).

Tactile:
- ☐ Difficulty telling what is in hands or what is touching him without looking.
- ☐ Must see object to use it.

[Continued on next page]

Sensory Discrimination Disorder, *continued*

Suggested Observations	Check box that applies			Suggested Materials	Comments
	No Prob.	Poss. Prob.	Yes Prob.		
Fails to actively explores tactile characteristics of objects.				Objects differing in shape, texture, size.	
Olfactory and Gustatory					
Cannot identify typical smells and tastes.				Vanilla, lemon juice, cinnamon, mint, etc.	
Has specific preference for different foods for his age (spicy, "pop rocks").				Query/observe.	
Proprioceptive					
Does not investigate objects with in hand manipulation or adjust to qualities of materials.				Penny, small peg, pencil; observe for manipulation.	
Poorly grades movements and applies inappropriate force.				Correct force on paper when writing.	
Cannot feel where feet/body are without looking.				Climbing stairs; moving through crowded space.	

BEHAVIORAL INDICATORS

Check all that apply

Vestibular:
- ☐ Difficulty sensing displacement of body center of gravity resulting in poor balance.
- ☐ Difficulty sensing speed and direction of his movement.
- ☐ Cannot balance without at least two of the following three systems: vestibular, visual, proprioception.

Proprioception:
- ☐ Holds pencil too tightly or loosely; not enough force to tear the scotch tape; kick a ball too hard/too soft.
- ☐ May have low muscle tone.
- ☐ Appears clumsy in body and/or extremity movement through space.

Postural Disorder

Suggested Observations	Check box that applies			Suggested Materials	Comments
	No Prob.	Poss. Prob.	Yes Prob.		
Cannot stabilize posture when challenged; sitting on stable or dynamic (unstable) surfaces.				Ask child to hold still as you try to push/pull their arms, legs, neck, trunk.	
Difficulty maintaining postural alignment and stability when standing/sitting at desk or in chair completing table top tasks.				Observe: bottom on the chair? Feet hooked around the chair? Head resting on the table? Body slumped?	
Does not automatically use non-dominant hand to assist dominant hand in fine motor tasks.				Stabilize paper while writing.	
Difficulty maintaining postural alignment and balance while moving body.				Observe getting on a swing; adjusting posture to account for swing movement; one-foot balance with reach.	
Difficulty with equilibrium, rotation, weight shift, crossing midline.				Observe during motor activities.	
Difficulty with stability on different surfaces e.g., climbing, walking on foam, walking on moving surfaces.				Observe. Query: e.g., walking on moving sidewalk at airport.	
Difficulty with bilateral symmetrical activities.				Clapping or jumping with two feet; rolling dough with rolling pin.	
Difficulty with bilateral reciprocal movements.				Clapping games in which the hands take turns moving; ride a trike or bike; swim using crawl stroke.	
Muscle tone and strength insufficient to accomplish antigravity activities and functional movement.				As age appropriate, sit up from lying on their back on the floor; note strength of hand shake.	
Facial expressions fixed during posturally challenging activities.				Observation.	
Difficulty with near/far gaze shift.				Look at Mom, back at toy; look at paper, back to chalkboard.	
Does not have developmentally expected physical fitness as evidenced by endurance, strength measures.				Observe or query: number of sit-ups, push-ups.	

BEHAVIORAL INDICATORS

Check all that apply

- ☐ Poor trunk stability at rest and/or during movement
- ☐ Tendency to fixate or stabilize the trunk using flexion or extension patterns resulting in poor fluidity of movement
- ☐ Difficulty stabilizing at shoulders and hips resulting in poorly refined movements of upper and lower extremities
- ☐ Tendency to avoid weight bearing in upper extremities
- ☐ Poor righting, equilibrium, trunk rotation, ocular control; difficulty isolating head and eye movements
- ☐ Avoids climbing; shows discomfort on uneven surfaces
- ☐ Avoidance or discomfort crossing the midline of the body

Dyspraxia

Suggested Observations	Check box that applies			Suggested Materials	Comments
	No Prob.	Poss. Prob.	Yes Prob.		
Has difficulty with action-based problem solving.				Do they look for new strategy if one in use does not work?	
Can figure out what to do but has trouble with how to do it.				Ask them to develop a plan of action.	
Appears clumsy and awkward in gross and/or fine motor tasks.				Observe/query.	
Has difficulty with motor imitation.				Postures, hand or mouth movements; rhythms.	
Unable to take small parts to make a whole.				Jigsaw puzzle without frame.	
Difficulty replicating space and form in 2D and 3D constructions.				Block building or figure drawing.	
Does not show joy in success; not motivated to persist with somewhat difficult activities requiring active problem solving.				Draw a person, block designs, figuring out grommet or maze use.	
Does not initiate activities, or initiates only when activity is familiar, or is he/she able to initiate creative and novel play.				Getting into and out of gross motor equipment like hanging inner tube, net swing.	
Is inefficient, ineffective in reaching goal of activity.				Observe strategies, frustration, success during task accomplishment.	
Pace/rate of activity is not age-appropriate.				Walk balance beam/step over stick. Make objects out of playdoh; observe pace and rate.	
Difficulty adapting to changes in task demand, new task demand, or novel situation.				Fold paper and put in envelope; various sizes of paper/envelopes.	
Difficulty sequencing tasks in an age appropriate manner.				Folding blanket or sheet.	
Talks self through motor sequences; tries to get out of doing by talking.				Plexiglas with toy under it; use stick to obtain toy; fishbowl with nerf ball that is too big; other activities above.	

BEHAVIORAL INDICATORS

Check all that apply

Ideational:
- ☐ Inability to formulate a goal (or idea) for action; may resort to rigid or inflexible behavior.
- ☐ May prefer fantasy games to doing.

Gross Motor:
- ☐ Tend to be accident-prone; trip, bump into objects or people.
- ☐ Generally poor in ball activities and other sports.
- ☐ Much trial and error; requires more time/practice to learn new skills.
- ☐ May break toys because of difficulty with planning and force modulation.
- ☐ Difficulty generalizing previously learned motor skills to new situations and contexts.
- ☐ May prefer sedentary activities such as watching TV, playing video games, reading a book, playing fantasy games.
- ☐ May try to mask their dyspraxia by acting like a clown.

(continued on next page)

Dyspraxia, *continued*

Suggested Observations	Check box that applies			Suggested Materials	Comments
	No Prob.	Poss. Prob.	Yes Prob.		

BEHAVIORAL INDICATORS

Check all that apply

Fine Motor:

- ☐ Difficulty with manipulative activities (using utensils; cutting, coloring, pasting, construction toys; [(pre)] handwriting).
- ☐ Often disorganized and may be disheveled looking.
- ☐ May perserverate or prefer simpler play activities.

Oral Motor:

- ☐ Difficulty with articulation, sucking, chewing, and swallowing sequences.
- ☐ Prolonged/excessive drooling.

Additional Materials and Activities Useful in Assessing RSPD

The materials and questions listed below are intended to offer options in addition to those listed on the record form. We suggest you "assemble a basket" which might include actual materials or questions you either answer through your own observation, or through caregiver query. The list is not intended to be all inclusive.

I. PATTERN ONE: SENSORY MODULATION CHALLENGES

Observe the child interacting with these materials, watching for indicators of over-responsiveness, under-responsiveness, or sensory seeking.

Tactile Basket

- Kinesio tape, band aids or coban lightly taping 2 or 3 fingers together
- Walking barefoot on various surfaces, e.g. fake grass
- Observe distinct preference for toys with specific characteristics (hard/without much tactile sensation; fuzzy or highly textured, etc.)

Visual Basket (many of these are visual and auditory)

- Spinning light show in a sphere (SRM Entertainment)
- Gyro spinning light show
- Stand up ball blast (Fisher Price)
- Fisher Price Sesame Street Shake Giggle and Roll
- Popcorn popping toy
- Turtle push and popcorn pops

Auditory Basket

- Drop coins in pan
- Spoon and pot lid
- Unpopped corn in plastic container, shake
- Fisher Price Sesame Street Shake Giggle and Roll
- Popping toy with push stick
- Turtle push and popcorn pops

Vestibular/Proprioceptive Basket

- Office chair that child can sit in and spin
- Tip child backward on a large therapy ball, or on parents' lap
- Lift child off the ground
- Have child wheelbarrow walk
- Observe or query caregiver on climbing: too high without fear? Fearful to climb?
- Walk up and down a ramp (integrate vestibular and visual)
- Observe or query response to bouncing on a trampoline (if available or something to jump on, such as a mattress or pillows
- Observe or query response to swinging and other playground equipment where child moves in space

PATTERN II. SENSORY DISCRIMINATION CHALLENGES

Tactile Basket

- Pick up pennies to put in bank
- Depending on age, identify objects or shapes by touch alone

Visual Basket

- **Figure – Ground** (Can the child discriminate a figure from a background?)
- Take a favorite cartoon figure and tape it to wall, see if he can find it
- Observe child in visually busy room as she searches for a toy she wants
- Puzzle edge pieces or finding pieces that represent a particular object in puzzle

- **Visual closure** (Can the child find partially hidden objects?)
- Observe or query caregiver: Is the child able to focus on the salient aspect of the object (e.g., in a gum ball machine, do they watch the gum ball come down or do they get stuck on the handle of the toy?)
- Observe visual search in both near and far space

Vestibular and Proprioceptive Basket

- Observe ability to grade movements during such things as: pushing a heavy door; push and pull activity with Theraband; push and pull resistance when swinging
- Finger-nose touching, eyes open and closed
- Balance on a piece of foam or a rounded foam form, balance beam, with eyes open and closed
- Walking up and down stairs, observe or query caregiver: does the child step on each stair or skip stairs?
- Ask child to walk or move with his eyes closed or covered
- Play with weighted balls: ask child to indicate which two are the same weight, which is lighter, and which is heavier
- In supine position, place on roll-up grid and place one limb then return it and then see if he can copy that placement with that arm
- Write on multi-sheet (no carbon required) paper so that you can see what is printed on the carbon copy
- During fine motor tool use, observe for correct gradation and specificity of movement as he explores objects in hand

Olfactory Basket

Many stimuli can be presented in a closed container (a contact lens case works well) and the child can be asked to name the smell. Sample should include pleasant, as well as unpleasant smells.

- Balsamic vinegar
- Garlic
- Horseradish
- Flavored salts

- Lemon juice
- Spices (e.g., cinnamon, clove)
- Perfume
- Mint
- Vanilla

PATTERN III. SENSORY-BASED MOTOR CHALLENGES

Dyspraxia Basket

Problem Solving

- Find a toy hidden under one of three cups
- Figure out how a container can open (use containers that open in different ways)
- Figure out which door the object is behind
- Use a clear plastic tube (e.g., a florescent light protector or paper towel tube), then use a stick or combination of sticks to push object which is in the center of the tube out of the tube

Imitation of Postures

- Imitate what you do with two sticks - toddler
- Imitate rhythms (e.g., rhythmic movements with both upper extremities)
- Imitate subtle emotional cues displayed by nonverbal motor behaviors

Complex Tasks Requiring Praxis (look for complexity and flexibility of action)

Fine Motor

- Figuring out how to use a grommet or maze
- Block designs
- Draw a person
- Origami

Gross Motor

- Getting into Lycra swing or tire swing
- Roll bolster at child asking him/her to step over it (projected action sequence)
- Observe child in spontaneous play in the OT Room or playground
- Walk line or balance beam and step over stick

Postural Basket

Muscle and Postural Tone

- Observe for laxity of the mouth, weakness when shaking hands, resistance when giving high fives

- In quadruped, can child resist while you push against him? ("I'm going to huff and puff and blow your house over..." as you push against his shoulder and hips). Can they be a statue as you try to wiggle arms, legs, neck, and trunk against resistance?

Static Postural Activities

- Observe posture during table top activities in an appropriately sized chair (not too deep a seat, height of chair enabling elbows to rest on table, and feet supported on the floor)
- Lie on back and lift head, hips and arms into little ball (i.e., assume and maintain supine flexion)

Dynamic Postural Activities

- Getting in and out of tire swing
- Stand with feet together and reach out for object and maintain balance
- Stand on one foot and reach out for object more than arms length to the side or forward
- Throw at target while lying prone on ball

Bilateral Activities

- Hold onto trapeze and kick ball with two legs (look at bilateral as well as balance aspects of this task)

Visual Vestibular Postural Activities

- Catch a ball while running
- Kick a ball while moving
- Walk up and down the stairs without holding onto banister
- Walk beam and step over stick
- Visual tracking of object moving in all planes
- Tracking a predictably moving object (e.g., ball swinging on string or rolling down incline)
- Observe visual saccades by having child sit at table and put objects in all four corners - child should name the objects while you stabilize her head

Selected References: Regulatory Sensory Processing Disorder

The focus of this reading list is on description of the Regulatory-Sensory Processing Disorder and supporting research. Intervention studies are not included in this document.

HISTORICAL PERSPECTIVES

Ayres, A.J. (1964). Tactile functions: Their relation to hyperactive and perceptual motor behavior. *American Journal of Occupational Therapy*, 18(1), 83-95.

Ayres, A.J. (1972). *Sensory integration and learning disabilities.* Los Angeles: Western Psychological Services.

Ayres, A.J. (1974). *The development of sensory integrative theory and practice: A collection of the works of A. Jean Ayres.* Dubuque, Iowa: Kendall/Hunt.

Ayres, A.J. (1975). Sensorimotor foundations of academic ability. In W. Cruickshank & Hallahan, D. (Eds.), *Perceptual and learning disabilities in children* (pp. 300-358).

Ayres, A.J. (1979). *Sensory integration and the child.* Los Angeles: Western Psychological Services.

Bergman, P., & Escalona, S. (1949). Unusual sensitivities in very young children. *The PSA study of the child*, Vol. III/IV. New York: International University Press.

Knickerbocker, B. (1980). A holistic approach to learning disabilities. Thorofare, NJ: Slack.

ASSESSMENT

Ayres, A.J. (1989). *Sensory Integration and Praxis Tests. Los Angeles:* Western Psychological Services.

Beery, K.E., Buktenica, N.A., & Beery, N.A. (2004). *The Beery-Buktenica Developmental Test of Visual Motor Integration*, 5th edition. Austin, TX: Pro Ed.

Bruininks, R.H. (1978). *Bruininks Oseretsky Test of Motor Proficiency.* Circle Pines, MN: American Guidance Service.

Cermak, S., & Murray, E. (1991). The validity of the constructional subtests of the Sensory Integration and Praxis Tests. *American Journal of Occupational Therapy*, 45(6), 539-543.

DeGangi, G. (1991). Part 1: Assessment of sensory, emotional, and attentional problems in regulatory disordered infants. *Infants and Young Children*, 3, 1-8.

DeGangi, G.A., Poisson, P., Sickel, R., & Wiener, A. (1994). *Infant/Toddler Symptom Checklist: A Screening Tool for Parents.* San Antonio, TX: Therapy Skill Builders.

Dunn, W. (1994). Performance of typical children on the Sensory Profile: An item analysis. *American Journal of Occupational Therapy*, 48, 967-974.

Dunn, W. (1997a). The impact of sensory processing abilities on the daily lives of young children and their families: A conceptual model. *Infants and Young Children*, 9(4), 23-35.

Dunn, W. (1997b). The Sensory Profile: A discriminating measure of sensory processing in daily life. *SISIS Quarterly*, 20(1), 1-3.

Dunn, W. (2002). *Infant Toddler Sensory Profile.* N.Y.: The Psychological Corporation.

Dunn, W. & Brown, C. (1997). Factor analysis on the sensory profile from a national sample of children without disabilties. *American Journal of Occupational Therapy*, 51, 490-495.

Dunn, W., & Daniels, D.B. (2002). Initial development of the Infant/Toddler Sensory Profile. *Journal of Early Intervention*, 25(1), 27-41.

Dunn, W. & Westman, K. (1997). The Sensory Profile: The performance of a national sample of children without disabilities. *American Journal of Occupational Therapy*, 51, 25-34.

Ermer, J. & Dunn, W. (1998). The Sensory Profile: A discriminate analysis of children with and without disabilities. *American Journal of Occupational Therapy*, 52, 283-290.

Harris, N. (1981). Duration and quality of the prone extension position in four-, six- and eight-year old normal children. *American Journal of Occupational Therapy*, 35, 26-30.

Henderson, S. & Sugden, D. (1992). Movement Assessment Battery for Children. Austin, TX: Psychological Corporation.

Koenig, K.P. (1996). Adaptability: The bridge to behavior. *Sensory Integration Quarterly*, June, 1-12.
Lai, J.S., Fisher, A.G., Magalhaes, L., & Bundy, A. (1996). Construct validity of the Sensory Integration and Praxis Tests. *Occupational Therapy Journal of Research*, 16(2), 75-97.
Miller, L.J., & Roid, G. (1994). *The T.I.M.E. Toddler and Infant Motor Evaluation: A Standardized Assessment.* San Antonio, TX: Therapy Skill Builders.
Miller, M.Q., & Quinn-Hurst, M. (1994). Neurobehavioral assessment of high-risk infants in the neonatal intensive care unit. *American Journal of Occupational Therapy*, 48(6), 506-513.
Murray, E., Cermak, S., & O'Brien, V. (1990). The relationship between form and space perception, constructional abilities, and clumsiness in children. *American Journal of Occupational Therapy*, 44(7), 623-628.
Royeen, C.B., & Fortune, J.C. (1990). TIE: Touch inventory for school aged children. *American Journal of Occupational Therapy*, 44, 155_160.
Van Waelvelde, H., De Weerdt, W., De Cock, P., & Smits-Engelsman, B.C.M. (2004). Aspects of the validity of the Movement Assessment Battery for Children. *Human Movement Science*, 23, 49-60.
Walker, K.F., & Burris, B. (1991). Correlation of Sensory Integration and Praxis Test scores with Metropolitan Achievement Test scores in normal children. *Occupational Therapy Journal of Research*, 11(5), 307-309.
Williamson, G.G. & Anzalone, M. (1997). Sensory integration: A key component of the evaluation and treatment of young children with severe difficulties in relating and communicating. *Zero-to-Three*, 17, 29-36.
Wilson, B., Pollock, N., Kaplan, B., & Law, M. (1994). *Clinical Observation of Motor and Postural Skills (COMPS).* San Antonio, TX: Therapy Skill Builders.
Wilson, B.N., Polatajko, H.J., Kaplan, B.J., & Faris, P. (1995). Use of the Bruiniks-Oseretsky Test of Motor Proficiency in occupational therapy. *American Journal of Occupational Therapy*, 49(1), 8-17.

SENSORY INTEGRATION THEORY AND CLINICAL-BASED DESCRIPTION

Anzalone, M.E., & Williamson, C.G. (Eds.) (2001). *Strategies to improve sensory integration and self-regulation in young children.* Washington, DC: Zero to Three.
Bakley, S. (2001). Through the lens of sensory integration: A different way of analyzing challenging behavior. *Young Children*, 56 (6), 70-76.
Bates, J.E., & Wachs, T.D. (1994). *Temperament: Individual differences at the interface of biology and behavior.* Washington, DC.: American Psychological Association.
Bundy, A.C., Lane, S.J., & Murray, E.A. (2002). *Sensory integration: Theory and practice (2nd ed.).* Philadelphia, PA: F.A. Davis Company.
Cermak, S.A. & Larkin, D. (2001). *Developmental coordination disorder.* Albany, NY: Thompson Delmar.
DeGangi, G. (2000). *Pediatric disorders of regulation in affect and behavior: A therapist's guide to assessment and treatment.* San Diego: Academic Press.
Dunn, W. (2001). The sensations of everyday life: Empirical, theoretical, and pragmatic considerations. *American Journal of Occupational Therapy*, 55(6), 608-620.
Frick, S. (1989). Sensory defensiveness: A case study. *Sensory Integration Special Interest Section Newsletter*, 12(2), 1-3.
Giordano, A. (2001, April 24). Sensory overload: For some kids, a shower feels like needles; is it SID, or just sensitivity? *The Boston Globe*, pp. C1, C3.
Greenspan, S.I. (1995). *The challenging child.* Reading, MA: Addison Wesley.
Greenspan, S., & Wieder, S. (1998). *The child with special needs: Encouraging intellectual and emotional growth.* Reading, MA: Addison-Wesley.
Greenspan, S., & Wieder, S. (1993). Regulatory disorders. In C.H. Zeanah (Ed.), *Handbook of infant mental health* (280-290). New York: Guildford.
Heller, S. (2002). *Too loud, too bright, too fast, too tight.* New York: Harper Collins Publishers.
Inamura, K.N. (1998). *SI for early intervention.* San Antonio, TX: Therapy Skill Builders.
Keefe, S. (2004). Sensory integration: Recognition in primary care settings. *Advanced Nurse Practitioner*, 12(1), 57-58.
Kinnealey, M. (1998). Princess or tyrant: A case report of a child with sensory defensiveness. *Occupational Therapy International*, 5(4), 293-303.

Kranowitz, C.S. (1998). *The out-of-sync child.* New York: Berkley Publishing Group.

Mailloux, Z., & Burke, J.P. (1997). Play and the sensory integrative approach. In Parham, L.D. & Fazio, L.S. (Eds.), *Play in occupational therapy for children.* (pp 112-125). St. Louis, Missouri: Mosby-Year Book, Inc.

Miller, L.J., Cermak, S.A., Lane, S., Anzalone, M., & Koomar, J. (2004, Summer). Position statement on terminology related to sensory integration dysfunction. *S.I. Focus*, pp. 6-8.

Miller, L.J. & McIntosh, D.N. (1998). The diagnosis, treatment and etiology of sensory modulation disorder. *Sensory Integration Special Interest Section Quarterly*, 21(1), 1-3.

Montagu, A. (1986). Touching: *The significance of the human skin.* New York: Harper & Row.

Mulligan, S. (1998). Patterns of sensory integration dysfunction: A confirmatory factor analysis. *American Journal of Occupational Therapy*, 52, 819-828.

Mulligan, S. (2000). Cluster analysis of scores of children on the sensory integration and praxis tests. *Occupational Therapy Journal of Research*, 20(4), 256-270.

Oetter, P., Richter, E., & Frick, S. (1995). MORE: *Integrating the mouth with sensory functions* (Revised ed.). Hugo, MN: PDP Press.

Parham, L.D., Mailloux, Z. (1996). Sensory integration. In Case-Smith, J., Allen, A.S., & Pratt, P. N. (Eds.), *Occupational therapy for children* (3rd ed., pp. 307-355). St. Louis, Missouri: Mosby-Year Book, Inc.

Pohl, P.S., Dunn, W., & Brown, C. (2003). The role of sensory processing in the everyday lives of older adults. *OTJR-Occupation, Participation, and Health*, 23(3), 99-106.

Sears, C.J. (1995). Recognizing and coping with tactile defensiveness in young children. In J.A. Blackman (Ed.) *Identification and assessment in early intervention, Infants and young children series* (pp. 188-197). Gaithersburg, MD: Aspen.

Smith, K.A., & Gouze, K. (2004). *The sensory-sensitive child: Practical solutions for out-of-bounds behavior.* New York: Harper Collins.

Smith Roley, S., Blanch, E.I., & Schaaf, R.C. (2001). *Understanding the nature of sensory integration with diverse populations.* USA: Therapy Skill Builders.

Spitzer, S., Roley, S., Clark, F., & Parham, D. (1997). Sensory integration: Current trends in the United States. *Scandinavian Journal of Occupational Therapy, 4.*

Trott, M.C., Laurel, M., & Windeck, S. (1993). *SenseAbilities, understanding sensory integration.* Tuscon, Arizona: Therapy Skill Builders.

Wilbarger, P. (1984, September). Planning an adequate "sensory diet": Application of sensory processing theory during the first years of life. *Zero to Three*, 7-12.

Wilbarger, P. (1995). The sensory diet: Activity programs based on sensory processing theory. *Sensory Integration Special Interest Section Newsletter*, 18(2).

Wilbarger, P., & Wilbarger, J.L. (1991). *Sensory defensiveness in children aged 2-12: An intervention guide for parents and other caretakers.* Santa Barbara, California: Avanti Educational Programs.

Williams, M.S., & Shellenberger, S. (1994). *How does your engine run? A leader's guide to the alert program for self regulation.* Albuquerque, NM: TherapyWorks.

Zuckerman, M. (1994). *Behavioral expressions and biosocial bases of sensation seeking.* New York: Cambridge University Press.

SELECTED RESEARCH ON THE CLINICAL DISORDERS: EMPIRICAL DESCRIPTION

Hotz, S.D., & Royeen, C.B. (1998). Perception of behaviours associated with tactile defensiveness: An exploration of the differences between mothers and their children. *Occupational Therapy International*, 5(4), 281-292.

Lee, C.Y., Lin, J.H., Sung, F.H., Shih, H.H., Hung, C.L., & Hung, T.M. (2004). Exploring the relationship between sensory integration, motor ability and emotion on preschool children. Journal of Sport & *Exercise Psychology, 26*, S116.

McIntosh, D.N., Miller, L.J., Shyu, V., & Hagerman, R.J. (1999). Sensory-modulation disruption, electrodermal responses, and functional behaviors. *Developmental Medicine and Child Neurology, 41*(9), 608-615.

Miller, L.J. (2003). Empirical evidence related to therapies for sensory processing impairments. *Communique, 31*(5), 34-37.

Ottenbacher, K. (1982). Sensory integration: Affect or effect? *American Journal of Occupational Therapy, 36*, 571-578.
Parham, D.L. (1998). The relationship of sensory integration development to achievement in elementary students: Four-year longitudinal study. *Occupational Therapy Journal of Research, 18*, 105-127.
Polatjko, H., Kaplan, B., & Wilson, N. (1992). Sensory integration treatment in children with learning disabilities: Its status 20 years later. *Occupational Therapy Journal of Research, 12*, 323-341.
Schaaf, R., Miller, L.J., Seawell, D., & O'Keefe, S. (2003). Children with disturbances in sensory processing: A pilot study examining the role of the parasympathetic nervous system. *American Journal of Occupational Therapy, 57*, 442-449.
Stephens, C.L., & Royeen, C.B. (1998). Investigation of tactile defensiveness and self-esteem in typically developing children. *Occupational Therapy International, 5*(4), 273-280.
Thomasgard, M. (2003). Working with challenging young children: Relations between child temperament, response to novelty and sensory processing. *Clinical Pediatrics, 42*(3), 197-204.
Tickle-Degnen, L. (1988). Perspectives on the status of sensory integration theory. *American Journal of Occupational Therapy, 42*(7), 427-433.
Zald, D.H. (2003). The human amygdala and the emotional evaluation of sensory stimuli. *Brain Research Reviews, 41*(1), 88-123.

Examples of Research Describing Sensory Processing Disorders with Different Clinical Populations

ATTENTION DEFICIT DISORDER

Ayres, A. J. (1964). Tactile functions: Their relation to hyperactive and perceptual motor behavior. *American Journal of Occupational Therapy, 18*(1), 83-95.
Cermak, S. (1988a). The relationship between attention deficit disorder and sensory integration disorders. Part 1: Theory. *Sensory Integration Special Interest Section Newsletter, 11*(2), 1-4.
Cermak, S. (1988b). The relationship between attention deficit disorder and sensory integration disorders. Part 2: Treatment. *Sensory Integration Special Interest Section Newsletter, 11*(3), 3-4.
Denckla, M., Rudel, R., Chapman, C., & Krieger, J. (1985). Motor proficiency in dyslexic children with and without attentional disorders. *Archives of Neurology, 42*, 228-231.
Dunn, W., & Bennett, D. (2002). Patterns of sensory processing in children with Attention Deficit Hyperactivity Disorder. OTJR: *Occupational Participation and Health, 22*(1), 4-15.
Gillberg, C. (1998). Hyperactivity, inattention and motor control problems: Prevalence, comorbidity and background factors. *Folia Phoniatrica et Logopaedica, 50*, 107-117.
Kadesjo, B., & Gillberg, C. (1998). Attention deficits and clumsiness in Swedish 7-year-old children. *Developmental Medicine and Child Neurology, 40*(12), 796-804.
Kadesjo, B., & Gillberg, C. (2001). The comorbidity of ADHD in the general population of Swedish school-age children. *Journal of Child Psychology and Psychiatry and Allied Disciplines, 42*(4), 487-492.
Landgren, M., Kjellman, B., & Gillberg, C. (1998). Attention deficit disorder with developmental coordination disorders. *Archives of Disease in Childhood, 79*(3), 207-212.
Lightsey, R. (1993). Tactile defensiveness in attention deficit/hyperactive disorder children. *Sensory Integration Quarterly, 21*(2), 6.
Mangeot, S.D., Miller, L.J., McIntosh, D.N., McGrath-Clarke, J., Simon, J., Hagerman, R.J., & Goldson, E. (2001). Sensory modulation dysfunction in children with attention-deficit-hyperactivity disorder. *Developmental Medicine and Child Neurology, 43*(6), 399-406.
Mulligan, S. (1996). An analysis of score patterns of children with attention disorders on the Sensory Integration and Praxis Tests. *American Journal of Occupational Therapy, 50*, 647-654.
Parush, S., Sohmer, H., Steinberg, A., & Kaitz, M. (1997). Somatosensory functioning in children with attention deficit hyperactivity disorder. *Developmental Medicine and Child Neurology, 39*, 464-468.
Pitcher, T.M., Piek, J.P., & Barrett, N.C. (2002). Timing and force control in boys with attention deficit hyperactivity disorder: Subtype differences and the effect of comorbid developmental coordination disorder. *Human Movement Science, 21*(5-6), 919-945.
Raggio, D.J. (1999). Visualmotor perception in children with attention deficit hyperactivity disorder-combined type. *Perceptual and Motor Skills, 88*(2), 448-450.

Rasmussen, P., & Gillberg, C. (2000). Natural outcome of ADHD with developmental coordination disorder at age 22 years: A controlled, longitudinal, community-based study. *Journal of the American Academy of Child and Adolescent Psychiatry, 39*(11), 1424-1431.

Tervo, R.C., Azuma, S., Fogas, B., Falls, S., Fiechtner, H. (2002). Children with ADHD and motor dysfunction compared with children with ADHD only. *Developmental Medicine and Child Neurology, 44*(6), 383-390.

AUTISM/PERVASIVE DEVELOPMENTAL DISORDER

Ayres, A.J. (1979). The autistic child. In A.J. Ayres *Sensory Integration and the Child* (pp.123-130). Los Angeles: Western Psychological Services.

Ayres, A.J., & Fisher, A.G. (1983). Sensory registration in autism and tactile defensiveness. *SISIS Newsletter*, 6, 179-180.

Ayres, A.J., & Heskett, W.M. (1972). Sensory integrative dysfunction in a young schizophrenic girl. *Journal of Autism and Childhood Schizophrenia, 2*(2), 174-181.

Ayres, A.J., & Mailloux, Z.K. (1983). Possible pubertal effect on therapeutic gains in an autistic girl. *American Journal of Occupational Therapy, 37*(8), 535-540.

Ayres, A.J., & Tickle, L.S. (1980). Hyper-responsivity to touch and vestibular stimuli as a predictor of positive response to sensory integration procedures by autistic children. *American Journal of Occupational Therapy, 34*, 375-381.

Baranek, G.T. (1994). Tactile defensiveness in children with developmental disabilities: Responsiveness and habituation. *Journal of Autism and Developmental Disorders, 24*, 457-471.

Baranek, G.T. (1997a). Sensory defensiveness in persons with developmental disabilities. *Occupational Therapy Journal of Research, 17*, 173-185.

Baranek, G.T. (1997b). Tactile defensiveness and stereotyped behaviors. *American Journal of Occupational Therapy, 51*, 91-95.

Baranek, G.T. (1998). Sensory processing in persons with autism and developmental disabilities: Considerations for research and clinical practice. *Sensory Integration Special Interest Section Quarterly, 21*(2), 1-3.

Baranek, G.T. (1999). Autism during infancy: A retrospective video analysis of sensory-motor and social behaviors at 9-12 months of age. *Journal of Autism and Developmental Disorders, 29*, 213-224.

Baranek, G.T. (2002). Efficacy of sensory and motor interventions for children with autism. *Journal of Autism and Developmental Disorders, 32*(5), 397-422.

Baranek, G.T. & Berkson, G. (1994). Tactile defensiveness in children with developmental disabilities: Responsiveness and habituation. *Journal of Autism and Developmental Disorders, 24*, 457-471.

Baranek, G.T., Chin, Y.K.H., Hess, L.M.G., Yankee, J.G., Hatton, D.D., Hooper, S.R. (2002). Sensory processing correlates of occupational performance in children with Fragile X syndrome: Preliminary findings. *American Journal of Occupational Therapy, 56*(5), 538-546.

Beadle-Brown, J. (2004). Elicited imitation in children and adults with autism: The effect of different types of actions. *Journal of Applied Research in Intellectual Disabilities, 17*, 37.

Case-Smith, J. & Miller, H. (1999). Occupational therapy with children with pervasive developmental disorders. *American Journal of Occupational Therapy, 53*, 506-513.

Cullen, L. & Barlow, J. (2002). 'Kiss, cuddle, squeeze': The experiences and meaning of touch among parents of children with autism attending a Touch Therapy Programme. *Child Health Care, 6*(3), 171-181.

Curcio, F. & Piserchia, E.A. (1978). Pantomimic representation in psychotic children. *Journal of Autism and Childhood Schizophrenia, 8*(2), 181-189.

DeMyer, M.K., Mann, N.A., Tilton, J.R., & Loew, L. H. (1967). Toy-play behavior and use of body by autistic and normal children as reported by mothers. *Psychological Reports*, 21, 973-981.

Dunn, W. & Fisher, A. G. I. (1983). *Sensory registration, autism and tactile defensiveness. Sensory Integration Special Interest Section Newsletter, 6*(2), 3-4.

Dunn, W., Myles, B.S., & Orr, S. (2002). Sensory processing issues associated with Asperger syndrome: A preliminary investigation. *American Journal of Occupational Therapy, 56*(1), 97-102.

Gal, E., Dyck, M., & Passamore, A. (2002). Sensory differences and stereotyped movements in children with autism. *Behavior Change, 18*, 207-219.

Gillberg, C., & Billstedt, E. (2000). Autism and Asperger syndrome: Coexistence with other clinical disorders. *Acta Psychiatrica Scandina Vica, 102*(5), 321-330.

Grandin, T. (1995). *Thinking in pictures and other reports from my life with autism.* New York: Doubleday.

Grandin, T. & Scariano, A. (1986). *Emergence labeled autistic.* Novato, CA: Arena Press.

Green, D., Baird, G., Barnett, A.L., Henderson, L., Huber, J., & Henderson, S.E. (2002). The severity and nature of motor impairment in Asperger's syndrome: A comparison with Specific Developmental Disorder or Motor Function. *Journal of Child Psychology and Psychiatry and Allied Disciplines, 43*(5), 655-668.

Hirstein, W., Iversen, P., & Ramachandran, V.S. (2001). Autonomic responses of autistic children to people and objects. *Proceedings of the Royal Society of London Series B-Biological Sciences, 268*(1479), 1883-1888.

Kientz, M. & Dunn, W. (1997). A comparison of the performance of children with and without autism on the Sensory Profile. *American Journal of Occupational Therapy, 51*, 530-537.

Korb, C.A. (2002). Music therapy, sensory integration, and the autistic child. *Arts in Psychotherapy, 29* (4), 235-236.

Leary, M.R. & Hill, D.A. (1996). Moving on: Autism and movement disturbance. *Mental Retardation, 34*, 39-53.

Lepisto, T. (2002). Auditory sensory processing in autism and Asperger's syndrome as reflected by event-related potentials. *International Journal of Psychophysiology, 45*, 39-40.

Libby, S., Powell, S., Messer, D., & Jordan, R. (1997). Imitation of pretend play acts by children with autism and Down Syndrome. *Journal of Autism and Developmental Disorders, 27*, 365-383.

Lincoln, A.J., Courchesne, E., Harms, L, & Allen, M. (1995). Sensory modulation of auditory-stimuli in children with autism and receptive developmental language disorder—Event related brain potential evidence. *Journal of Autism and Developmental Disorders, 25*(5), 521-539.

Mailloux, Z. (2001). Sensory integrative principles in intervention with children with autistic disorder. In S. Smith Roley, E.I. Blance, & R.C. Schaaf (Ed.), *Understanding the nature of sensory integration with diverse populations* (pp. 365-384). San Antonio: Therapy Skill Builders.

Miller, H. (1996). Eye contact and gaze aversion: Implications for persons with autism. *Sensory Integration Special Interest Section Newsletter, 19* (2), 1-3.

Miller-Kuhaneck, H. (2004). *Autism: A comprehensive occupational therapy approach.*(2nd ed.). Rockville, MD: American Occupational Therapy Association.

Myles, B.K., Cook, N., Miller, L., Rinner, L., & Robbins, L. (2000). *Asperger syndrome and sensory issues: Practical solutions for making sense of the world.* Shawnee Mission, KS: Autism Asperger Publishing.

O'Neil, M. & Jones, R. (1997). Sensory-perceptual abnormalities in autism: A case for more research? *Journal of Autism and Developmental Disabilities, 27*, 283-293.

Ornitz, E.M. (1974). The modulation of sensory input and motor output in autistic children. *Journal of Autism and Childhood Schizophrenia*, 4, 197-215.

Ornitz, E.M. (1989). Autism at the interface of sensory processing and information processing. In G. Dawson (Ed.), *Autism: Nature, diagnosis, and treatment* (pp. 174-207). New York: Guilford.

Ornitz, E.M., Guthrie, D., & Farley, A.J. (1978). The early symptoms of childhood autism. In G. Sebman (Ed.). *Cognitive deficits in the development of mental illness* (pp. 24-42). New York: Bruner-Mazel.

Restall, G., & Evans, J. (1994). Play and preschool children with autism. *American Journal of Occupational Therapy, 48*(2), 113-120.

Rimland, B. (1990). Sound sensitivity in autism. *Autism Research Review International, 4*(1), 6-12.

Rogers, S.J., Bennetto, L., McEvoy, R., & Pennington, B.F. (1996). Imitation and pantomime in high-functioning adolescents with autism spectrum disorders. *Child Development, 67*, 2060-2073.

Rogers, S.J., Hepburn, S.L., Stackhouse, T., & Wehner, E. (2003). Imitation performance in toddlers with autism and those with other developmental disorders. *Journal of Child Psychology and Psychiatry and Allied Disciplines, 44*(5), 763-781.

Rogers, S.J., Hepburn, S.L., & Wehner, E. (2003). Parent reports of sensory symptoms in toddlers with autism and those with other developmental disorders. *Journal of Autism and Developmental Disorders, 33*, 631-642.

Seal, B.C. & Bonvillian, J.D. (1997). Sign language and motor functioning in students with autistic disorder. *Journal of Autism and Developmental Disorders, 27*, 437-465.

Shore, S. (2001). Beyond the wall: Personal experiences with autism and Asperger syndrome. Shawnee Mission, KS: Autism Asperger Publishing.

Smith, M.D. (1986). Use of similar sensory stimulation in the community-based treatment of self-stimulatory behavior in an adult disabled by autism. *Journal of Behavior Therapy and Experimental Psychiatry, 17*, 121-124.

Smith, I.M. & Bryson, S.E. (1994). Imitation and action in autism: A critical review. *Psychological Bulletin, 116*, 259-273.

Smith, I.M. & Bryson, S.E. (1998). Gesture imitation in autism I: Nonsymbolic postures and sequences. *Cognitive Neuropsychology, 15*, 747-770.

Smith, T. & Antolovich, M. (2000). Parental perceptions of supplemental interventions received by young children with autism in intensive behavior analytic treatment. *Behavioral Interventions, 15*, 83-97.

Stevens, S. & Gruzelier, J. (1984). Electroderman activity to auditory stimuli in autistic, retarded, and normal children. *Journal of Autism and Developmental Disorders, 14*(3), 245-260.

Sturm, H., Fernell, E., & Gillberg, C. (2004). Autism spectrum disorders in children with normal intellectual levels: Associated impairments and subgroups. *Developmental Medicine and Child Neurology, 46*, 444-447.

Talay-Ongan, A. & Wood, K. (2000). Unusual sensory sensitivities in autism: A possible crossroads. International *Journal of Disability, Development, and Education, 47*, 201-212.

Waterhouse, L., Fein, D., & Modahl, C. (1996). Neurofunctional mechanisms in autism. *Psychological Review, 103*(3), 457-489.

Watling, R., Deitz, J., Kanny, E.M., & McLaughlin, J.F. (1999). Current practice of occupational therapy for children with autism. *American Journal of Occupational Therapy, 53*, 498-505.

Watling, R., Deitz, J., & White, O. (2001). Comparison of Sensory Profile scores of young children with and without autism spectrum disorders. *American Journal of Occupational Therapy, 55*, 416-423.

Watson, L.R., Baranek, G.T., & DiLavore, P.C. (2003). Toddlers with autism- Developmental perspectives. *Infants and Young Children, 16*(3), 201-214.

Williams, D. (1998). *Autism and sensing: The unlost instinct.* London: Jessica Kingsley Publishers.

Williamson, G.G. & Anzalone, M. (1997). Sensory integration: A key component of the evaluation and treatment of young children with severe difficulties in relating and communicating. *Zero-to-Three*, 17, 29-36.

ENVIRONMENTAL DEPRIVATION

Ames, E.W. (Ed.). (1997). *The development of Romanian orphanage children adopted to Canada.* Burnaby, British Columbia: Simon Fraser University.

Carlson, M., & Earls, F. (1997). Psychological and neuroendocinological sequelae of early social deprivation in institutionalized children in Romania. *Annals New York Academy of Sciences, 807*, 420-428.

Casler, L. (1961). Maternal deprivation: A critical review of the literature. *Monographs of the Society for Research in Child Development, 26*(2),

Casler, L. (1968). Perceptual deprivation in institutional settings. In G. Newton, & S. Levine (Eds.), *Early experience and behavior.* Springfield: Charles C. Thomas.

Cermak, S. (1994). Romanian children demonstrate sensory defensiveness. *Attachment Newsletter.* Evergreen, CO: The Attachment Center at Evergreen.

Cermak, S. & Daunhauer, L. A. (1997). Sensory processing in the post-institutionalized child. *American Journal of Occupational Therapy, 51*, 500-507.

Cermak, S., & Groza, V. (1998). Sensory integration in post-institutionalized children: Implications for social workers. *Child and Adolescent Social Work Journal, 15*(1), 5-37.

Fisher, L., Ames, E.W., Chisholm, K., & Savoie, L. (1997). Problems reported by parents of Romanian orphans adopted to British Colombia. *International Journal of Behavioral Development, 20*(1), 67-82.

Harandon, G., Bascom, B., Dragomir, C., & Scripcaru, V. (1994). Sensory functions of institutionalized Romanian infants: A pilot study. *Occupational Therapy International, 1*, 250-260.

Kadlec, M.B. & Cermak, S. (2002). Activity level, organization, and social-emotional behaviors in post-institutionalized children. *Adoption Quarterly.* 6(2), 43-57.

Kraemer, G.W. (1992). A psychobiological theory of attachment. *Behavior and Brain Sciences, 15*, 493-511.

Kraemer, G.W. (1994). Significance of social attachment in primate infants: The infant-caregiver relationship and volition. In C.R. Pryce, R.D. Martin, and D. Skuse (Eds.). *Motherhood in human and non-human primates*, 3rd Schultz-Biegert Symposium (pp. 152-161). Basel: Karger.

Lin, S.H., Cermak, S., Coster, W., & Miller, L.C. (in press). The relationship between length of institutionalization and sensory integration in children adopted from Eastern Europe. *American Journal of Occupational Therapy, 59.*

Spitz, R. (1945). Hospitalism: An inquiry into the genesis of psychiatric conditions in early childhood. *The Psychoanalytic Study of the Child, Vol. 1.* New York: International Universities Press, 53-74.

Sweeney, J.K., & Bascom, B.B. (1995). Motor development and self-stimulatory movement in institutionalized Romanian children. *Pediatric Physical Therapy, 7*, 124-132.

Tizard, B., & Hodges, J. (1978). The effect of early insitutional rearing on the development of eight year old children. *Journal of Child Psychology and Psychiatry, 19*, 99-118.

Tizard, B., & Joseph, A. (1970). Cognitive development of young children in residential care: A study of children ages 24 months. *Journal of Child Psychology and Psychiatry, 11*, 177-186.

Tizard, B., & Rees, J. (1975). The effects of early institutional rearing on the behavior problems and affectional relationships of four-year-old children. *Journal of Child Psychology and Psychiatry, 16*, 61-73.

INFANT AND PRETERM

Barnard, K.E., & Brazelton, T.B. (Eds.) (1990). *Touch: The foundation of experience.* Madison, CT: International Universities Press.

Case-Smith, J., Butcher, L., & Reed, D. (1998). Parent's report of sensory defensiveness and temperament in preterm infants. *American Journal of Occupational Therapy, 52*(7), 547-555.

Cochrane, C.G. (1986). Vestibular-proprioceptive and tactile-kinesthetic intervention for premature infants. *Physical & Occupational Therapy in Pediatrics, 6*(2), 87-94.

DeGangi, G.A., DiPietro, J.A., Greenspan, S.I., & Porges, S.W. (1991). Psychophysiological characteristics of the regulatory disordered infant. *Infant Behavior and Development,14*, 37-50.

DeGangi, G.A., & Greenspan, S.I. (1989). The development of sensory functions in infants. *Physical & Occupational Therapy in Pediatrics, 8*(4), 21-34.

DeGangi, G.A., Sickel, R., Kaplan, E., & Wiener, A. (1997). Mother infant interaction in infants with disorders of self-regulation. *Physical & Occupational Therapy in Pediatrics, 17* (1), 17-44.

DeGangi, G.A., Sickel, R., Weiner, A., & Kaplan, E. (1996). Fussy babies: To treat or not to treat. *British Journal of Occupational Therapy, 59*(10).

DeSantis, A.M. (1994). Sensory, motor, and regulatory problems: Behavior and early intervention strategies. In D. Clark & G. Ensher (Eds.), *Newborns at risk*, pp. 295-322. Aspen.

Diamond, M.C. (1990). Evidence for tactile stimulation improving CNS function. In K.E. Barnard, & T.B. Brazelton (Eds.), *Touch: The foundation of experience* (pp.73-96). Madison, WI: International Universities Press.

Greenspan, S., & Wieder, S. (1998). *The child with special needs: Encouraging intellectual and emotional growth.* Reading, MA: Addison-Wesley.

Holloway, E. (1994). Parent and occupational therapist collaboration in the neonatal intensive care unit. *American Journal of Occupational Therapy, 48*(6), 535-538.

Kinnealey, M. & Wilbarger, P. (1993). Outcomes of SIPT testing of children born at risk. *Sensory Integration Quarterly*, 21(1), 1-6.

Korkman, M., Liikanen, A., & Fellman, V. (1996). Neuropsychological consequences of very low birth weight and asphyxia at term: Follow-up until school-age. *Journal of Clinical Neuropsychology, 18*(2), 220-233.

Korner, A.F. (1984). Interconnections between sensory and affective development in early infancy. *Zero to Three.* Washington, DC: National Center for Clinical Infant Programs.

Korner, A. (1996). Reliable individual differences in preterm infants' excitation management. *Child Development, 67*(4), 1793-1805.

Kuhn, C.M., Schanberg, S.M., Field, T., Symanski, R., Zimmerman, E., Scafidi, F., & Roberts, J. (1991). Tactile-kinesthetic stimulation effects on sympathetic and adrenocortical function in preterm infants. *Journal of Pediatrics, 119*, 434-440.

Lane, S., Attanasio, C., & Huselid, R. (1994). Prediction of preschool sensory and motor performance by 18-month neurological scores among children born prematurely. *American Journal of Occupational Therapy, 48*(5), 391-396.

Largo, R.H., Kundu, S., & Thun-Hohenstein, L. (1993). Early motor development in term and preterm children. In A.F. Kalverboer, B. Hopkins, & R. Geuze (Eds.), *Motor development in early and later childhood: Longitudinal approaches* (pp. 245-265). Cambridge: Cambridge University Press.

Liaw, J. (2000). Tactile stimulation and preterm infants. *Journal of Perinatal and Neonatal Nursing, 14*(1), 84-103.

Lester, B.M., McGrath, M.M., Garcia-Coll, C., Brem, F.S., Sullivan, M.C., & Mattis, S.G. (1995). Relationships between risk and protective factors, developmental outcome, and the home environment at four years of age in term and preterm infants. In H.E. Fitzgerald, B.M. Lester, & B. Zuckerman (Eds.), *Children of poverty: Research, health, and policy issues* (pp. 197-231). New York: Garland Publishing.

Litovsky, R. (1990). Stimulus differentiation by preterm infants can guide caregivers. *Pre- and Peri-Natal Psychology Journal, 5*(1), 41-67.

Majnemer, A., Rosenblatt, B., & Riley, P. (1994). Predicting outcome in high-risk newborns with a neonatal neurobehavioral assessment. *American Journal of Occupational Therapy, 48*(8), 723-732.

Mangelsdorf, S., Shapiro, J.R., & Marzolf, D. (1995). Developmental and temperamental differences in emotion regulation in infancy. *Child Development*, 66, 1817-1828.

Matthews, C. L. (1994). Supporting suck-swallow-breath coordination during nipple feeding. *American Journal of Occupational Therapy, 48*(6), 561-562.

Michelsson, K., & Lindahl, E. (1993). Relationship between perinatal risk factors and motor development at the ages of 5 and 9 years. In A.F. Kalverboer, B. Hopkins, & R. Geuze (Eds.), *Motor development in early and later childhood: Longitudinal approaches* (pp. 266-285). Cambridge: Cambridge University Press.

Mouradian, L., & Als, H. (1994). The influence of neonatal intensive care unit caregiving practices on motor functioning of preterm infants. *American Journal of Occupational Therapy, 48*(6), 527-533.

Neisworth, J.T., Bagnato, S.J., & Salvio, J. (1995). Neurobehavioral markers for early regulatory disorders. *Infants and Young Children, 8*(2), 8-17.

O'Callagan, M.J., Burns, Y., Gray, P., Harvey, J.M., Mohay, H.I., Rogers, Y., & Tudehope, D.I. (1995). Extremely low birth weight and control infants at 2 years corrected age: A comparison of intellectual abilities, motor performance, growth, and health. *Early Human Development, 40*(2), 115-128.

O'Callagan, M.J., Burns, Y., Gray, P., Harvey, J.M., Mohay, H.I., Rogers, Y., & Tudehope, D.I. (1996). School performance of ELBW children: A controlled study. *Developmental Medicine and Child Neurology, 38*(10), 917-926.

Olson, J.A. & Baltman, K. (1994). Infant mental health in occupational therapy practice in the neonatal intensive care unit. *American Journal of Occupational Therapy, 48*(6), 499-505.

Piek, J.P. (1998). The influence of preterm birth on early motor development. In J.P. Piek, (Ed.). *Motor behavior and human skill*, pp. 233-252. Champaign, IL: Human Kinetics.

Porges, S. W. (1996). Physiological regulation in high-risk infants: A model for assessment and potential intervention. *Developmental Psychopathology, 8*, 43-58.

Riese, M. L. (1998). Patterns of reactivity to an aversive tactile stimulus in fullterm and preterm infants. *Merrill-Palmer Quarterly, 44*(1), 97-113.

Strelau, J. (1998). Temperament: *A psychological perspective.* New York: Plenum.

Thoman, E.B., & Graham, S.E. (1986). Self-regulation of stimulation by premature infants. *Pediatrics, 78*(5), 855-860.

Thoman, E.B., Ingersoll, E., & Acebo, C. (1991). Premature infants seek rhythmic stimulation and the experience facilitates neurodevelopment. *Developmental and Behavioral Pediatrics, 12*, 11-18.

Vergara, E. R. & Bigsby, R. (2005). *Developmental and therapeutic interventions in the NICU.* Towson, MD: Brookes Publishing Co.

Wallace, I. F., Rose, S.A., McCarton, C., Kurtzberg, D. , & Vaughan, H.G. (1995). Relations between infant neurobehavioral performance and cognitive outcome in very low birth weight preterm infants. *Journal of Developmental and Behavioral Pediatrics, 16*(5), 309-317.

Weatherston, D.J., Ribaudo, J., & Globak, S. (2002). Becoming whole: Combining infant mental health and occupational therapy on behalf of a toddler with sensory integration difficulties and his family. *Infants and Young Children, 15*(1), 19-28.

Weiss-Salinas D, Williams N. (2001). Sensory defensiveness: A theory of its effect on breastfeeding. *Journal of Human Lactation, 17*(2), 145-51.

Williamson, G.G., & Anzalone, M.E. (2001). *Sensory integration and self-regulation in infants and toddlers: Helping very young children interact with their environment.* Washington, DC: Zero to Three.

White-Traut, R.C., Nelson, M.N., Silvestri, J.M., Patel, M.K. , Kilgallon, D. (1993). Patterns of physiologic and behavioral response of intermediate care preterm infants to intervention. *Pediatric Nursing, 19*(6), 625-629.

Wiener, A., Long, T., DeGangi, G., & Battaile, B. (1997). Sensory processing of infants born prematurely or with regulatory disorders. *Physical and Occupational Therapy in Pediatrics, 16*(4), 1-17.

LEARNING DISABILITIES

Ayres, A.J. (1965). Patterns of perceptual-motor dysfunction in children: A factor analytic study. *Perceptual and Motor Skills, 20*, 335-368.

Ayres, A.J. (1969). Deficits in sensory integration in educationally handicapped children. *Journal of Learning Disabilities, 2*(3), 160-168.

Ayres, A.J. (1971). Characteristics of types of sensory integrative dysfunction. *American Journal of Occupational Therapy*, 25(7), 329-334.

Ayres, A.J. (1972b). *Sensory integration and learning disorders.* Los Angeles: Western Psychological Services.

Ayres, A.J. (1972c). Types of sensory integrative dysfunction among disabled learners. *American Journal of Occupational Therapy, 26*(1), 13-18.

Ayres, A.J. (1977a). Cluster analyses of measures of sensory integration. *American Journal of Occupational Therapy, 31*, 362-366.

Beyer, R. (1999). Motor proficiency of boys with attention deficit hyperactivity disorder and boys with learning disabilities. *Adapted Physical Activity Quarterly, 16*(4), 403-414.

Bundy, A.C. (1989). A comparison of the play skills of normal boys and boys with sensory integration dysfunction. *Occupational Therapy Journal of Research, 9*, 84-100.

Burdette, J.H. (2002). Functional MR imaging to evaluate sensory processing in dyslexia. *Academic Radiology, 9*(9), 1062-1063.

Byl, N., Byl, F., & Rosenthal, J. (1989). Interaction of spatial perception, vestibular function, and exercise in young school age boys with learning disabilities. *Perceptual and Motor Skills, 68*, 727-738.

Cermak, S. (1985). Developmental dyspraxia (chapter 10). In E. Roy (Eds.), *Advances in Psychology: Neuropsychological Studies of Apraxia and Related Disorders* New York: Oxford.

Cermak, S., & Ayres, A. J. (1984). Midline crossing in learning disabled children. *American Journal of Occupational Therapy, 38*, 35-39.

Cermak, S., Coster, W., & Drake, C. (1980). Representational and nonrepresentational gestures in boys with learning disabilities. *American Journal of Occupational Therapy, 34*, 19-26.

Cermak, S., Trimble, H., Coryell, J., & Drake, C. (1990). Bilateral motor coordination in adolescents with and without learning disabilities. *Physical and Occupational Therapy in Pediatrics, 10*(1), 5-18.

Cermak, S., Trimble, H., Lebby, M., Kinsbourne, M., Coryell, J., & Drake, C. (1991). The persistence of motor deficits in older students with learning disabilities. *Japanese Journal of Sensory Integrative Dysfunction, 2*, 17-31.

Cermak, S., Ward, E., & Ward, L. (1986). The relationship between articulation disorders and motor coordination in children. *American Journal of Occupational Therapy, 40*, 546-550.

Clark, F., Mailloux, Z., & Parham, D. (1989). Sensory integration and children with learning disabilities. In P. N. &. A. Pratt A.S. (Eds.), *Occupational Therapy for Children* (pp. 457-509). St. Louis: C.V. Mosby.

Conrad, K E., Cermak, S.A., & Drake, C. (1983). Differentiation of praxis among children. *American Journal of Occupational Therapy, 37*, 466-473.

Dietz, J., Richardson, P., Crowe, T., & Westcott, S. (1997). Performance of children with learning disabilities and motor delays on the Pediatric Clinical Test of Sensory Interaction for Balance (P-CTSIB). *Physical and Occupational Therapy in Pediatrics, 17*, 1-22.

Fanchiang, S. P. (1996). The other side of the coin: Growing up with a learning disability. *American Journal of Occupational Therapy, 50*, 277-285.

Feldman, D. (1994). Somatosensory processing abilities of very low-birth weight infants at school age. *American Journal of Occupational Therapy, 48*(7), 639-646.

Grimwood, L. M., & Rutherford, E. M. (1980). Sensory integration therapy as an intervention procedure with grade one "at risk" readers - a three year study. *Exceptional Child, 27*, 52-61.

Humphries, T., Wright, M., McDougall, B., & Vertes, J. (1990). The efficacy of sensory integration therapy for children with learning disability. *Physical and Occupational Therapy in Pediatrics, 10*, 1-18.

Kalverboer, A.F. (1990). Neurobehavioural studies of sensory-motor development and its origins. In H. Bloch, B. Bertenthal (Eds.), *Sensory-motor organizations and development in infancy and early childhood. NATO Advanced Science Institutes series D: Behavioural and Social Sciences*, Vol 56 (pp. 97-104). Dordrecht, Netherlands: Kluwer Academic Publishers.

Koves, L. (1994). The relationship between tactile defensiveness and temperament style in children with learning disabilities. *Sensory Integration Quarterly, 22*(1), 6.

Lane, S., Attanasio, C.S., Huselid, R.F. (1994). Prediction of preschool sensory and motor performance by 18-month neurologic scores among children born prematurely. *American Journal of Occupational Therapy, 48*(5), 391-396.

Liu, Y.L., & Paul, S. (2002). Simultaneous assessment of the sensory integration subcommands: A study on preschool children with learning disabilities. *Research Quarterly for Exercise and Sport, 73*(1), A105-A106.

Polatajko, H. (1985). A critical look at vestibular dysfunction in learning-disabled children. *Developmental Medicine and Child Neurology, 27*, 283-292.

Polatajko, H.J., Kaplan, B.J. & Wilson, B.N. (1992). Sensory integration for children with learning disabilities: Its status 20 years later. *Occupational Therapy Journal of Research, 12*, 323-341.

Reynolds, D., Nicholson, R.I., Hambly, H. (2003). Evaluation of an exercise-based treatment for children with reading difficulties. *Dyslexia, 9*(1), 48-71.

Schaffer, R. (1984). Sensory integration therapy with learning disabled children: A critical review. *Journal of Occupational Therapy, 51*(2), 73-77.

Szklut, S., Cermak, S., & Henderson, A. (1995). Learning disabilities. In D. Umphred (Eds.), *Neurological Rehabilitation*, 3rd ed. New York: Mosby. (312-359).

Tickle-Degnen, L., & Coster, W. (1995). Therapeutic interaction and the management of challenge during the beginning minutes of sensory integration treatment. *Occupational Therapy Journal of Research, 15*(2), 122-141.

Varney, N., & Sivan, A. (1985). Pantomime recognition in normal and dyslexic children. *Developmental Neuropsychology, 1*, 49-52.

Wallen, M., & Walker, R. (1995). Occupational therapy practice with children with perceptual motor dysfunction: Findings of a literature review and survey. *Australian Occupational Therapy Journal, 42*(1), 15-25.

DEVELOPMENTAL COORDINATION DISORDER/ DYSPRAXIA

Barnhard, R.C., Davenport, M.J., Epps, S.B., & Nordquist, V.M. (2003). Developmental coordination disorder. *Physical Therapy, 83*(8), 722-731.

Candler, C. & Meeuwsen, H. (2002). Implicit learning in children with and without developmental coordination disorder. *American Journal of Occupational Therapy, 56*, 429-435.

Cantell, M.H., Smyth, M.M., & Ahonen, T.P. (2003). Two distinct pathways for developmental coordination disorder: Persistence and resolution. *Human Movement Science, 22*, 413-431.

Case-Smith, J., Heaphy, T., Marr, D., Galvin, B., Koch, V., Good Ellis, M., & Perez, I. (1998). Fine motor and functional performance outcomes in preschool children. *American Journal of Occupational Therapy, 52*(10), 788-796.

Cermak, S., & Larkin, D. (2002). (Eds.), *Developmental coordination disorder.* New York: Delmar Thomson.

Chen, H.F., & Cohn, E.S. (2003). Social participation for children with developmental coordination disorder: Conceptual, evaluation and intervention considerations. *Physical & Occupational Therapy in Pediatrics, 23*(4), 61-78.

Dewey, D., Kaplan, B.J., Crawford, S.G., & Wilson, B.N. (2002). Developmental coordination disorder: Associated problems in attention, learning, and psychosocial adjustment. *Human Movement Science, 21*(5-6), 905-918.

Geuze, R.H. (2003). Static balance and developmental coordination disorder. *Human Movement Science, 22*, 527-548.

Geuze, R. H., Jongmans, M. J., Schoemaker, M. M., & Smits-Englelsman, B. C. M. (2001). Clinical and research diagnostic criteria for developmental coordination disorder: A review and discussion. *Human Movement Science, 20*, 7-47.

Gillberg, C., & Kadesjo, B. (2003). Why bother about clumsiness? The implications of having developmental coordination disorder (DCD). *Neural Plasticity, 10*, 59-68.

Kadesjo, B., & Gillberg, C. (1999). Developmental coordination disorder in Swedish 7-year-old children. *Journal of the American Academy of Child and Adolescent Psychiatry, 38*, 820-828.

Karatekin, C., Markiewicz, S.W., & Siegel, M.A. (2003). A preliminary study of motor problems in children with attention-deficit/hyperactivity disorder. *Perceptual & Motor Skills, 97*, 1267-1280.

Kimball, J.G. (2001). Developmental coordination disorder from a sensory integration perspective. In S. Cermak & D. Larkin (Eds.) *Developmental coordination disorder* (pp. 210-220). Albany, NY: Delmar.

Lee, C.Y., Lin, J.H., Sung, F.H., Shih, H.H., Hung, C.L., & Hung, T.M. (2004). Exploring the relationship between sensory integration motor ability and emotion on preschool children. *Journal of Sport & Exercise Psychology, 26*, S116.

Macnab, J. J., Miller, L. T., & Polatajko, H. J. (2001). The search for subtypes of DCD: Is cluster analysis the answer? *Human Movement Science, 20*, 49-72.

Mandich, A., & Polatajko, H.J. (2003). Developmental coordination disorder: Mechanisms, measurement and management. *Human Movement Science, 22*, 407-411.

Mandich, A.D., Polatajko, H.J., & Rodger, S. (2003). Rites of passage: Understanding participation of children with developmental coordination disorder. *Human Movement Science, 22*, 583-595.

Miller, L.T., Missiuna, C.A., Macnab, J.J., Malloy-Miller, T., & Polatajko, H.J. (2001). Clinical description of children with developmental coordination disorder. *Canadian Journal of Occupational Therapy, 68*(1), 5-15.

Poulson, A.A., & Ziviani, J.M. (2004). Can I play too? Physical activity engagement of children with developmental coordination disorders. *Canadian Journal of Occupational Therapy, 71*, 100-107.

Rodger, S., Ziviani, J., Watter, P., Ozanne, A., Woodyatt, G., & Springfield, E. (2003). Motor and functional skills of children with developmental coordination disorder: A pilot investigation of measurement issues. *Human Movement Science, 22*, 461-478.

Sigmundsson, H., Hansenc, P.C., & Talcottc, J.B. (2003). Do 'clumsy' children have visual deficits. *Behavioral Brain Research, 139*(1-2), 123-129.

Smits-Engelsman, B.C., Wilson, P.H., Westenberg, Y., Duysens, J. (2003). Fine motor deficiencies in children with developmental coordination disorder and learning disabilities: An underlying open-loop control deficit. *Human Movement Science, 22*, 495-513.

Smyth, M.M., & Anderson, H. I. (2000). Coping with clumsiness in the school playground: Social and physical play in children with coordination impairments. *British Journal of Developmental Psychology, 18*, 389-413.

Smyth, T.R. (1994). Clumsiness in children: A defect of kinesthetic perception. *Child: Care, Health and Development, 20*, 27-36.

Tervo, R.C., Azuma, S., Fogas, B., Falls, S., & Fiechtner, H. (2002). Children with ADHD and motor dysfunction compared with children with ADHD only. *Developmental Medicine and Child Neurology, 44*(6), 383-390.

Visser, J. (2003). Developmental coordination disorder: A review of research on subtypes and comorbidities. *Human Movement Science, 22*, 479-493.

Wann, J. P., Mon-Williams, M., & Rushton, K. (1998). Postural control and co-ordination disorders: The swinging room revisited. *Human Movement Science, 17*, 491-513.

Watkinson, E.J., Dunn, J. C., Cavaliere, N., Calzonetti, K., Wilhelm, L., & Dwyer, S. (2001). Engagement in playground activities as a criterion for diagnosing developmental coordination disorder. *Adapted Physical Activity Quarterly, 18*, 18-34.

Zoia, S., Pelamatti, G., Cuttini, M., Casotto, V., & Scabar, A. (2002). Performance of gesture in children with and without DCD: Effects of sensory input modalities. *Developmental Medicine and Child Neurology, 44*(10), 699.

MENTAL RETARDATION/ DEVELOPMENTAL DISABILITIES

Baranek, G.T., Chin, Y.K.H., Hess, L.M.G., Yankee, J.G., Hatton, D.D., & Hooper, S.R. (2002). Sensory processing correlates of occupational performance in children with fragile X syndrome: Preliminary findings. *American Journal of Occupational Therapy, 56*(5), 538-546.

Baranek, G.T., Foster, L.G., & Berkson, G. (1997). Sensory defensiveness in persons with developmental disabilities. *Occupational Therapy Journal of Research, 17*(3), 173-185.

Berkson, G., Gutermuth, L., & Baranek, G. (1995). Relative prevalence and relationships among stereotyped and similar behaviors. *American Journal of Mental Retardation, 100*, 137-145.

Cermak, S. (1988). Sensible integration. *American Journal of Mental Retardation, 92*, 413-414.

Clark, F.A., & Shuer, J. (1978). A clarification of sensory integrative therapy and its application to programming with retarded people. *Mental Retardation, 16*, 227-232.

Dura, J.R., Mulick, J.A., & Hammer, D. (1988). Rapid clinical evaluation of sensory integrative therapy for self-injurious behavior. *Mental Retardation, 26*(2), 83-87.

Edelson, S. (1984). Implications of sensory stimulation in self-destructive behavior. *American Journal of Mental Deficiency, 89*, 140-145.

Friefeld, S. J., & MacGregor, D. (1994). Sensorimotor coordination in boys with Fragile X syndrome. *Occupational Therapy International, 1*(i), 174-182.

Goldson, E. (2001). Sensory integration and Fragile X syndrome. *Revista De Neurologia, 33*, S32-S36.

Harris, S., Stewart, K., Berkey, S., Fewell, R. R., & Jenkins, J. R. (1984). The relationship between tests of sensory-motor integration, tactile sensitivity and gross motor skills in normal and developmentally delayed preschool children. *Physical and Occupational Therapy in Pediatrics, 4*, 5-18.

Hill, E.L., Bishop, D.V.M., & Nimmo-Smith, I. (1998). Representational gestures in developmental coordination disorder and specific language impairment: Error-types and the reliability of ratings. *Human Movement Science, 17*(4-5), 655-678.

Hyman, S.L., Fisher, W., Mercugliano, M., & Cataldo, M.F. (1990). Children with self-injurious behavior. *Pediatrics, 85*, 437-441.

Iwasaki, K., & Holm, M.B. (1989). Sensory treatment for the reduction of stereotypic behaviors in persons with severe multiple disabilities. *Occupational Therapy Journal of Research, 9*(3), 171-183.

Kinnealey, M. (1973). Aversive and nonaversive responses to sensory stimulation in mentally retarded children. *American Journal of Occupational Therapy, 27*, 464-471.

Larrington, G.G. (1987). A sensory integration based program with a severely retarded/autistic teenager: An occupational therapy case report. *Occupational Therapy in Health Care, 4*(2), 101-117.

Larson, K. (1982). The sensory history of developmentally delayed children with and without tactile defensiveness. *American Journal of Occupational Therapy, 36*, 590-596.

Lemke, H. (1974). Self-abusive behavior in the mentally retarded. *American Journal of Occupational Therapy, 28*(2), 94-98.

Luiselli, J.K. (1994). Oral feeding treatment of children with chronic food refusal and multiple developmental disabilities. *American Journal on Mental Retardation, 98*(5), 646-655.

Martini, R. & Polatajko, H.J. (1998). Verbal self-guidance as a treatment approach for children with developmental coordination disorder: A systematic replication study. *Occupational Therapy Journal of Research, 18*(4), 157-181.

Miller, L.J., McIntoch, D.N., McGrath, J., Shyu, V., Lampe, M., Taylor, A.K., Tassone, F., Neitzel, K., Stackhouse, T., & Hagerman, R.J. (1999). Electrodermal responses to sensory stimuli in individuals with Fragile X syndrome: A preliminary report. *American Journal of Medical Genetics, 38*, 268-279.

Schaaf, R. (1985). The frequency of vestibular disorders in developmentally delayed preschoolers with otitis media. *American Journal of Occupational Therapy, 39*, 247-252.

Shuer, J., Clark, F., & Azen, S. P. (1980). Vestibular functions in mildly mentally retarded adults. *American Journal of Occupational Therapy, 34*, 664-670.

Stackhouse, T. (1994). Sensory integration concepts and Fragile x syndrome. *Sensory Integration Special Interest Section Newsletter*

Wells, M.E., & Smith, D.W. (1983). Reduction of self-injurious behavior of mentally retarded persons using sensory-integrative techniques. *American Journal of Mental Deficiency, 87*(6), 664-666.